Becoming
Psychiatrists

Donald Light

Becoming Psychiatrists

The Professional Transformation of Self

W·W·NORTON & COMPANY

NEW YORK   LONDON

Permission has been obtained and is acknowledged for reprinting portions of the following publications. Table 1-15.1 from Robert R. Holt and Lester Luborsky, *Personality Problems of Psychiatrists* (New York: Basic Books, 1958), from Imago Publishers. A table from Robert Plutchik, Hope Conte, and Henry Kandler, "Variables Related to the Selection of Psychiatric Residents, *The American Journal of Psychiatry*, vol. 127, pp. 1504–1508, 1971, copyright 1971, the American Psychiatric Association; reprinted by permission. The table in Leo Srole, "errata," *Journal of Health and Social Behavior*, vol. 17, no. 2, p. 192. Passages from my article, "Treating Suicide: The illusions of a Professional Movement," *International Social Science Journal*, vol. XXV, no. 4, 1973, pp. 475–488; copyright UNESCO 1973. Passages from my article, "The Impact of Medical School on Future Psychiatrists," *The American Journal of Psychiatry*, vol. 132, no. 46, pp. 607–610, 1975; copyright 1975, the American Psychiatric Association; reprinted by permission. Passages from my article, "Work Styles Among American Psychiatric Residents," pp. 101–108 in Joseph Westermeyer, editor, *Anthropology and Mental Health* (The Hague: Mouton, 1976). Passages from my article," Professional Problems in Treating Suicidal Persons," *Omega*, vol. 7(1); copyright 1976, Baywood Publishing Company, Inc. Passages from my article, "Psychiatry and Suicide: The Managing of a Mistake," *American Journal of Sociology*, vol. 77, pp. 821–838; copyright 1972 by The University of Chicago; all rights reserved. Passages from my article, "The Sociological Calendar: An Analytic Tool For Fieldwork Applied to Medical and Psychiatric Training," *American Journal of Sociology*, vol. 80, pp. 1145–1164; copyright 1975 by the University of Chicago; all rights reserved. The tables on pp. 688 and 690 in Darrell A. Regier, Irving D. Goldberg, and Carl A. Taube, "The De Facto U.S. Mental Health Services System," *Archives of General Psychiatry*, vol. 35; copyright 1978, American Medical Association.

Library of Congress Cataloging in Publication Data
Light, Donald, 1942–
Becoming psychiatrists.
Includes index.
1. Psychiatry—Study and teaching (Residency)
2. Psychiatrists. I. Title. [DNLM: 1. Psychiatry.
WM21 L723b]
RC336.L53   1979   616.8′9′023   79–20256
ISBN 0-393-01168-2

1 2 3 4 5 6 7 8 9 0

To
Nancy Catherine Louise,
Holly Grace
and
Peter Richmond

CONTENTS

APPENDICES

Preface

No profession is so ridiculed or worshipped, so suspected or trusted as psychiatry. The very same individuals who put down "shrinks," with their imprecise methods and high fees, will also describe in glowing, vague terms the marvelous way *their* therapist has pulled them through the worst moments and somehow understands them totally. Psychiatrists make a deep impression on patients and their relatives, and they want to know more about them. In this book they will learn how psychiatrists are trained and witness their struggles toward professional identity.

The influence of psychiatry in American life has been steadily growing. Kids who act up in school, once called "cut-ups," are now diagnosed as "hyperactive" and controlled by drugs. As we shall see, the range of human quirks, habits, and upsets that now are given psychiatric labels and treated as forms of mental illness is much greater than it was a generation ago. Who is this small company of physicians, less than 10 percent of the medical profession, that is so influential, and how are they trained? How is the training organized, and to what effect?

Embodied in the training of any profession are the profession's ideals about itself and its relations to the public. Answers to such questions as what work is worthwhile, which patients or clients are "crocks" or "duds," what treatment procedures are the best or worst, and how should professional work be organized are contained implicitly or explicitly in the training program. If we want to know, for example, why psychiatrists abandoned the community mental health movement, we must look to the values instilled in psychiatric residency programs.

In addition to the implications which psychiatric training has for the organization and nature of services to clients, it also resonates with the struggles for professional identity in other programs—in law school, military academies, business school and medical school. Virtually everyone aspires to be a professional today: the quintessential mark of "modern man" is to command technical knowledge and translate it into solutions for practical problems. Yet in becoming this symbol of technological society, most professionals do not take notice of what happens to their values and to the way they treat clients. These values, this moral order of rights and obligations, are as much embedded in a profession's procedures as in its technical knowledge, and through examining psychiatrists in training, we will gain insight into the transformations of self experienced by other professions as well.

This book examines the training program at University Psychiatric Center, part of what we shall call Distinguished Medical School. In order to protect professionals and patients whose confidential relations I observed, their names and the names of the institutions (including citations bearing their names) have been changed. Of necessity, I have also eliminated those references and notes which would identify persons and institutions in question. University Psychiatric Center is one of the largest and most influential training programs in American psychiatry. It has produced an extraordinary number of psychiatry's leaders and leaders of mental health services in the United States. At the Center, I had the rare opportunity to observe residents in all phases of their training, including individual supervision, the sensitivity group for residents, regular rap sessions among them, and private meetings with the chief of service. Even senior psychiatrists can rarely enter these confidential settings, and to my knowledge no other investigator of residency training has drawn upon them.

Uniting this rich, voluminous information with numerous studies of other training programs in psychiatry, I examine what kinds of people choose to become psychiatrists, how their training experience alters their sense of illness, treatment, and responsibility, how they cope with suicidal patients, and how they overcome the uncertainties of their work. Underlying these lessons is the organization of the program, the moral transformation it puts residents through, and the tendencies toward omnipotence it embodies.

The larger and ever-changing context of this study is psychiatry itself. The profession constantly vacillates between the psychological and physiological explanations of mental problems, but in no country have the psychoanalytic schools of Freud and his successors influenced the profession so deeply and broadly as in the United States. The psychoanalytic theories of pathology and therapy have dominated training not only in elite residencies, where graduates can reasonably expect to find clients sufficiently articulate and affluent to make this kind of therapy feasible, but these theories have served as the models for training in half-filled residencies at state mental hospitals, where the trainees aspire to psychoanalytic therapy as they shock, drug or isolate hundreds of back ward patients. This prevalence was illustrated when investigators developed scales to measure three basic orientations in psychiatry: the psychoanalytic, the somatic or biological, and the sociotherapeutic, with its emphasis on group, milieu and family therapy. When they sampled residents in the early 1960s, they found so few with either a somatic or sociotherapeutic viewpoint that they had to draw special, biased samples just to test the scales, even though the revolution in psychopharmacology was fully established and community psychiatry was ascending.[1] During the 1960s, fashion turned completely to community psychiatry and to being "eclectic." Yet most psychiatrists teaching at residencies which described themselves in these terms were psychoanalysts, and the core program changed little, except to add elective courses and perhaps brief orientations in social psychiatry, community psychiatry, family therapy and the like.

Today the leading edge of psychiatry—the departments in medical schools—is shifting toward biology and physiology with a seriousness and depth that are neither cosmetic nor ephemeral. This orientation is still combined with basic training in the psychoanalytic model of mental disorders and their treatment, and graduates of psychoanalytic institutes still hold many senior posts. But there are basic differences between the two groups in how they go about their work, in the model of pathology they use, and in the values they hold.[2] This being the case, incompatibility may force psychoanalysis to the periphery. The new biopsychiatry, then, constitutes a basic shift in how psychiatrists are trained and go about their work. The vast majority of practicing psychiatrists, however, were trained in residencies with orientations like the one described in these pages, "eclectic" but fundamentally psychoanalytic. Thus our study describes how today's leading psychiatrists were trained—before the new mandarins ascended.

Acknowledgments

Few studies of how psychiatrists are trained have benefitted from such intimate observation of their activities as this one, and I am indebted to those who made it possible. Larry Rosenberg developed the project, invited me to carry it out, and taught me invaluable lessons in the subtleties of participant-observation. Dr. Black, then director of University Psychiatric Center, approved of the project and lent it support at critical moments. The director of a research institute there provided me with a field office and became my chief adviser as the study and its challenges unfolded. His steadfast support and constructive criticism greatly aided my work. Finally, the residents themselves introduced me to their world and took me to the most confidential corners of their work. A number of them provided valuable insights into the nature of their training. Without the support and good counsel of all these people, this project would not have been possible.

The intellectual debt I owe to Everett Cherrington Hughes and to Morris S. Schwartz is made clear in these pages. This study carries on the seminal ideas of Hughes about the professions, extending and modifying them in light of new information about professional training. There is also an important parallel between this book and the classic work which Morris Schwartz wrote with Alfred Stanton, *The Mental Hospital*. Stanton and Schwartz found that patients' aberrant behavior reflects latent conflicts among staff members. In a similar pattern, I found that residents' behavior, which is often interpreted psychologically, reflects the structural forces latent in the training program. Professors Schwartz and Hughes also provided me with valuable advice, and Morris Schwartz was especially generous with his support.

Renée C. Fox has strongly influenced and improved this study. From our first meeting early in the project to the present, she has been the source of important ideas and good advice. Two of the chapters, on the sociological calendar and training for uncertainty, rest directly on her pioneering work.

A number of other colleagues have provided valuable suggestions and criticisms. I am grateful to Samuel W. Bloom, Marvin Bressler, Rose Laub Coser, Arlene K. Daniels, Erving Goffman, Daniel J. Levinson, Rachel Kahn-Hut, Robert K. Merton, Frederick C. Redlich, Robert A. Scott, Robert C. Tucker, and Irving K. Zola for all their help.

This book has benefitted from two exceptional editors. In a time of corporate publishing and hasty editing, James Mairs has worked with the manuscript every step of the way, from initial draft through revisions, design, and production. This meticulous, personal way of publishing is now more the exception than the rule. Jim's encouragement, patience, and good judgment have measurably improved the book. I was doubly fortunate to have Luna Carne-Ross as copyeditor. She went far beyond the technical polishing of the text to sharpen its arguments.

I would probably have not developed an interest in the psychiatric profession had NIMH not awarded me a fellowship early in my career (7-FL-MH-25, 333-04). The Department of Labor generously provided a grant to carry out this research (91-23-68-46). Princeton University and the Sophie Davis School for Biomedical Education both provided valuable time for developing this book and secretarial staff for typing it.

PART I

Becoming a Psychiatrist

1.

The Psychiatric Domain

Studying how psychiatrists are trained has taken on a significance it did not once have. Before the mid-sixties, sociologists and investigators focused primarily on the patient, who was presumed "mentally ill." They studied the prevalence of various disorders and tried to single out what social or personal attributes might account for different rates. They investigated patients' behaviors with therapists and in hospitals. They looked at the organization of hospitals or wards to see how differences might affect treatment, and in general they tried to "help psychiatrists understand how social events impinge upon psychiatric events."[1]

Few of these studies questioned psychiatry itself and its model of mental illness. Even when Thomas Szasz argued that, except for mental disorders having a physiological basis, "mental illness" is an unjustifiable extension of medical thinking which gives psychiatrists license to violate patients' civil rights,[2] the full implications were not understood for several years. But now, besides investigating the prevalence of mental illness, researchers ask how it is that some people get labeled mentally ill, while the vast majority with similar symptoms do not. Besides examining patients' behavior, studies look at how that behavior is interpreted by the professional and what consequences flow from such interpretation. They doubt the expertise underlying profes-

3

sional judgment. And besides just describing health care organizations, investigators analyze the ways in which a profession's values and ambitions lead to having services organized the way they are instead of another way. Today nearly all professions are coming under the harsh scrutiny of this perspective.

Clearly psychiatrists wield great power over who is regarded as "sick" and over the organization of services available to the public. This view of professionals ruling over a domain of institutions, subordinates, research, services and money makes their training all the more important, because it is in these formative years that their ideas about psychiatric practice are shaped, which will influence the institutions they will later direct. This view also requires that a book on professional education, unlike previous studies, begin with an analysis of the profession's domain and consider the relations between that domain and how the profession trains new members to do their work.

Professional Origins

To appreciate the relations between values, ambitions or models of work and the organization of services, one must understand the social contract which gives a profession its power. The profession claims to apply an esoteric, complex body of knowledge to important problems. The people in general and the state in particular grant it the autonomy to choose and train its own members, the monopoly over its domain of services, and the privileges necessary to carry out those services, in return for a guarantee that these powers will be used to help others and that the profession will monitor the quality and integrity of its members.

As any reader of the newspapers knows, abuses of this contract abound. Professions have a terrible record of monitoring their members. Their privileges are used when duties do not require them. Each profession has a complex body of knowledge, but whether that can be applied effectively is often doubtful. Professional monopoly over services is widely used for power and profit.

Psychiatry, of course, has been an easy profession to attack for breaching this social contract. In England, for example, the profession began when some physicians in the eighteenth century took over madhouses for profit. By keeping inmates on a minimal budget and by advertising for new customers, profits could be large.[3] When William Tuke and other reformers attacked the foul, brutal conditions of these institutions and founded competing ones based on Christian morality in the 1790s, medical directors started generating esoteric knowledge at a rapid rate, founded "scientific" journals, and then used them to show Parliament that they had sophisticated knowledge which lay reformers could not claim.[4] It worked. Moral treatment by Tuke and others was both more humane and more successful. However, it was based on a *rejection* of expertise or science as relevant to treatment, and thus provided no basis for professional status. This sociological flaw proved fatal, and the medical profession slowly gained legal control over the asylums.

While the origins of psychiatry in America were more honorable and stemmed from a missionary desire to cure lunatics in the newly built mental hospitals, a similar drive to gain control took place. In retrospect, the ideologies of the tightknit group of superintendents "were but rationalizations of existing conditions within mental hospitals as well as popular attitudes."[5] Charismatic and prolific, these leaders found the causes of insanity in almost every institution and practice of the day. Some said schools drove young people mad by being too strict; others, by being too lenient. They saw the advance of civilization as increasing mental illness. The amorphous nature of modern life (in 1851!) was seen to produce great mental strain, because ambitions were not confined by stable values and social hierarchies. These stresses caused lesions of the brain and were thus similar to other physiological disorders.[6]

Conflicting theories and the moral assessment of social life were not the only similarities between the early profession and the present one. Legislatures and public officials were the greatest obstacles to professional autonomy, for they felt that mental health services must be in the hands of public officials responsive to the community.[7] In subsequent waves of public criticism up to the present, it has been legislatures which have repeatedly called the profession to account for itself, to show that its techniques are effective and that its commitment to service is genuine.

Ironically, the early profession suffered from its own rhetoric. It raised expectations of cure so much and "proved" its techniques so "effective" that everyone sent their worst cases to the new mental asylums. In a few short decades, the asylums filled to overcrowding with chronic cases. By the 1870s, the cure rate had dropped, legislators became disillusioned, and the profession suffered humiliation. The psychiatrists "unwittingly transformed their own occupation into an administrative and managerial specialty. . . ."[8] Thus, professional entrepreneurship eventually led to professional humiliation. In the twentieth century, this part of psychiatry has initiated several reforms to regain its prestige, the latest being the community mental health movement, but it has never recovered its initial elan and charisma within the profession.

The cycle of exaggerated claims followed by disillusionment has continued to characterize the claim of cures in psychiatry. Reviewing psychiatric therapies from 1800 to 1968, G. Tourney found that each new "cure" fit cultural expectations. At first it developed with moderate claims of success; then its use expanded dramatically as very high success rates were "demonstrated"; and finally disillusionment set in as success rates were found to be low.[9]

One therapy, psychoanalysis, shaped the psychiatric domain during the twentieth century. It took the profession out of the asylum. Besides his intellectual contributions, Sigmund Freud gave psychiatry a new social base: upper-class patients who could pay. It is difficult for a profession to attain high status with lowly clients. Psychoanalysis not only provided a new, prestigious clientele outside the asylum, but it also created a new awareness that functioning, competent people could be neurotic. The potential was unlimited. Culturally, psychoanalysis appealed to Americans. According to Peter Berger, they believed in their country as the land of opportunity; yet it was quite stratified.[10] In addition to this frustrating disparity, industrialization and the spread of bureaucracy sharpened the division between public and private spheres of life, and Berger claims it fostered an impersonal, emotionally controlled public manner. Thus, a theory that emphasized repressed primitive drives, the experience of being controlled by unconscious forces, and sexual sublimation responded to needs which many Americans felt. Around this new therapy and clientele arose what is now the upper half of the profession, which treats a quarter of those seeking help and earns an average of $10,000 to $20,000 more yearly than the other half.[11]

In terms of the profession, the psychoanalytic movement brought wealth and prestige, and in time it came to dominate that older part of the profession located in large public mental hospitals. Psychiatry already had the vital power of legal monopoly. To this was added a strong affiliation with universities, the institutions in modern society which bestow prestige and legitimation on a profession. The psychoanalytic interpretation of personality became the doctrine in which everyone was trained and by which other, nonanalytic therapies were measured. For example, when a new generation of drugs dramatically improved large numbers of mildly and severely disturbed people in the 1950s, psychiatrists considered them as providing surface relief to symptoms but leaving untouched the root of the symptoms, which could only be treated by psychodynamic therapy. At the same time, psychoanalysis was applied to the full spectrum of patients. In particular, to treat schizophrenics psychoanalytically became the ultimate professional challenge at which most psychiatrists tried their hand. Since little evidence has appeared to show that this approach is more effective than other methods, one can best understand this preoccupation sociologically, as a vehicle by which the new psychoanalytically based profession could keep control over the old asylums, which were heavily populated by schizophrenics. Thus, in state mental hospital residencies, where the masses of chronic patients made psychotherapy almost impossible and where staff overwhelmingly used physical or chemical treatments, psychodynamic therapy was given predominant emphasis.

To summarize a lot of data, there is a privileged half of the profession. They earn more, work with healthier and wealthier patients, have a more diverse work life, are better trained, and include few foreign medical graduates. Within this half is a much smaller group, the psychoanalysts, who until recently enjoyed all these privileges to an even greater degree.[12] Some might object that the other half of the profession, who work in public institutions and hospitals, are not less privileged but prefer such work. Doubtless a number of individuals do, and with the increasing portion of jobs in public institutions, more will have to find fulfillment there. But so far, the evidence suggests that this half of the profession is less well-trained, earns less, works with sicker patients, is forced to use "inferior" forms of therapy (though no one has shown them to be inferior), and has a more restricted work life. Institutional psychiatrists seem to constitute an underculture of the profession. Rogow concludes: "Indeed it is difficult to resist the suggestion that in terms of theoretical influence and cultural level, psychoanalysts can be regarded as the highbrow, private practice psychiatrists can be regarded as the middlebrow, and public mental hospital psychiatrists as the lowbrow element in American psychiatry." [13]

This brief portrait does not convey the variety of factions and splinter groups within the psychoanalytic framework that have torn at the profession's identity. Nor does it consider the challenges of behavioral psychiatry and biopsychiatry, which are based on fundamentally different theories of mind and which use a scientific precision that the rest of psychiatry lacks. But it does convey the two basic kinds of patients and treatment which characterize the profession, and which are oddly mixed in the study at hand, where an elite program turning out psychoanalytically oriented psychiatrists trains them at a state mental hospital on the edge of Boston's black ghetto.

The Psychiatric Domain

Besides understanding the nature of the psychiatric profession, one must know about the domain in which the profession works. Its outer boundaries include all people with psychiatric problems, but these boundaries are unclear and changing. Leo Srole, in his "Midtown Manhattan Study," persuasively argues that psychiatry has not yet developed a clear, consistent set of diagnoses. [14] Moreover, psychiatric terms have greatly expanded, even to include phrases like "conditions without manifest psychiatric disorder" and "nonspecific conditions." Expanding one's clientele by enlarging the definition of pathology is a well-known technique for getting more business, [15] and this is a constant tendency in psychiatry.

Srole and his colleagues devised a scale of symptoms that was reliable and ranged across six points from "well" to "incapacitated." In the original 1954 study, and the restudy twenty years later, the distribution was about the same. Only one-fifth of the people were assessed as psychologically well. Forty percent manifested mild symptoms, 20 percent moderate, and nearly 20 percent had serious symptoms. (See Appendix I, table 1.) Srole's figure for serious symptoms matches the median percent of "functional psychiatric disorders" in eleven other studies, all of which probably underestimate psychiatric problems in the nation. [16] Even at that we are talking about 35 million Americans.

The cost of mental illness was estimated conservatively to be

$20.9 billion in 1968 and $36.8 billion in 1974. In 1968, $4 billion went to direct services, and the rest consisted of lost productivity and other social costs to society. By 1974, direct costs had risen to $14.5 billion—they more than tripled in six years.[17] While due in part to inflation, this dramatic increase indicates an important set of trends which few people recognize. (See Appendix I, table 2.) First, state mental hospitals were being emptied under a policy known as "deinstitutionalization." This has led to the belief that inpatient services for mental patients have decreased. But while they have decreased in state mental hospitals, inpatient services in general hospitals, VA hospitals, and community mental health centers have skyrocketed, so that over a twenty-year period *there has been a significant increase of inpatient services despite deinstitutionalization.*

Second, discharging wards of the state did not accomplish the goals of lowering costs and transferring funds to outpatient services. "Between 1968 and 1974 the cost of the traditional mental hospital system increased from $1.7 to $2.8 billion. There is little indication that the reduction in the population of large institutions has freed funds for less restrictive services."[18] The old pattern of custodial care for chronic patients gave way to intermittent care, which becomes more expensive each time a patient is seen. Inpatient services at other facilities are also more expensive (and probably better) than services in state mental hospitals. At community mental health centers, for example, where inpatient services grew from nothing to a quarter of a million, the occupancy rate was only 64 percent, making the cost per bed high.[19] In sum, aside from the proliferation of new therapies outside the traditional institutions, the entire mental health system has become much larger and more expensive.

The major shift in the psychiatric domain over the past twenty years is commonly attributed to modern psychopharmacology. David Hamburg, current director of the Institute of Medicine, and his colleagues reflect the prevailing myth when they write: "Drug treatments for psychiatric disorders have sharply decreased the number of severely ill patients in state and county mental hospitals."[20] While the drugs introduced in the mid-fifties have been an important tool for health administrators, and while the patient population began to decline in 1956, table 2 shows that the number of episodes in state and county hospitals declined by less than 2 percent in the first ten years after the drugs were introduced. As Andrew Scull has effectively shown, "decarceration" is mainly the product of policy, not phar-macology.[21] The new drugs facilitated the process, but many custodial patients could have been discharged without them because they were capable of living in homes or on their own. On the other hand, thou-sands of patients who have been discharged continue to be so disorga-nized and disruptive even with medication that irate citizens have been protesting for years against the policies of massive discharges. The Task Panel on Deinstitutionalization for the President's Commission on Mental Health observes, "It is now widely acknowledged that dein-stitutionalization has, in fact, often aggravated the problems of the chronically mentally disabled."[22] These major shifts are the product of professional and social policies affecting the psychiatric domain. For example, the sharp decline in episodes for state and county hospitals occurred as a result of the human rights movement and efforts to reduce welfare costs.[23] Meanwhile, the dramatic rise of community mental health centers during that time reflected the profession's new image of itself as a crusader against mental illness in the community. The average length of stay declined, partly due to drugs, but signifi-cantly affected by insurance, reimbursement policies and administra-tive ambitions. When one learns, for example, that the average stay declined by 41 percent (to twenty-six days) during the four short years from 1971 to 1975,[24] one knows the drug revolution of the 1950s or other new forms of therapy play almost no part in the decline.

Another myth is that the community mental health movement has been dead for several years. Ideologically, this is true for the psychia-tric profession, which abandoned the movement when it threatened professional identity by deemphasizing the medical aspects of care and giving nonphysicians a prominent role. But throughout the 1970s, community mental health centers have been growing. In 1975, these centers accounted for 34.3 percent of all outpatient care episodes, and for 28.5 percent of all episodes, inpatient and outpatient. (See Appen-dix I, table 2.) The number of centers and the services they offer keep expanding. Ever since 1971, when the glow began to fade from the community mental health movement, to the most recent figures in 1977, expenditures rose from $300 million to $1,500 million, and pa-tient care rose from 750,000 episodes to over 2 million.[25] At the same time, all other outpatient services have been expanding, particularly since 1971. Whereas outpatient services constituted 23 percent of the total in 1955, they now account for 72 percent of all services, even though inpatient services have not declined!

In this expanding range of services, how many people with emotional problems get treated and where? Of the estimated 32 million people with such problems in 1975, the best figures show that one-fifth are seen by psychiatrists, psychologists, mental hospitals and clinics or other facilities specializing in mental health.[26] This is the usual figure cited—that over three-quarters of the people which community surveys find have serious emotional difficulties (and not just problems of living) receive no treatment from mental health specialists. But what has not been appreciated until recently is that *three times this number are seen by medical people outside mental health facilities*—doctors' offices, outpatient and emergency rooms of hospitals, nonpsychiatric wards of medical hospitals, nursing homes and the like (figure 2, table 3 in Appendix I).

While approximately 19.2 million of the 32 million people are estimated to have come in contact with nonpsychiatric health personnel, this does not mean they were recognized or treated for emotional problems. Studies estimate that 15 percent of the patients in a general practice have serious emotional problems. But without special training or coaching, general practice physicians diagnose 4 to 5 percent of their patients as having mental problems. With such coaching, however, they "see" mental problems in 10 percent of their patients. And if they are also sensitized to consider psychosocial stresses in their patients' lives, they designate 15 percent as having mental problems. Thus a new generation of sensitized physicians could quickly end up providing most of the outpatient mental health services, unless psychiatrists increased their productivity. Canadian psychiatrists, for example, see five times as many patients a year as American psychiatrists do.[27]

Within this context of institutions and services, the psychiatric profession does its work. About 20,000 psychiatrists are active in clinical practice in the United States, and their number has been growing much more slowly than that of psychologists and social workers during the last two decades.[28] Moreover, the influx of foreign medical graduates (FMGs) has accounted for much of this growth. FMGs end up in the unfilled residencies, and psychiatry has had plenty. Before immigration laws recently cut out FMGs, they had increased to fill 40 percent of all psychiatric residencies. Yet, with their language and cultural barriers, psychiatry is the worst specialty for them and for their patients. FMGs are concentrated in state and county hospitals, making up over 50 percent of the staff, in an unholy alliance that allows them to stay in the United States unlicensed if they will work for low salaries. This underclass of the profession reaches back to training programs as well. About three-fourths of the residencies are affiliated with universities, and FMGs constituted 29 percent of these residents in 1975. In the unaffiliated programs, 68 percent were FMGs.

Describing what psychiatrists do is difficult because studies come up with divergent figures. About half the nation's psychiatrists have primarily office-based, private practices, though three-quarters see some patients in private practice. The trend, however, has been shifting as government programs and hospitals create more and more salaried positions. A study of psychiatrists in Maryland found that in 1974, 45 percent did some work in a general hospital, 33 percent in a medical school, and 26 percent in community mental health centers, though only 4 percent said that community psychiatry was their area of specialty. Most psychiatrists try to work in more than one setting, the ideal being a private practice with a hospital affiliation, some consulting with schools or a community center, some hospitalized patients, and possibly some supervision of residents. Virtually all psychiatrists work with patients, diagnosing them and administering some combination of psychotherapy and chemotherapy. Family therapy, behavioral therapy, shock and other modalities run far behind these two forms of therapy. With the growing role of third-party payments, the difference between patients seen in private practice and those seen at a public clinic is diminishing. A recent study found patients in both groups had about the same diagnoses and were seen if anything more often in the public clinic. Those in private therapy received considerably more electroshock treatments on one hand, and significantly more individual psychotherapy on the other, than those at the clinics, which used group and family therapy more.[29]

For their efforts, psychiatrists receive about the same income as general practitioners, and earn 10 or 15 percent less than the average for other specialties. Geographically, psychiatrists concentrate in metropolitan areas and near centers of psychiatric training. Two-thirds of all counties in the United States have no psychiatrist, making the profession probably the most unequally distributed of any medical specialty. Mental health services follow suit, with adequate coverage only in the Northeast, the Great Lakes, the Pacific Coast, and Hawaii. Sociologically, psychiatrists tend to treat patients who are like themselves—white, middle-class, college-educated adults.[30] Institutionally, psychiatrists make up less than 5 percent of the overall staff in mental health facilities, and less than 2 percent of the full-time staff (Appendix I, table 4). This preference for part-time positions has led to the profession's diminished power, as psychologists and social workers have assumed more of the full-time positions. State and county hospitals, general hospitals, outpatient clinics and CMHCs have been the principal institutions for work and training. Only in the first of these do psychiatrists tend to work full-time more than part-time, again because they often cannot choose to do otherwise.

The Power and Influence of Psychiatry

The extent of power and influence which psychiatrists exercise has yet to be studied well. However, they have had great power over the structure of mental health facilities and over the modes of treatment delivered. They direct virtually all mental hospitals, public and private, the psychiatric wards of general hospitals, private clinics, and the outpatient facilities which these institutions provide. Clinical psychologists, their chief rivals, generally work under psychiatrists in hospital settings as test-giving diagnosticians and some-time therapists. Clinical psychologists have assumed an increasing number of administrative posts and are successful in private practice, but they generally lack some prestige by not being physicians, even though their psychological training is often more comprehensive.

Psychiatrists also wield direct power through their control over how state and federal monies will be spent, and they have an increasingly important monopoly over prescribing drugs. Another center of power is the universities, where psychiatry's dominance has grown to virtual monopoly. Psychology, its main competitor, has lost power as experimental psychologists have squeezed clinicians out of departments of psychology and as clinical psychology has been internally torn between being an academic or a service profession. In addition, psychiatrists control the legal aspects of mental health. While psychiatrists are, on the whole, politically liberal, they exercise these various powers (with some exceptions) in a conservative way.[31]

Although less tangible than power, the *influence* of psychiatry over the other half million staff who care for patients assures its dominance. For example, nearly all social workers, nurses, and psychiatric aides learn their skills at facilities directed by psychiatrists. Psychiatrists often shape their training program and write much of the literature from which they learn mental health care. Significant numbers of residents are trained at all the major service institutions, and chances are that most of these have training programs for social workers, nurses, psychologists and other staff as well. Over one-third of all psychiatrists teach![32] Thus the small number of psychiatrists in these facilities belies the extent to which the profession's ideas determine how people are diagnosed and treated. It is therefore of major importance to know how psychiatrists learn their ideas.

Diagnosis and the Power of Labeling

Nothing so clearly illuminates the power and influence of psychiatry on its clients than labeling theory. Taking cognizance of the disparity between the 36 million people with serious symptoms and the 5 million people who get treated in mental health facilities, labeling theorists argue that the critical issue is to understand how those 5 million were singled out. In other words, primary deviance is much more widespread than social—particularly professional—reaction to that deviance.[33] And it is psychiatry more than any other group which controls that social reaction which leads to some people being labeled "mentally ill."

Research shows that a number of *social* characteristics determine who gets labeled mentally ill and who does not.[34] First is the kind of deviant behavior involved. If the symptoms are socially invisible, neither the person involved nor others are as likely to define that person as "sick" and begin the procedure which would lead to making this official; for "being sick" is society's way of containing and managing psychologically aberrant behavior. A second influence is the cultural context in which the symptoms occur. Expectations of normal behavior vary widely by social class, ethnicity and region. They also change over time. Homosexuality, for example, was defined *per se* as a mental illness, until the American Psychiatric Association voted in 1973 that it was not.[35] Third, having power and status makes a difference, not only in how successfully people can resist a label of mental illness, but in how likely they are to be diagnosed as ill in the first place. Thus measures of status such as age, race, income, and education all correlate with diagnostic labels.[36] Finally, how people were labeled in the past affects how they will be labeled in the present. Rosenhan's study is one of many to show that once a patient has been designated as mentally ill—even if s/he is actually normal—ordinary daily behavior will be reinterpreted by professional staff to conform to that label.[37]

Once a person gets a diagnostic label, it tends to affect what kind of treatment s/he will receive and how likely s/he is to "get better." Getting better is, itself, another label which seems to be a matter of professional psychiatric judgment but is in fact heavily influenced by social forces.[38] Because diagnosing schizophrenia characterizes a person's whole being much more than diagnosing kidney stones, psychiatric labels are particularly powerful. They allow a psychiatrist to deprive people of their civil rights and to incarcerate them for years in hospitals where no treatment takes place. For example, the civil liberties lawyer, Bruce J. Ennis, writes of an innocent man who was fingered by the police so that they could close a murder case, and was then declared incompetent to stand trial so that the false charges would not have to be proven. For twenty years he remained in Mattawan State Hospital, where 20 percent of the inmates have been waiting for more than twenty years to stand trial. A psychiatrist saw Ennis's client briefly every eighteen months or so. Describing a patient in Florida State Hospital, Ennis writes, "Only rarely during his first four years did a doctor or nurse so much as pass through Donaldson's ward. Doctors were seen in their offices, by invitation only. . . . It was not uncommon for patients to go two, three, or even four years without speaking to a doctor. Life on the wards was governed by untrained and occasionally brutal attendants . . . many of the attendants could neither read nor write."[39]

Once in these hospitals, the psychiatrists who direct them have made the patients work for wages as low as three-quarters of a cent to three cents an hour.[40] Only recently have a spate of law suits forced psychiatrists to restrict involuntary commitment, to guarantee that treatment takes place, and to stop slave labor.[41] But the broader significance of labeling theory is that social variables predict improvement as well as or better than psychiatric diagnosis.[42] This has led some investigators to conclude that when one compares the illness careers of people in Africa or Ceylon, where cultural beliefs about illness do not put so great an onus on the person with symptoms and where mental health care is loosely organized, with the illness careers of Americans or Englishmen, the former are defined as sick less often and lose their symptoms faster, because they are allowed to return to their normal activities with no stigma.[43] Nancy Waxler concludes that "the more comprehensive and available the treatment system, the more likely it will be that patients will receive illness-confirming messages and will thus remain in the sick role."[44]

To summarize, psychiatrists have considerable power and influence over mental health services dispensed by themselves and others. At the heart of this power are diagnostic labels which set off a chain of secondary reactions for the people being labeled, a chain which may affect their home or job, which influences what kind of treatment they get, and which contributes to how long they are considered sick. One would be glad for such professional intervention if psychiatrists knew what they were doing. Unfortunately, one is forced to conclude, on the basis of serious investigations, that too often they do not.

The fundamental problem is diagnosis. A recent authoritative overview concludes that while psychiatrists have tried for over a century to develop a "hard" diagnostic system, they have largely failed, because they lack disease-specific pathogenesis on which all good diagnostic systems are based.[45] As another observer puts it, "For the major mental illness classifications, none of the components of the medical model has been demonstrated: cause, lesion, uniform and invariate symptoms, course and treatment of choice."[46] Yet this has not stopped the profession from producing an official nomenclature. Most psychiatrists and a much larger number of social workers, nurses, psychologists, psychiatric aides, and other professionals use the established terms without serious question even though research shows that large numbers of patients do not have the symptoms which fit into the diagnostic categories used to characterize them.[47] The result is a low level of agreement between individuals on how a given case should be diagnosed. The evidence of low reliability is overwhelming—and is ignored in practice.[48]

This conclusion indicates that the psychiatric domain of mental health care is based on unreliable, unsubstantiated criteria for treatment. Far worse is the confidence which each clinician has in his/her own knowledge and judgment. Each understands the terms in his/her own way, and services are arranged so that people do not have to confront each other's differences. The same is true of involuntary commitment, perhaps the most serious deprivation of civil rights in the

United States. In the critical decision of involuntary commitment, psychiatrists have time and again demonstrated that they cannot predict with any accuracy who will be dangerous. Age and prior ciminal activity predict potential dangerousness better than professional diagnosis.[49] Yet courts continue to defer automatically to psychiatric assessment.[50] A survey of psychiatrists found that virtually all of them were confident they knew the laws concerning commitment, but in fact a large percentage did not.[51] The criteria they used to commit someone varied considerably.

> One psychiatrist proposed simply "mental alienation." Another indicated that he would only commit on the basis of "solid criteria of psychiatric diagnosis." A third stated, "if the patient has symptoms of behavior which require treatment and he refuses this voluntarily."[52]

The practical results are the same: each of these psychiatrists has the right to commit patients on his own criteria, which usually go unexamined. When lawyers are introduced prior to probate court appearance, the discharge rate is increased by one-half.[53] Psychiatrists, on the other hand, have asked for decades to be allowed full explanation of their assessment in court, rather than to be confined to a few narrow questions of law. Judge David Bazelon gave them that freedom with the Durham ruling. Twenty years later, Judge Bazelon summarized how psychiatrists used that freedom.

> Psychiatrists continued adamantly to cling to conclusory labels without explaining the origin, development, or manifestations of a disease in terms meaningful to a jury. . . . I regret to say that they [the diagnostic labels] were largely used to cover up a lack of relevance, knowledge, and certainty in the practice of institutional psychiatry.[54]

In contrast with the reckless speed of court psychiatrists in committing large proportions of their "clients"[55] stands the great reluctance of military psychiatrists to diagnose someone as mentally disturbed. A military psychiatrist describes a "reasonable" or "honorable" breakdown this way:

> A man should have been in combat for probably nine, ten months. . . . He's had to see probably a lot of his friends get killed. Or he might have had to be wounded himself quite severely. . . . And he also has to be a good soldier up until that time.
> Then . . . finally he is triggered by this trauma of someone else get-

ting killed, a close friend, or his unit may be overrun or himself getting severely wounded. It sets off a severe combination of anxiety, usually G.I. (gastro-intestinal) symptoms, anorexia, sometimes nausea, vomiting and bad dreams.[56]

Psychiatrists interviewed said that if a soldier comes in with the same symptoms after just one or two traumas in the first months of battle, he is considered to be either malingering or just immature. Characterological weakness is *not* assumed; therefore quick recovery is expected. Hospitalization is considered dangerous; in five to seven days, hospital life might turn a soldier's head away from the battlefield. He might begin to think that something has happened to him for which he is not responsible.[57] It is noteworthy that military psychiatrists deemphasize their medical status, speak of "counseling" rather than "diagnosis" or "treatment," and wear battle dress rather than white coats.

The sharp contrast between the assumptions, diagnoses and treatments of these two groups of psychiatrists illustrates a more universal truth: that psychiatry is always socially, culturally and politically embedded in the institution or community where it is practiced. In the nineteenth century, masturbation was considered sick, and in Freud's Vienna, women of independent mind were diagnosed as having a "masculinity complex." American psychiatry considered homosexuality a mental illness until recently, and Soviet psychiatry considers political dissent a sign of insanity.[58] Not only do cultural and political values profoundly affect the application of presumably universal criteria for diagnosis from one institutional setting to another within the psychiatric domain, but cultural shifts have also changed how psychiatrists use the same terms over time. In a paper which breaks through the limitations of both labeling theory and official diagnostic nomenclature, Nakagawa, Osborne, and Hartmann have argued that changing expectations by psychiatrists and a widening of cultural values in society have led to an increasing number of presenting complaints among patients first admitted to a hospital over the past twenty-five years.[59] Thought disorder, the traditional image of mental illness, has steadily decreased, but problems of social adjustment (as opposed to physiological and psychic symptoms) have risen sharply. Bruce Dohrenwend has found a similar expansion in the rate of people diagnosed as psychiatrically impaired in fifty-three studies over the past several decades. He concludes: "The tremendous increase is not a function of the increasing stresses and strains of the times in which we live.

Rather, it is a function of the tremendous expansion of psychiatric nomenclatures on the basis of experiences with psychiatric screening during World War II. This expansion has led not only to an increase in the types of disorders included in diagnostic manuals, but also to a broadening of the definition of previously included types."[60] As I. K. Zola points out, this is part of a larger process whereby "medicine is becoming a major institution of social control, nudging aside, if not incorporating, the more traditional institutions of religion and law. It is becoming the new repository of truth, the place where absolute and often final judgments are made by supposedly morally neutral and objective experts."[61]

This expansion of diagnostic nomenclature is about to make a quantum leap with the publication of the third Diagnostic and Statistical Manual of Mental Disorders (DSM-III). It is an old technique for a profession to enlarge its clientele by expanding its criteria for treatable problems; this is how agencies serving the blind, for example, "made" more blind people.[62] A review of the new manual concludes, "DSM-III widens the orbit of psychiatry, staking claims to a wide new territory of human problems."[63] At the same time, it does so with much more precision by using explicit, descriptive criteria instead of theoretical concepts.[64] Ironically, the effort to enhance psychiatry's professional stature by making diagnosis more scientific and precise may backfire. For in the process, the new diagnostic systems become less dependent on the clinical judgment or theoretical models of interpretation that distinguish a profession. As the President's Commission on Mental Health observes, these new diagnostic instruments "can be administered by nonpsychiatrists, and diagnosis is made by computer in a systematic fashion rather than relying on the interviews or interpretations of a psychiatrist."[65] Yet the new diagnostic system is more organic, which favors physicians, and it is hard to imagine that clinical judgment or personal interpretation can be eliminated in any diagnostic approach to emotional problems.

If we turn from diagnosis to treatment, we find again that psychiatrists tend to have a "style" which they use on a wide range of problems, though there is no good evidence to show that it is more effective than other techniques, or better than no professional treatment. In studies of therapeutic effectiveness, "The controls [in experimental studies] are getting better because they are getting help from persons untrained in formal psychotherapy, who practice a kind of natural therapy. It could be that these agents of personality integration are actually more effective as a group than trained therapists.''[66] ''In terms of drug research, it would be like testing responsiveness to a drug when allied substances are freely available and no record is kept of what else has been ingested by the patient.''[67] Thus the methodological problem of controls reveals a major pattern, namely that ''the vast majority chose non-mental-health professionals, and generally they felt more satisfied with the help received than did those who chose psychiatrists and psychologists.''[68]

If one looks behind average results to variability, those in psychotherapy tend to improve or get worse more than those not in therapy. Just as in medicine,[69] treatment—institutional, chemical, surgical and individual—creates new disorders as well as improving old ones.[70] ''Evidently there is something unique about psychotherapy which has the power to cause improvement beyond that occurring among controls, but equally evident is a contrary deteriorating impact that makes some cases worse than they were to begin with. When these contrary phenomena are lumped together in an experimental group, they cancel each other out to some extent, and the overall yield in terms of improvement . . . is no greater than the change occurring in a control group via 'spontaneous remission factors'.''[71]

Overall, the studies of therapeutic effectiveness have been inconclusive because the techniques and criteria of success are so vague. This is not only true for psychoanalytic therapies but for behavior therapy, group therapy and the like. Only certain drugs seem to demonstrate clear benefits. One is forced, therefore, to conclude that while psychiatrists have been granted a great deal of legal and cultural power, they exercise that power without reliable expertise. Leaders of biopsychiatry, however, believe all this will change in the next generation.

Training Psychiatrists

The confusion caused by vague diagnostic categories and a multiplicity of largely unproven treatments is reflected in not knowing how to train residents. The Commission of the American Psychiatric Association on the Education of Psychiatrists states:

In the recent past, conferences on psychiatric education have reached few conclusions as to the role of faculty and so faculty have been urged to remain flexible—expected to teach everything, not teach anything. The result has been that some students know next to nothing and have a resultant identity crisis and role confusion. The coming decade is going to call for a decision which will necessitate a delineation of psychiatry's role.[72]

It seems rather late for psychiatry, being over 130 years old, to start delineating its role and responsibilities. In fact, while this quotation accurately reflects the national situation, at the local level curricula are shaped around the knowledge and values of each residency's faculty and therefore can have a distinct character. Given that there is little scientific basis for choosing one approach over another, a local faculty's choice is more a matter of ideological closure than anything else. The major issues of training are not well understood, and in fact there are few actual descriptions of what training entails. Beyond local folk theories, for example, little is known about how future psychiatrists are selected. Each program works out its own ways, and the APA commission concludes that almost anyone can get in.[73] There is a high rate of psychopathology among residents. After selection, the commission found that the training process itself is also not well understood:

. . . a review of the education literature in psychiatry, and discussions with faculty and residents, suggests that whatever a program's emphasis may be—whether it is psychoanalytically oriented psychotherapy, community psychiatry, biological psychiatry, or whatever else (in whatever combination), the theme of role modeling (and the related phenomenon of professional socialization) is most consistently present and, unfortunately, usually least explicitly dealt with.[74]

The study which follows does explicitly address role modeling and a number of other aspects of psychiatric training. How does training affect the values of young psychiatrists? How do psychiatrists learn to cope with the uncertainties of their trade? Are psychiatrists well equipped to treat suicidal cases? What effect does the organization of the training program have on the psychiatric residents? In answering these questions, a number of theoretical issues in sociology are addressed: the nature of professional socialization, the interplay of social structure and personality on moral careers and omnipotent tendencies, the structural characteristics of diagnosis, treatment and training, and the organization of time. In examining these topics, the book brings together findings from a wide range of studies of other psychiatric residencies; thus we can obtain as comprehensive a picture as possible of how psychiatrists at leading schools are trained.

If psychiatry is the elite of the mental health team, the training program run by University Psychiatric Center is one of the elite of psychiatry. It has produced at least as many powerful and distinguished members of the profession as any other. In recent years, its graduates have continued to hold senior positions in the federal government and to direct major institutions in psychiatry. It is reasonable to suppose that their primary training as psychiatrists at this program shaped the values and practices by which they lead these institutions and direct national policy.

Although a leader, University Psychiatric Center was ideologically close to the norm. It was analytic-eclectic, meaning that it had deep commitments to psychoanalysis but was surrounded by projects and research in community and social psychiatry, behavior therapy, drug experiments and so forth. In professional politics it might be called enlightened orthodoxy, reflecting the pattern in most residencies of psychoanalytic dominance tolerating eclectic forays into other approaches.[75] Therefore, this study concerns an influential but ideologically normal program.

Finally, this research is fixed in time. Any study is an episode in history and should be regarded that way. The rapid changes occurring in psychiatry force upon us the question of history but also leave no choice: one must present the findings of research as true for their time. This study occurred in the late 1960s, at the height of community psychiatry's commitment to reach poor clients on their own turf, make clients partners in therapy, and change their stressful environment. More important, it documents the kind of training which leaders of psychiatry today experienced, a kind of training that may change fundamentally in the years to come.

2.

Getting into Psychiatry

Although educational institutions emphasize their effect on the people they train, their graduates closely resemble the candidates they admitted at the start. Because psychiatry, which emphasizes psychotherapy, considers one's personality the principal tool, to be honed and refined, *who* gets selected into the profession is no small matter. As residents and staff often said at the University Psychiatric Center, "It's not what you know but who you are that counts."[1] Although the purport of this aphorism was to emphasize the importance of self-knowledge, it echoed the widespread public fascination with psychiatrists. Do they have psychiatric symptoms themselves? Are all those stories about neurotic psychiatrists true? Personality is usually neglected in studies of socialization.[2] But suppose that psychiatrists tend to score high as authoritarians (which they do not). Without quite knowing why, patients[3] would find themselves heavily dependent on such therapists and would feel inferior. This relation could be quite damaging to a person who already feels beaten down in daily life. Or suppose that students going into psychiatry express more anxiety about death than other medical students (which they do); what are the chances that they can help a suicidal person with the supporting strength that such an individual needs?

The layman's concern over neurotic psychiatrists parallels an intricate web of professional attitudes on the same subject. On one hand, the ideal candidate for training is a person anyone can admire. On the other hand, older residents and training staff will often say: "Most of us are in here to learn about ourselves. To get through premed and med school you have to be pretty compulsive, and we're not quite sure how to handle our emotions." While the staff tries to screen out anyone with serious mental problems, a continuous theme in training is that a therapist cannot "go with" patients as they take him[4] into their emotional turmoil nor work through therapeutic problems unless he can empathize with the patients' craziness. To have empathy, it is believed, one must have experienced or at least be able to imagine what the patient is going through. In this context, of course, psychoanalysis for the therapist is a way for him to go crazy in a controlled way, to open up repressed fantasies and deep injuries so that he can become a more effective therapist.

The implications of this outlook are highlighted by a case where a respected therapist-resident treated a woman who drowned her two little children in their bath water. After many months of effort, he doubted he could help her because, "when she gets to that scene, I just can't go with her." What kind of therapist could? The theory assumes that within even the most healthy resident lie feelings of murder, rape, autism, great sadness, despair, rage and inferiority. An intense professional training which aims to elicit and give expression to such feelings may well produce emotional disturbances and sanction neurotic mannerisms.*

Taken as a whole, the views which psychiatry expresses about the therapist's personality are probably ambivalent and possibly heroic. The profession seeks "healthy" candidates, yet assumes that neurosis accompanies application. It encourages the resident to explore the depths of his psyche so that his capacity for empathy will grow, yet it disciplines him against projecting his own feelings onto the patient (countertransference). Possibly this is the heroic quest of Faust: to know everything, to have no horror or secret or fantasy of the human psyche barred, yet to keep full possession of one's soul. Even Faust could not do that.

Although the public, sociology, and psychiatry itself wish to know who enters psychiatry, studies of the subject are fragmentary.

---

*Ironically, the profession is worried about the prevalence of emotionally disturbed residents but does not consider its mode of training a cause.

This means that the psychiatric profession (and everyone else) knows little about those who will inherit its position in mental health. However, if we labor over the pieces, we can puzzle together a plausible design. Yet this puzzle is made of cardboard, not solid wood; for almost every piece is a case study of one group at one time. Thus, the picture which emerges in the following pages should be taken as a series of tentative conclusions to be investigated more systematically when either the profession or interested parties decide to do so.

Does Medical School Discourage Psychiatrists?

Professional training (or countertraining) for psychiatry begins in medical school. One reason for starting here is that we know almost nothing about the earlier years—the adolescent commitment to set one's course, the struggles with organic chemistry or biology in college, the parents who ache to have their child become a doctor but who feel betrayed if the child decides to become a psychiatrist. Another reason for starting with medical school is to examine the relations between these two professions when they are closely intertwined.

Every profession has an ideal of itself. In recruiting, a profession seeks candidates who come closest to that ideal. In training, a profession shapes and polishes its recruits, putting forward its finest examples for the next generation to emulate. Most of us naturally assume that recruitment and training complement each other, but this is not always the case.[5]

In psychiatry, for example, medical school is both a source of recruitment and a training experience. This double function makes it important to examine the impact of the medical school experience on potential or future psychiatrists. Because it intertwines the two professions, this relationship mingles the ideals and goals of medical recruitment and training with those of psychiatric recruitment and training.

The ideal doctor has not changed much over time. In *Samhita,* the Hindu book of medicine, the ideal student is "born of a good family, possessed of the desire to learn," and having "strength, energy of action, contentment, character, self-control, a good retentive memory, intellect, courage, purity of mind and body, and a simple and clear comprehension."[6] Recent descriptions of the ideal doctor differ only slightly. For example, one author stated that the ideal physician is "compassionate, sympathetic, perceptive and understanding and he likes human beings. He is a man of culture."[7] The qualities of the ideal psychiatrist are strikingly similar, suggesting an enviable compatibility between general medicine and psychiatry.

In practice, however, a different picture of the medicine-psychiatry relationship emerges. Medical schools select students primarily on the basis of science grades and test scores. A recent study showed once again that America's physicians are chosen on criteria that have no relation to their clinical competence. These criteria emphasize science, and those with high scores tend to have narrower interests, be less adaptable, and feel less comfortable with other people.[8] By contrast, psychiatry begins with a pool of technically competent medical students and concentrates on selecting those who manifest qualities that distinguish a good clinician.

This picture suggests that medical schools recruit against the best interests of both medicine and psychiatry, particularly in terms of primary care. A sensible remedy would be for medical schools first to screen out only candidates whose science scores are so low they will flunk out and then to use psychological tests and interviews for making the final decision. This would balance technical skills with the clinical ideals of the profession.

The impact of the experience of medical school on potential psychiatrists was measured in a study at Tufts Medical School,[9] where 58 percent of the freshmen expressed a high interest in psychiatry and 21 percent listed psychiatry as their first choice for a specialty, putting psychiatry in a tie for first place with surgery. However, by the fourth year, only about 10 percent of a given class entered psychiatry. The ironic inference is that *psychiatry rests its claims for professional status on a profession that is hostile toward it.*

Influences of Pressure and Personality

The pressures of medical school and its atmosphere have long been known to require or generate qualities in medical students quite at odds with the profession's ideal of the physician. Successful students "are usually obsessive, compulsive, orderly, highly organized, responding primarily to the dictates of their own conscience."[10] One study found that the most frequent ideal among first-year medical students was to be a critical-sadistic person.[11] Four common patterns of "adjustment" to medical school are: 1. emotional constriction; 2. a fierce concentration on grades; 3. manipulation of others to get ahead; and 4. high anxiety.[12] Personal pathology severe enough to require psychiatric assistance runs from a minimum of 20 to a maximum of 46 percent of a class. Summarizing fifty-three articles and books, one reviewer concludes:

> The brief historical and social portrait of the student from the beginnings of medicine onward, plus the personal and professional expectations of him, are presented to indicate the massive stress that is placed on an ego that is still in the process of becoming. The rapid technological advances and social demands constantly increase the stress and inexorably produce emotional turmoil in every student."[13]

Several authors have focused on the rise of cynicism over the four years of medical school.[14] This has been interpreted by Becker and Geer as the process of medical students realistically adjusting their initial idealism to life in medical school,[15] but the cynicism scales used have little to do with such adjustment and are tapping a more basic outlook on life. Moreover, general cynicism does not appear to increase in other training programs such as nursing or law,[16] and thus it is not simply part of "maturity."

Since psychiatry depends so heavily on the personal strengths and resources of its practitioners, the assault by medical school on these qualities considerably affects who goes into psychiatry. As Donald Winnecott, a noted psychoanalyst, wrote, "The doctor's long and arduous training does nothing to qualify him in Psychology and does much to disqualify him. It keeps him so busy from eighteen to twenty-five that he finds he is middle aged before he has the leisure in which to discover himself."[17] Even if cynicism goes down after the student gets in psychiatry,[18] considerable damage may have been done.

Faculty Influence

Does the problem lie with medical school faculty? Somehow it must, yet a careful study of faculty influence could find little evidence to this effect. When a large sample of students from eight medical schools were asked about the greatest influence on their career decisions, 54 percent mentioned informal faculty influence.[19] Each student named faculty members who were most influential in various ways.

When these were organized by specialty, professors of internal medicine were named six times more often than psychiatrists as someone a student would talk to about choosing a specialty, and nine times more often as the person who had most influenced the student's view of medicine. Professors of psychiatry were chosen least often in every category of influence and psychiatry ranked as the lowest specialty in prestige.[20] However, when the investigators tried to pin down just how these faculty had been influential, they did not succeed.[21]

Nevertheless, just as racial prejudice is difficult to document scientifically, though both black and white observers have no doubt of its existence, so psychiatrists and other physicians widely acknowledge an antipsychiatric prejudice in medical school, even though it eludes scientific investigation. For example, a psychiatrist captured the experience of many when he wrote about "the subtle and snide remarks that come from other members of the medical profession. While many professors of medicine and surgery will make pompous statements about the need for psychiatry and, at times, even support its place in the curriculum, a raised eyebrow or a gesture sometimes convey more to a student than does an official statement."[22]

The Curriculum

Just as there is no evidence that faculty overtly discourage medical students from psychiatry, so the curriculum seems to give psychiatry its fair share of time with the students. Virtually all medical students take a required course in the first year, with lectures and readings on normal and abnormal development, as well as a survey of psychopathology, and such courses usually include a clinical seminar where students can see, if not interview, people with emotional problems. In many medical schools—there is much individual variation among them—students must also take courses introducing them to clinical medicine or teaching them to interview, where the psychiatric sensitivity to interpersonal relations makes its contribution. Another course, introduction to clinical psychiatry, is also required in some schools. In the third year many students must take a full-time clerkship in psychiatry for four to six weeks, where they work directly with patients, usually in psychiatric wards or clinics, but increasingly on medical services such as pediatrics or internal medicine. Beyond that, most schools offer several electives in psychiatry.[23]

Yet a general disregard if not hostility to matters psychiatric pervades the curriculum. As early as 1949, Karl Menninger and Bernard Hall found a great interest in psychiatry among medical students mixed with the following opinion:

> Psychiatry is vague, ethereal, and mystical; it is divorced from good medicine; it is too subjective; there is a lack of personal gratification in the practice of psychiatry; . . . psychiatry is irreligious; psychiatry does not help anyone; psychiatry is concerned only with diagnosis and not with treatment.[24]

A recent study found that when students were asked to rate "myself," "doctor," surgeon," "psychiatrist," and "patient" on a variety of general qualities such as foolish/wise, clean/dirty, they rated themselves highest and psychiatrists at the bottom, just above patients. Taking the basic psychiatry course did not change these ratings; the students learned about psychiatry but did not change their attitudes toward it. Most interesting was the discovery that the faculty gave the same ratings to psychiatry as did the students! Even some psychiatrists downgraded other members of their profession—but not themselves.[25]

These matters are also reflected in the medical school curriculum, where the psychological dimension of physical medicine remains largely segregated and ignored. The psychiatrist Iago Gladston writes:

> The now prevailing philosophy in medical education is Cartesian in derivation and atomistic in character. It fosters the dismemberment of man. What we need is a philosophy of medicine and of medical education that perceives man and understands him holistically, ecologically, and existentially. These may be odd terms, but they do encompass what is requisite for the modernization of medical education and medical service.
>
> The young medical man who comes to us for his residency training in psychiatry all too often brings with him a quantum of attitudes and beliefs which impede his learning of psychiatry.[26]

The Teaching of Psychiatry in Medical School

The general problem of training humane doctors and the specific tensions between psychiatry and medicine have not gone unnoticed. In a time of community practice, these problems go to the heart of good medicine. Over the past two decades, everyone has agreed that a technological emphasis pushed humane care into the shadows of medical training. In response, scores of programs have been launched to bring psychiatric insights and humanistic values into the center of medical education. A mood of optimism prevails, suggesting that the inhumane, antipsychiatric days are over. But studies of what medical students actually learn are discouraging. A survey of five medical schools in Philadelphia revealed that half the students believed that if a person talks about suicide he will not do it; half believed that masturbation frequently causes mental illness; two-thirds thought a psychotic could not hold a job; and a third believed that neurosis is diagnosed by excluding organic factors.[27] Even when students do learn psychiatry, some studies show they do not apply the knowledge in practice.[28]

Medical Students' Opinions of Psychiatry

The reasons are not hard to find. Psychiatry is rated as one of the worst taught specialities.[29] Specific comments from graduates of forty-one American and Canadian medical schools are revealing: no detectable purpose, poor organization, uncoordinated clinical experiences, poor teachers. Much of the teaching is done by lecture, and 20 percent said their clinical experience amounted to observing demonstrations. The majority never began or completed the treatment of their clinical cases. Thirty-six percent reported little or no supervision, and 38 percent felt they had received no guidance from supervisors. Yet despite such discouraging experiences, half the physicians said they needed more psychiatry to practice medicine well, and three-quarters said they enjoyed trying to understand a patient's problems. Again, we find a stifling of widespread interest, but with a clear mandate: make psychiatry a living, clinical experience with excellent supervision.[30]

The experience of psychiatry and its image in medical school influence students' perspective on the profession and therefore affect who decides to enter it. In general rankings of medical specialties, psychiatry rates low.[31] Thus students rarely give it as a second choice; it is either a first choice (for some) or a third or lower choice (for most). To be more specific about psychiatry's image, students deem psychiatrists to be less competent but more likeable than surgeons or internists. For example, medical students in one study considered psychiatrists to be less clear-thinking, less realistic and not so alert as the other two specialties—but they also thought psychiatrists were less rigid, less arrogant, more easy-going and more sensitive. A three-week clerkship in psychiatry reinforced both halves of this perspective. "The greatest changes were in the students' perceptions of the *style of relationships* that psychiatrists form. Not only were the psychiatrists . . . seen as more considerate, friendly, gentle, and informal, but they were also perceived as being more appreciative, calm, humorous, and relaxed."[32]

The point is that such qualities, which give psychiatry a low rating among medical students who esteem competence and boldness, are in fact the marks of competence in the profession! Thus, students perceive psychiatry accurately, but from the hostile perspective of technical medicine.

Other studies reflect an even more negative image of psychiatry among medical students. One researcher followed a small group of students over four years and found that their evaluation of a full range of psychiatric treatments, from electroshock to psychotherapy, worsened significantly.[33] Another examined students' medical opinions of various specialties at the University of Oklahoma and found that psychiatrists alone were characterized as deeply interested in intellectual problems, yet confused thinkers and emotionally unstable.[34] More clinical experience led these students to see psychiatrists as less intellectual and more confused than before. Overall, their views were similar to the public's stereotype of psychiatry, even though they had worked closely with practitioners.

What Kinds of Students Choose Psychiatry?

Given these reports of bad teaching, low status, and poor imagery, what kind of person retains an interest in psychiatry? He or she claims a great interest in intellectual problems and research, though his/her academic record may not be distinguished.[35] In one study, psychiatric students scored high on complexity of thought and on introversion.[36] Students with a strong interest in psychiatry are also less committed to medicine and more likely to have considered another career than other medical students. Their decision is more likely to have been their own rather than one encouraged by their family.[37]

As a group, potential psychiatrists are divided between those who decide early to become psychiatrists and those who want to become physicians but then find they like psychiatric work more than medical practice. The first kind is intellectual, probably captivated by the psychoanalytic theory of man, and enters medical school only as a means to becoming a psychiatrist. S/he is less likely to be uncertain and anxious than the other kind, who vascillates and essentially changes his or her career and self-image in midstream.[38] However, the early deciders may be more anxious, cynical about what they see happening in medicine, and therefore may isolate themselves from the general student culture.[39]

In psychological tests, candidates for psychiatry score as having little prejudice and few authoritarian attitudes.[40] Low authoritarianism in turn is linked to low scores on aggression and orderliness, and high scores on intraception and nurturance. Moreover, authoritarianism relates inversely to admiration for psychiatry. Thus, nonauthoritarian students score high on qualities valued in psychiatry, are more likely to admire it as a specialty, and also emphasize understanding as an important attribute of a good physician. By contrast, most medical students do not like psychiatric patients because they are not friendly and cooperative, and most prefer not to treat patients with emotional illnesses.[41]

Besides scoring lower on authoritarianism than other medical students, candidates for psychiatry score low on measures of racism.[42] This does not mean, however, that blacks do not have problems when they train to be psychiatrists. As a group of them recently wrote, they enter an ethnocentric white middle-class, psychoanalytic world that is foreign to blacks and the needs of the black community. In training, race was simply not mentioned. In a society filled with racial tension, they found this omission amazing. Residents tended to incorporate and identify with this form of "white institutional racism." "The black resident chosen for these training programs must demonstrate a willingness to accept the institution's values and biases."[43] White residents tried to show the black resident that he was accepted by telling him he was not thought of as a Negro and by assuring him that he could talk to white people too. Black residents interpreted such efforts as "latent antiblack sentiment." This was also reflected in the effort of training programs to screen out black patients, so that the residents could have "good," "interesting" cases.[44] Given the colorblind, class-biased nature of psychiatric theory and the great position of power bestowed upon the psychiatrist, one is not sure what low scores on racism and authoritarianism mean.[45]

While medical students going into psychiatry are low on the authoritarian scale, they are high on the Machiavellian scale, which measures how much people endorse manipulating moral standards.[46] Religiously, nonbelievers are five times more likely, compared to Protestants, to enter psychiatry than other specialties.[47] The importance of religion (which cuts across several faiths) has a strong negative relation to the Machiavellian scale and a strong positive relation to the authoritarian scale.

A final trait found among potential psychiatrists is high death anxiety, which is inversely related to being authoritarian. In an excellent study, Livingston and Zimet discovered that the defense which medical students have for working around dying people comes not from learning detached concern, but from their own personality. Death anxiety does not decrease but actually increases in the third year, indicating that early work with cadavers and experimental animals does not prepare sensitive students for working with human patients. Rather, different kinds of personalities sort themselves out by specialty, with psychiatry and pediatrics getting a preponderance of nonauthoritarian students with high scores on death anxiety. The authors add that extremely nonauthoritarian as well as authoritarian personalities can prevent stable, anxiety-free relations. "Too much authoritarianism distorts the physician's sense of reality and renders him incapable of a beneficial relationship with his patients; too little makes the physician liable to doubts, extreme introspectiveness, and a pathologic sensitivity that makes him unable to retain the detachment necessary for useful service to a suffering human being."[48]

The implications of these studies are important. As Livingston and Zimet state, "the inability of a medical student to view a patient as a 'whole man,' as psyche and soma, is not an isolated trait but part of a whole personality syndrome characterized as authoritarian."[49] This has a number of implications for selection into both medicine and psychiatry. First, aside from extreme cases, the students who would be the best practicing physicians ironically are the most likely to be turned off by medical school and to be oriented toward psychiatry. Second, at a time when psychosocial functions of medical care are seen as very important, medical schools tend not to select students by personality, and therefore may be admitting numbers of students who will not carry out these functions well.[50] (Note, however, that when medical schools choose women over men, they are more likely to get students who are independent but not aggressive, sensitive and emotionally expressive, yet strong.[51]) Finally, it appears that psychiatry gets many of the candidates it wants only because they slip into medical school on other merits.

In conclusion, by insisting on a medical degree, psychiatry finds itself in the awkward position of letting *another* profession select its pool of candidates on different—if not counterproductive—grounds and then discourage many of those interested in psychosocial problems from choosing psychiatry. Beyond psychiatry, medical school emerges as a punishing, technologically preoccupied institution which selects students on the wrong criteria and belittles an interest in the patient as a person. In recent years these problems have received increasing attention, and many educators are working to overcome them. But for psychiatry the question is whether its "return to medicine" means that future psychiatrists will be selected increasingly for scientific rather than clinical ability.

Selecting the Psychiatric Elite

As the dominant profession in mental care, psychiatry has a duty to recruit and train practitioners by the highest standards. This is true of any profession; for society grants a profession its privileges in return for excellence. Thus we expect psychiatry to search for and find the most successful way to select and train candidates.

If psychiatry did this, there would exist careful, longitudinal studies of different selection procedures and how well they chose people who provided good patient care. Instead, we find (again) half-completed bits of research by individuals in different residencies. Clearly, selection into this powerful profession is a folk art. Despite the fact that the American Psychiatric Association has long-term committees on training and manpower, there appears to be no centralized, coordinated effort to analyze these matters. Moreover, most of the information we have comes from famous residencies, perhaps because the pressure to publish leads a staff psychiatrist or ambitious resident to research. Nevertheless, some important insights emerge from these materials, though they necessarily pertain to only the elite programs. Most of these elite centers represent the psychoanalytic segment of the profession, with its distinctive ideology and career patterns.[52]

Selection is a two-way process, of choosing and being chosen.

From the selection process we learn about both the candidates and the psychiatric profession. The first half of this present chapter analyzed the relationships between the personalities of psychiatric candidates and the social structure of medical schools from which they emerge. We found them largely in conflict, and for that matter we found medical training in conflict with its own image of the ideal physician. The same questions now apply to psychiatric residencies. Who are the ideal candidates? How are they selected? What is the character of those finally chosen?

The Great Study

Amidst the studies that fill the literature lies dormant and dust-covered one great work, *Personality Patterns of Psychiatrists,* by Robert R. Holt and Lester Luborsky.[53] The study covered six years of residencies at the Menninger School of Psychiatry and took another four years to write. Although the work is far from perfect, especially in its lack of control groups, it sets a standard of examination no other work has matched. Yet, strangely, it is neglected in current literature; authors merely refer to it for support on a minor point. More important, it has been neglected in a second sense: its startling implications have been overlooked. Perhaps it was too admired when it came out and too uncritically read; yet it contains striking discoveries.

The question, of course, is whether it is still valid today. In many ways I think it is, and I will draw on it in the pages to come. It is so much more thorough than other studies that on some questions it is all we have. But one is struck by how well its conclusions stand up against more recent research; rarely have its findings been reversed or seriously altered by newer studies. Does this mean that much of the selection and training process has remained unchanged in twenty years? One would think not from reading residency brochures, which herald a new, eclectic approach that is multidisciplinary and socially oriented. But this "new" rhetoric is old: from its beginning the Menninger School claimed that it offered training in all adjunct therapies, that it had a first-rate staff in social work and other professions, and that it emphasized the team approach, drawing upon the entire therapeutic milieu to help the patient. Even the juxtaposition of ideology and practice remains similar: eclectic on the surface and stubbornly psychoanalytic at root.

Defining the Good Psychiatrist

The selection criteria and procedures for recruitment into psychiatry are not openly discussed. The quick silence or vague answers which characterize conversations on this topic imply either embarrassment or a conviction that this is a most private matter. Unable to obtain specific information on how the staff at the University Psychiatric Center[54] selected its residents, I turned to other studies 'of selection and was impressed by how consistently psychiatrists have used the same criteria for judging candidates.

Personal characteristics so dominate the literature on choosing good candidates that one almost overlooks the larger point. Hardly any writer refers to a technical or medical skill. One would not know that all candidates must have gone through medical school and internship. Here is a striking paradox, a scientific profession whose entire screening apparatus is geared to the personality of the candidate. Candidates see professional training in a similar light. One of few ideas they share as they begin a psychoanalytic residency is that supervisors should focus on residents' personality traits.[55]

Beyond this single unity, specific traits sought in the ideal candidate are extremely diffuse, though they do not cover the entire spectrum of human qualities. However, some patterns emerge among them, and since they are so important to the profession, they deserve a closer look.

The most comprehensive survey of expert opinion on criteria was conducted by Karl Menninger in 1950, when he asked directors of the largest residencies what qualities are most important for deciding whom to accept.[56] No reports since that time have altered the list; it is so wide-ranging that none could! Yet despite the lack of overlapping criteria from center to center, the list (table 2.1) has an underlying continuity. Nearly all the qualities would be universally embraced as admirable. The ideal candidate is intelligent, empathetic, has a sense of humor, is interesting and interested in others, has the capacity for growth but is already a man of breadth and accomplishment, is sincere, honest, and mature. Other lists are similar.[57]

A few disagreements surfaced in the Menninger survey. Some training directors explicitly preferred candidates in the bottom third of their medical school class, because they were less likely to be grinds or overintellectualized individuals. Others preferred brighter students, by which they only meant the upper third of the class. In contrast to colleges and medical schools, psychiatry does not appear to seek the brilliant student who might make fundamental contributions to the field.

A second area of disagreement concerned whether extroverts or introverts make better psychiatrists. While the Menninger study found that introverted, quiet people whose warmth was subdued made the best therapists, Abel and his colleagues found the extroverts to be rated higher.[58] This disagreement stands for a larger one on the desirability of neurotic candidates. The distinguished analyst, Ives Hendrick, complained that the profession was suffering from including "more matter-of-fact, common-sense well-adjusted individuals" than in years before. The profession seemed to prefer, he wrote, very normal, not too bright, all-around people, though many of its pioneers were "primarily introspective individuals, inclined to be studious and thoughtful, and tended to be highly individualistic and to limit their social life to clinical and theoretical discussions with colleagues."[59]

Another interesting difference is that between the qualities believed desirable in psychiatry, psychotherapy and psychoanalysis. Besides the general qualities mentioned above, psychiatrists are seen as needing administrative and leadership ability, a sense of humor, and a likeable personality. On the other hand, psychotherapists and psychoanalysts, but not psychiatrists, are seen as needing *"introspectiveness, insight into one's self, creativity, sublimated voyeurism, grasp of cultural implications and of the relativity of behavior. . . ."*[60] What these differences show is that psychiatrist refers to an administrator who needs the qualities of a manager and diplomat, while psychotherapist is nearly synonymous with being psychoanalyst. These differences persist today in residents who have a managerial as opposed to a therapeutic approach toward their work.[61]

Overall, however, "the degree of overlap in discussions of the personalities of psychiatrists, psychoanalysts, and psychotherapists is impressive."[62] Of particular note is the similarity, in table 2.1, between the prescriptions for good psychoanalytic candidates and the qualities of good psychotherapists. Since these are personal characteristics, the similarity implies that the most important skills of this profession are not acquired by training. The resident learns new knowledge and gets supervised practice in refining interpersonal skills, but "if a man is not all of these things by the time he has entered medical

TABLE 2.1   Summary of Expert Opinion on Personality Requisites for Psychiatry*

Qualities to be Sought in Applicants for Psychiatric Training	Qualities Characterizing the Trained (Effective) Psychiatrist

I. ABILITIES AND CAPACITIES

A. Intellectual

1. Superior intelligence	1. Intelligence
	2. Common sense
	3. Observational ability
	4. Imagination

B. Interpersonal: Receptive

1. Intuitiveness	1. Intuition
2. Capacity for understanding	2. Sensitivity to subtle dynamics of human behavior
3. Empathy	3. Empathy
4. Psychological-mindedness	

C. Interpersonal: Interactive and Relational

1. Verbal facility	
2. Capacity to attract friendship	2. Likeability: ability to win affection
3. Ability to interrelate with many types of people	
	4. Ability to win respect and trust
5. Ability to work harmoniously with institutional colleagues	5. Ability to work as member of a team; absence of annoying traits
6. Leadership ability	6. Ability to raise morale, maintain serene atmosphere

II. ATTITUDES, INTERESTS, AND VALUES

A. General Characteristics of Attitudes and Values

1. Breadth of (nonmedical) interests	1. Breadth of interests

B. Interest in Psychiatry

	1. Interest in subject-matter
	2. Preference for dynamic concepts

C. Attitudes toward Patients and People Generally

1. Interest in people	
2. Concern with human problems in their universal aspects	

3. Respect for the dignity and integrity
of the individual

4. Tolerance

5. Sense of social responsibility
6. Therapeutic optimism

7. (*Negative quality*) *Communist beliefs*

V. OTHER TRAITS OF PERSONALITY

A. Adjustment and Health

1. Maturity
2. Emotional stability   2. Emotional stability
3. Relative freedom from symptoms

A . *Psychopathology (Negative Indications)*

1. *Addiction*   1. *Alcoholism*
2. *Overt homosexuality*
3. *Psychopathic tendencies*   3. *Sleeping with nurses in the hospital*
    4. *Egocentric traits*

B. General Evaluative Traits

1. Integrity of character   1. Integrity; truthfulness
2. Sincerity
3. Stature and breadth of personality
4. Acceptance of responsibility   4. Dependability
5. General appearance and manner   5. General appearance and manner

C. Emotional and Interpersonal Traits

1. Emotional warmth   1. Warmth
    2. Sympathy, kindliness, considerateness
    3. Co-operativeness

D. Inner-personal Traits

1. Independence without hostility to authority

    2. Inner confidence

3. Extraversion

*Where a corresponding quality is lacking in a column, the number is omitted.
Source: Holt and Luborsky, table I-15.1.

school, it is probably too late for him to acquire them. . . . The psychiatrist as a person is more important than the psychiatrist as a technician or scientist. What he *is* has more effect upon his patients than anything he *does*."[63]

Selecting the Best Candidates

Having defined the ideal resident, the profession must go on to select him (or sometimes her). Although this selection process may seem psychological because of the profession's emphasis on personal qualities, it is really sociological, because it concerns the profession's self-concept and its methods for self-perpetuation. The quality of this process varies considerably from the top to the bottom of the profession, where "undesirable" residencies scramble to fill their quota with any suitable candidate who applies.[64] Here, for lack of data, we must concentrate on famous residencies which choose candidates from a large pool of applicants.

Besides written applications, which sometimes require an essay by the applicant, psychiatric residencies rely on personal interviews by their staff. Although they are selecting for personality, only a few use psychological tests. The results are obvious. First, this means that most programs do not know precisely what they are looking for. After listing the criteria which residencies seek, Bernard Riess writes, "The disparate nature of these qualities and the difficulty of measurement are too obvious to make comment necessary. It would appear that there is a need to specify experimentally the factors involved in selection."[65]

Second, most programs, whether happy with their procedures or not, do not evaluate it. In one study, "A majority of the eleven [residencies] reported that they were dissatisfied with 20 percent or more of the applicants accepted. . . . Actually, however, no one *knew* how good a job of selection was being done anywhere."[66]

Finally, since the criteria are both diffuse and vague, the psychiatrists who do the interviewing only agree some of the time. Holt and Luborsky found the reliability among interviewers to be 0.4. Moreover, interviewing psychiatrists often gave similar ratings to applicants they accepted and applicants they rejected.[67] Essentially, each interviewer picked candidates he liked. As Bucher has suggested, these are candidates whom the interviewer would like to have (and perhaps will have) as a long-term patient. For the qualities of a good patient—sensitive, articulate, insightful, responsive—are the qualities of a good therapist.[68]

The results of selection usually go unmeasured, but from those programs which do so, it appears that residencies have mixed successes in choosing good psychiatrists. Holt and Luborsky found that the residents who earned high ratings from the faculty had scored higher on scales of genuineness and social adjustment, and lower on preoccupation with status than residents who earned lower ratings. Nevertheless, the admissions committee had chosen them as well.

More recently, a team at the Albert Einstein College of Medicine in New York City designed a thirty-two-item rating scale based on what faculty members told them were the criteria for selecting residents.[69] The candidates chosen did indeed score better on these criteria than those rejected, though there was considerable overlap. Table 2.2 shows which items did or did not discriminate between those accepted and those rejected. As a group, the items which discriminated are qualities which everyone admires, and while some such qualities did not discriminate, most of the nondiscriminating items are negative. This implies that while the interviewers told the team that they did *not* want people who were dependent or who complained, they directed their attention in the interview toward finding out which applicants had more of the *good* qualities. In addition, items pertaining to academic record or specific interests in certain psychiatric fields did not discriminate. This adds further support to the idea that the psychiatric profession selects on personality and not on items pertaining to the profession.

The same team used tests to measure the emotional style and values of candidates. The results give an insightful portrait of people going into psychiatry which finds corroboration in other studies. On the whole, they are "sociable and enjoy being with people but do not go out of their way to meet new people."[70] While they are "interested in relating to people in a friendly way, they are ambivalent about allowing their involvement to become very deep . . . their sociability frequently conflicts with strong tendencies toward individualism and self-sufficiency."[71] Two clinicians, looking at average profiles of those accepted and rejected by Einstein, agreed that those accepted were more friendly but also more distrustful and tended to look for hidden motives in others. Thus, while psychiatric residents have the personal qualities which the profession deems valuable, they are not unalloyed.

TABLE 2.2   Rank Order of the Discriminating Power of RAS Items Discriminating Between Accepted and Rejected Applicants

ITEM	MEAN SCORES	
	Accepted	Rejected
Discriminating items		
Creativity	26	35
Curiosity	23	30
General range of knowledge	24	31
Intellectual grasp of psychiatry	26	35
Lack of anxiety	25	33
Problem-solving ability	26	32
Independence	25	31
Sense of humor	35	40
Sensitivity to others	22	29
Cheerfulness	29	34
Appropriate response to supervision	27	40
Impressiveness of outside interests	31	38
Cooperativeness	21	25
Self-insight	25	32
Appropriate reactions to criticism	27	37
Nondiscriminating items in terms of interviews		
Overempathetic tendencies	29	38
Dependency	24	30
Likableness	27	31
Emotional instability	25	33
Emotional rigidity	27	32
Number of outside interests	31	35
Tendency to complain	23	27
Interest in psychoanalytic training	43	50
Inhibition	24	29
Past academic record	34	39
Passive response to supervision	24	27
Submissive reactions to criticism	30	32
Preoccupation with self	28	29
Interest in group and family therapy	44	43
Exhibitionistic tendencies	29	28
Personal appearance	22	21
Interest in social and community psychiatry	43	43

Other signs of inner tension come from a study by Domino, who found future psychiatrists flexible but restless, intolerant of routine, intensely interested in others but self-centered. Domino's study is important because of its thoroughness and because it studied both practicing psychiatrists and current students from the medical school at the University of California, San Francisco. He concluded that psychiatrists are "spontaneous and sensitive, excitable and restless. Perhaps the main theme that can be discerned is that of an inner restlessness, colored by the lower mean on Achievement, indicating somewhat of a dissatisfaction with one's current status, and by the lower mean on Dominance, indicating a relative avoidance of situations requiring an action-centered approach."[72] Domino found that psychiatrists scored on the Strong Vocational Interest Blank like salesmen, psychologists and lawyers. They were person-centered "not because of humanistic or affiliative tendencies, but because the other person can gratify one's needs."[73]

Looking at psychiatrists sociologically, a national study found that 15 percent of those surveyed grew up in cities, 67 percent in the surrounding metropolitan area.[74] Over 40 percent came from Eastern European families, largely second-generation. Half were Jewish. They had improved their class position significantly over their parents' and tended to be less religious than their parents—psychological determinism being their new faith. The less religious they were, the more immersed they became in psychotherapy. The portrait is one of a group estranged from its roots by its own ambitions, treating the estrangements and reconnecting the roots of others. In all of these matters, psychiatrists were different from other physicians.

Does psychiatry choose the best candidates? No one knows. But we do have figures on the number of psychiatric candidates who have emotional problems. A national survey of trainees during 1971–72 found that "eight percent of the residents exhibited emotional illness and/or failing performance."[75] A longitudinal study of graduates over twenty-five years at one residency found that 13 percent of them had been psychotic, severely neurotic, or addictive.[76] And a survey comparing psychiatric trainees with trainees in other medical specialties found that 22 percent of the psychiatric residents appear to have emotional but nonpsychotic problems, compared to 3 percent among residents in other specialties.[77]

Do Good Candidates Become Good Psychiatrists?

Despite the hours of interviewing and discussion which training staff devote to selecting the best people, most of them do not know

how successful they have been in choosing good psychiatrists. This is
more true of other professions than they would like to admit. Some
programs keep an eye on what happens to their better and worse students, but almost none compares those they accepted with those they
turned down. Holt and Luborsky, however, did this, and found that in
professional terms the Menninger candidates did better than rejected
applicants. For example, 4 percent of the Menninger residents left psychiatry, while 26 percent of the rejects left psychiatry. On passing
specialty boards, 73 percent of the residents at Menninger received
their diploma, compared to 37 percent of those not accepted to the program.[78] These differences, of course, may be compounded by the impact of being rejected and the possible effects of going to a less reputa-
ble residency than the Menninger Clinic.

But Holt and Luborsky went much further to find out which candidates made good psychiatrists and produced the first and perhaps the
last effort of such thoroughness. The basic finding was that the qualities which interviewers identified as foreshadowing good clinical work
and by which they selected candidates for the program were not confirmed by the ratings of clinical supervisors two or three years later.

Besides this major conclusion, the report contains important insights implicit in the attempt to determine the qualities of a good psychiatrist, so that they could have a standard by which to measure the
performance of residents.[79] At first, Holt and Luborsky wanted to conduct a job analysis of practicing psychiatrists, certaintly the most accurate and objective way to establish their standard. Finding this too expensive, they settled for interviewing psychiatrists. However, they
write, "the more we consulted psychiatrists (in Topeka and in Boston), the more apparent it became that there were no criteria of success
that could command widespread agreement in the profession. . . ."[80]
Given that psychiatrists today are wont to look back nostalgically on
the 1950s as a time when psychiatry had cohesion and knew its mis-
sion, the lack of consensus is probably even worse today. It makes one
wonder—if the profession cannot agree on the qualities of a good practitioner, what are the chances that it can monitor the quality of care
the public receives?

Having failed to establish by observation or interview measures of
good professional work, Holt and Luborsky settled for determining
what constituted good work in the residency program. Here they found
considerable agreement on what a resident should do and what quali-

ties distinguished his performance. These included the ability to establish good relations with patients, to accept responsibility, to be tolerant toward aggression and pressure, to be sensitive but firm, and to have no problems of countertransference—that is, problems of projecting their own troubles onto the patient. Then supervisors were asked to select the best and worst residents for more detailed study. The main point is buried in the question. Here as elsewhere throughout the literature, the measure of quality is the opinion of colleagues or supervisors. *At no time in the 786 pages of this exhaustive study, nor in others, is the effectiveness of a psychiatrist considered in terms of how well his patients do.*

Another insight comes from the supervisors' ratings of the best and worst residents. While they had a general sense of who was good and bad, their ratings of residents in specific functions such as diagnosis, management, and administration overlapped heavily with each other and with the overall rating. Holt and Luborsky hoped that their study of the best and worst residents would enable them to overcome this problem. But they conclude, "In the wisdom of afterthought this seems rather absurd. A better lesson to have learned would have been that most judges have great difficulty in making judgments of psychotherapeutic, diagnostic, and other competencies independently of their impression of a man's general 'goodness.' "[81]

Besides the inability of training psychiatrists to evaluate specific skills, overall competence was seen only in terms of psychotherapeutic ability. This reflected the heavy bias in the program, despite its claims to being eclectic: ". . . some of the Lows were doing adequately in other work-functions, but were considered poor psychotherapists."[82] Peer ratings by fellow residents showed the same pattern, but more strongly. Reliability for these ratings was high. All of these facts found in the methodological appendix form a coherent picture: while few agree on what makes a good psychiatrist in the profession at large, within a given training center there may arise a homogeneous, quite inarticulate and almost intuitive subculture based on psychoanalysis or some other school of thought which measures all psychiatrists by its sense of worth. This subculture is shared by supervisors and residents alike. Either someone is a good man or he is not. As for the others, evidence indicates that many supervisors did not know many of the less highly rated residents.[83]

None of this answers the question of how successfully candidates are chosen. Rather, in preparation for that answer, it clarifies important features of the profession which pertain both to successful recruitment and to the quality of professional work. As for the answer, correlations between supervisors' ratings and initial tests and interviews were made and came out in the .2 to .4 range. Thus, like others, Holt and Luborsky found that elaborate tests and careful interviews cannot very well select which applicants would, if accepted in the program, later be regarded as successful residents, that is, "good men" in the eyes of the supervisor.

Being Liked: The Key to Professional Success

In the last stages of their long work, Holt and Luborsky asked judges who were predicting how residents would do to say how much they liked the candidate from his test scores and file before they interviewed him. This enabled them to control for "initial bias." Bias indeed. "Liking" turned out to correlate higher with supervisors' ratings (.6–.7) and peers' ratings (.5–.7) than any other variable![84] Being likeable also correlated with most of the personality traits originally considered important for practicing good psychiatry.[85] Given the attractiveness of the traits, this is no surprise. Thus, after years of painstaking research, Holt and Luborsky uncovered one vague, universal trait that predicted being selected and performing well better than any of the following: credentials, the Rorschach Test, a word association test, the Wechsler-Bellevue Scale, the Szondi Test, the Strong Vocational Interest Blank, a dream interpretation test, the Thematic Apperception Test, the Classification Test, a literary sensitivity test, a picture reaction test, an autobiography, a biography test, a social attitude questionnaire, a psychiatric attitude questionnaire, and interviews.

Holt and Luborsky concluded, "all of these results make sense if we consider likeableness (in our special meaning) intrinsically related to aptitude for psychiatry." That is, "psychiatry is an occupation in which the general impression the practitioner makes on other people may be important for his effectiveness."[86] Being liked is important for getting ahead with colleagues and supervisors; it even seems to help patients get better, because patients have more faith in someone they like and gain from the nurturant relationship.

3.

Graduate Training in Psychiatry

It is no accident that physicians refer to medical students as "under-graduates," for medical school today merely prepares one for clinical work and specialty training. Traditionally, graduates of medical school have taken a year of internship, where they work as apprentice physicians in a hospital, before beginning residency training in their chosen specialty. Usually this year of internship has not been graduate training *in* psychiatry, but whether one can consider it graduate training *for* psychiatry (or any other specialty) has been subject to intense debate. To appreciate the importance of this debate for psychiatrists' professional identity and for the structure of graduate training requires a brief historical background.

Internship: The Creation of an Educational Anomaly

In 1905, the American Medical Association's Council on Medical Education recommended that graduates take "an internship in a hospital to complete their basic training."[1] By 1914, about 75 to 80 percent of the graduates were taking one; but those two phrases, "in a hospital" and "to complete their basic training," created problems that remained unresolved until recently. Although the council recom-

47

mended from the beginning that internships be affiliated with medical schools, the majority were established in unaffiliated hospitals. These quickly grew dependent on the inexpensive apprentice physicians, and internship increasingly became a requirement for receiving a medical license. But as specialty training grew in the form of residencies, internship made less and less sense. It was not really the capstone to basic training for general practice, because hospital patients and procedures are not typical of office practice. Nor was it part of a graduate training program. Moreover, the quality of internships varied greatly, and no professional body like the council had control over them. Thus, a power struggle emerged between educators who wanted to reduce the number of internships, increase their quality, and tie them to graduate training, and practicing physicians who wanted as many internships as possible, particularly in community hospitals, and who recommended a rotating internship, where the young physician would be exposed to a number of specialties. At issue were two views of medicine—practice in the community versus a growing concentration of power by the scientific elite in medical schools. This power increased, as evidenced by the large decline in rotating internships, the increasing percentage of internships at hospitals affiliated with medical schools, and the large number of unfilled internships elsewhere.[2]

Regardless of the kind or quality of internship, that period of a year has had a special significance for psychiatry. Unlike internal medicine or surgery, psychiatry has not been very "medical," particularly in the United States, where a psychodynamic rather than a biological view of psychopathology has reigned. Thus, many of the psychiatric residents studied here vividly remembered their internship as the one year when they were "real doctors." According to senior residents, internship formed an important preparation for psychiatric training, largely because it deeply imprinted on medical students responsibility for their patients—something the rival profession of psychology was said not to have. Internship also exposed one to the psychological dimensions of medicine, even if this was not an explicit focus of instruction. Whether this view of internship is romantic, whether psychiatric residency actually capitalizes on a foundation of medical responsibility and psychiatry-in-medicine, is a question we shall examine. Nevertheless, all psychiatric residencies required their trainees to intern for a year.

Abolishing the Requirements for Internship

In 1969, without prior consultation with the profession or with anyone else, the American Board of Psychiatry and Neurology suddenly announced that internship would no longer be required of candidates for psychiatry. No one exactly knows why the board made this decision—it does not have to explain its actions to anyone—but one can make reasonable guesses. There was widespread concern over how long medical training had become, and efforts were being made to shorten it.[3] Colleges and medical schools were combining into six- or seven-year programs, and in some schools the fourth year resembled internship, with its emphasis on supervised clinical experience. Besides shortening medical education, abolishing the requirement for internship also eliminated an educational anomaly and got students directly into graduate training. In addition, large segments of the psychiatric profession did not value internship. Psychoanalysts, the most powerful intellectual and academic force, had members who openly doubted the relevance to psychiatric work of apprenticing in general hospital medicine, and the surging popularity of community psychiatry shifted the profession's focus even further away from medical care to issues of social injustice and community action. For these groups, the board's decision meant that trainees could more quickly get down to the business of psychiatry.

However, everyone was angered by the high-handed manner of the board, and important segments of the profession thought the decision was a mistake. Some residency programs continued to require internship as a graduate year in preparation for psychiatry, and most programs admitted candidates both with and without the experience. Educators immediately began to compare the two kinds of residents. The early seventies were years of turmoil, when the profession struggled with the implications of having embraced community psychiatry so fully in the sixties. Residents and educators alike confessed at each annual meeting that they did not know what to teach psychiatrists; almost any thoughtful model made sense in a profession now ranging from biochemistry to radical community organization in its effort to reduce mental disorders.

Professional Consolidation: Taking Over Internship

With equal suddenness and without prior consultation, the American Board of Psychiatry and Neurology reinstated the requirement for internship as of 1977. Again the profession expressed its fury over the board's arbitrary action. Again one can guess at the larger forces behind this decision; the romance with community mental health was fading, and the importance of biochemical advances in psychiatry had become increasingly apparent. Of greater significance, however, was the integration of internship with residency training, for the board now requires that the internship year be "planned, sponsored and supervised" by approved residencies.[4] It still allows the three previous types of internship: a "straight" year in one specialty, either internal medicine, family practice, or pediatrics; a rotating internship with a focus in one of these three specialties; or the old rotating internship, now called "a flexible first year."

In two strokes, the board had stripped hospitals of their independent control over the old internship by abolishing it, and had gained control over it by reinstating it under the direction of psychiatric residencies. In the process, the board reaffirmed the importance of learning general medical care as a foundation for psychiatric training, but in a way that now allowed departments of psychiatry to shape it and contribute to it. This handily coincided with a powerful concern by Congress that physicians have training in primary care at the same time that it lengthened residency training to four years. Two classic signs of a profession's power and prestige are the amount of prerequisite training it can require of its candidates and the length of this training. Psychiatry and other medical specialties now have more of both than at any time in their history.

While the recent abolition and reconstruction of the internship requirement deepen one's appreciation of its role in graduate training, they did not affect the education of most psychiatrists active today or those studied here, because they all took internships. What was it like? According to the residents studied here and to observers of interns, one works very hard getting a lot done at a gruelling, if not exhausting, pace. For the first time one is in charge of patients, discussing diagnosis, treatment plans, patient reaction to treatment with the attending physician, and one makes a hundred other serious judgments. According to one study of internship at about the time our residents were interns, this work, plus all the visiting rounds, consulting rounds, lectures, conferences and lab research and seminars, is overwhelming.[5] One intern said, "I knew I had to work hard, but I didn't know what hard was. I just had no idea. I kept thinking to myself, I know there's a routine here somewhere, and once I learn it, everything will be okay."[6] There is a routine, but not one the intern had in mind.

Initially interns try to do everything, but within a month or two they find it impossible. Out of their crisis of time and fatigue emerges a clinical perspective in which they emphasize their responsibility to their patients over academic conferences and believe that they will learn the most medicine by taking care of their patients.[7] They custom-build their education by drawing selectively on what interests them in the academic program. They cut conferences, limit reading to what the resident and consultant recommend, and drop seminars of peripheral interest. As one intern put it, "Running around doing all those things doesn't add anything to what you already know, but taking care of a sick patient is a valuable experience."[8] The routine grinds on, and increasingly, interns feel most of it is irrelevant to their future work.

After half a year interns feel used and no longer think that treating the kind of medically uninteresting patients a public hospital receives is an educational experience. But in a good program, the residents and attending physicians show how there are interesting aspects to even the most routine of patients, and the grind takes on more meaning. What is of great personal importance is that interns often finish their year genuinely confident that they can take care of patients and can stand up to the pressure of intense medical work. They have also learned some useful professional tricks: how to pose a problem so that it will interest (if not impress) a consulting physician; how to present a patient in a medically challenging way; how to give nurses the illusion of social equality and get along with them.[9]

Not all internships are like the one just described. Until the reconstruction of internship, most were not affiliated with a medical school but with a city, county, or voluntary hospital. The residents who came to the University Psychiatric Center for psychiatric residency, however, had strong academic records at good medical schools and applied for the best internships. Medical students use four key criteria to judge the best internships: prestige, professional contacts, the quality of teaching, and the amount of responsibility the intern gets.[10] By these measures, internships affiliated with the great medical schools are the best, particularly when located in a city hospital, because interns get more responsibility there than at hospitals with private patients.

Going to an academic internship also leads to a different educational experience.[11] The program is more academic and specialized because more patients are selected for clinical research and the staff have very specialized training. One's fellow interns, by dint of high achievement and an interest in academic medicine, are more alike in talents and interests than interns at the greatly diverse nonacademic hospitals. While internship at a community or voluntary hospital may be just an interim year before residency somewhere else, interns at academic programs often hope to stay on for residency nearby and act accordingly. In academic programs, the norm of learning throughout one's life is more deeply ingrained than in nonacademic internships, and this is supported by the constant exploration of medicine's frontiers. Interns work more as a team, which includes residents, researchers, faculty, and consulting physicians. The prestige and power of this professional network are so good for one's future career that interns (and residents) take care to nurture relationships and prepare for residency.[12]

Types of Psychiatric Residents

Over the past twenty years, researchers have classified different types of residents by the various psychiatric schools of treatment they believe in. A major book and widely cited articles are based on these measures of psychotherapeutic, somatic, and sociotherapeutic beliefs;[13] yet for technical reasons explained in Appendix III, I discovered they had never really worked well in discriminating between types of beginning residents, whose beliefs were not well formed. Could another way be found to identify types of residents?

Watching new residents treat patients, give nurses orders, and talk about their cases, I noticed that they differed in how they approached their work. These differences in work style seemed to underlie and help explain their beliefs, values, comments, preferred modes of treatment, and ways of relating to other staff. They probably exist in other branches of medicine and in clinical professions such as law, though no one yet has tried to find out.

In the field work and interviews, three quite distinct work styles became evident: the therapeutic, the managerial, and the intellectual.

Therapeutic psychiatrists want very much to help their patients. Ideologically they are open-minded and eclectic. They will employ whatever techniques promise results. They are not usually committed to a certain approach before they begin, but if they come to believe that a specific approach works—and many are channelled into thinking so—then they will incorporate it into their therapy. These are the residents who suffer the most anxiety and who experience the transition from medicine to psychiatry most intensively. As a group, they loved medical school and internship. They always wanted to be doctors, friendly family doctors. Since they attended sophisticated medical schools in the era of modern medicine, they realized that family doctors went the way of roadside towns. "I couldn't go the boondocks," said one resident, 80 percent of whom are from metropolitan homes. They could have become general practitioners in the suburbs, but they thought the work would be dull and would lack prestige. In addition, many echoed a resident who said that at some point in the final years of medical school, "I realized that I would much rather talk to [a hospitalized mother] about her kid than her kidney."

Another study of recruitment into psychiatry also found a therapeutically-oriented group of residents. They had majored in the natural sciences, but unlike most medical students, also took a number of college courses in the humanities and social sciences.[14] They had long planned to become physicians and their plans did not waver. In contrast with the first group, "They came to medical school expecting to work very hard and to learn everything, not primarily for intellectual pleasure, but for the benefit of their future patients."[15] These students did not consider psychiatry before medical school, but many admired the leaders of psychiatric discussions for their appreciation of the patients' problems. As might be expected, they particularly liked the clinical years of medical school of which "the psychiatric clerkship was a highlight."[16] They enjoyed direct care of patients. "Their consideration, tact, and friendliness with patients was usually outstanding."[17]

Out of this second group of medical students came what is called here the therapeutic psychiatrist. Significantly, about half of them did not decide to enter psychiatry but pursued other forms of clinical medicine. Nemetz and Weiner characterize them as having "a broad humanitarian and pragmatic concern for the problems of an individual, in a family and a society."[18] However, they found the house staff "cruel, mechanical, and callous," and overconcerned with specialized work. To maintain their identity as personal, caring doctors, all of this group thought seriously about psychiatry, even though half of them eventually chose another speciality. The Sharaf team discovered a similar group at another medical school whom they described as "more concerned . . . with directly helping patients, with 'results,' and less concerned with the subtle, sensitive understanding and theoretical mastery of intrapsychic conflicts."[19]

Managerial psychiatrists share many background traits with therapeutic residents. They wanted to become doctors, they enjoyed medical school and internship, and now they want to get patients better. However, their work style is quite different. They do not become so personally concerned about their patients, and from the start they prefer the administrative techniques of therapy. On hospitalized patients they use restrictions, drugs, ECT, perhaps behavioral therapy, and they may organize a therapeutic milieu for a patient with nurses and attendants. In short, they manage their patients. Emotionally they are less expressive, less (apparently) neurotic. In their second and third years, they tend to become administrators or to choose an administrative form of psychiatry such as community psychiatry. Given the psychoanalytic tone of the program at University Psychiatric Center, they may still go into psychoanalysis and even attend the Psychoanalytic Institute, but they speak of the decision in terms of connections, power, and "the right thing to do." They also gain satisfaction from simply organizing and running things. Unlike the therapeutic residents, they do not become emotionally involved in identifying with certain psychiatrists as therapeutic models.

Intellectual psychiatrists distinguish themselves by approaching patients as cases which illuminate theoretical aspects of the psyche. This style is supported by another study which concluded, "In the clinical years, the relative lack of interest in therapeutics . . . is consonant with their tremendous interest in psychology as an intellectual, rather than an instrumental discipline."[20] Many of these residents hated medical school, which seemed to demand obedience, dependence, strained enthusiasm about everything medical, and a mechanistic view of treatment. They suffered through it in order to reach their goal of theoretical psychiatry (in this case usually psychoanalysis). As a result, they incorporated less of the medical model and entered psychiatry *not* expecting to cure patients. In addition, they have read and talked psychoanalysis over the years, so that they do not find it frustratingly vague. Therefore, they do not suffer the initial anxiety which other residents experience. They approach their patients cognitively, less to cure them or to understand them as persons than to understand their intrapsychic dynamics. This approach has its advantages: such residents seem less reluctant to probe intimate details of patients' lives and less frustrated by the passivity of psychoanalytic therapy. Seemingly unaware of it, they talk about their patients as case studies in psychoanalytic theory and are very intellectual, though not necessarily brighter than their peers. Unlike other residents, they do not resist early suggestions of countertranference, and they can easily talk about their neurotic tendencies. Their greatest and most terrifying moment comes when they apply to the Psychoanalytic Institute, a moment beautifully described by Sharaf and Levinson.[21] They feel as if their whole life, their worth as a person, are being judged. In the balance rests their career, and after all those painful years of premed courses, medical school and internship, some do not make it.

These three work styles may well reflect personal characteristics that were apparent in college or earlier. In a retrospective study of medical students, Funkenstein identified three types of candidates with qualities similar to those observed among psychiatric residents.[22] For example, psychologically-minded students usually majored in the humanities, wanted to be psychiatrists, were very oriented to people, and expressed themselves well—traits reflected in therapeutic residents. A partial but less perfect match are managerial residents and Funkenstein's student practitioners, who majored in extracurricular activities, wanted to work with people and were not very introspective. Intellectual residents may once have been among Funkenstein's student scientists, who are strong in research and science but weak in clinical understanding and patient care. A major difference between the two studies, however, is that Funkenstein explicitly says that student practitioners and scientists have trouble learning psychiatry. Nevertheless, a small number of them may end up in psychiatry for personal reasons.

Another personal characteristic of these different residents may be how they learn and solve problems. In a dissertation on learning styles among medical students, Plovnick used two axes by which to identify learning styles: feeling vs. thinking, and acting vs. doing.[23] Three of his four styles parallel the work styles we observed in residents, as is described in figure 3.1.

It is worth emphasizing again the narrow, intense, uniform grind of early medical school, which takes no cognizance of these differences but rather trains everyone on the assumption that they are

Figure 3.1   Professional Work Styles and Their Antecedents

Types of Psychiatric Residents by Work Style (Light)	Orientation in College of Medical Students (Funkenstein)	Learning Styles (Plovnick)
1. THERAPEUTIC a) Eclectic. Uses what works b) Involved in his patients.	PSYCHOLOGICALLY-MINDED a) Majored in humanities b) Oriented to people c) Verbal	DIVERGING a) Prefers concrete experiences b) Reflective rather than active
2. MANAGERIAL a) Eclectic. Uses what works b) Manages patients rather than personally get involved	PRAGMATIC a) Active, not introspective b) Likes working people	ACCOMMODATING a) Prefers concrete experiences b) Active rather than reflective
3. INTELLECTUAL a) Works by a theory or therapeutic ideology b) Treats patients as cases of analytic hypothesis	SCIENTIFIC a) Likes science and research b) Less interested in patient care	ASSIMILATING a) Prefers abstract to concrete b) Reflective rather than active

Funkenstein's student scientists or Plovnick's assimilators. Educators find this assumption convenient; for the burden of adjustment then falls on all those who deviate from a uniform curriculum. It comes as no surprise that Funkenstein's psychologically-minded medical students and student practitioners had the most academic trouble in medical school, or that about 50 percent of Plovnick's divergers and accommodators were dissatisfied with their course work, which is taught largely by a faculty of assimilators. This approach injures the very medical students who are most likely to become good clinicians and psychiatrists.[24]

The Training Program at University Psychiatric Center

The twenty-five students who each year arrived at this famous residency entered a program whose structural ambivalence[25] reflected basic tensions in the profession itself. On one hand it embodied the elitism to which the rest of the profession aspired, while on the other hand it was the cradle of community psychiatry located in a state hospital on the edge of a black ghetto. Most of the faculty and supervisors who taught the residents had training in psychoanalysis, the prestige therapy of the profession.[26] They belonged to or were affiliated with the Psychoanalytic Institute, the area's most distinguished network of practitioners treating its most desirable patients. They also belonged to a powerful and prestigious department of psychiatry whose graduates had colonized[27] a number of other departments, and they did intellectual work, a valued activity in psychiatry. Best of all, they combined these activities in what the profession regards as an ideal career:[28] some private patients, some research and writing, affiliation with a good department of psychiatry, and, perhaps, some community service.

Yet the training for this model took place at an old, ugly state hospital where the rats foraged through the basement at night. For decades, however, the arrangement had worked well. Distinguished Medical School gained a hospital and training facility paid for by the state, and in return staffed the hospital with talented professionals as well as bright, energetic trainees in psychiatry, psychiatric social work, psychiatric nursing, psychology and research. A key provision of this pact was that, in the tradition of academic medicine, the center could draw from all over the state to obtain interesting acute cases that would make good teaching material. But out of the sixties, with its urban violence and drive for civil and economic rights, a national program in community mental health was formed which defined catchment areas to be served by community mental health centers. Thus, just before the residents of this study became involved, University Psychiatric Center had to confine its patient load to one catchment area, which included a black ghetto as well as more middle-class and white working-class neighborhoods. The director of the center, Dr. Black, had played a leading role in developing the community mental health program for the United States. And nearby the hospital was a well-known institute of community psychiatry.

In theory, this emphasis on community service and the elite character of the program had compatibilities. For example, community psychiatry was the new intellectual fashion. Assuming the posture of *noblesse oblige* which characterizes professionals' concerns about the

poor, faculty could go forth and analyze urban sources of psychopathology, obtain research grants, and train the next generation of psychiatrists to serve the people.[29] This is almost what they did. No decision-
making power was given to citizens of the catchment area, but community psychiatry provided a new large source of research grants and service funds. Otherwise, these activities stayed on the periphery of inpatient and outpatient services. Local residents, particularly blacks, did
not use the hospital and its clinics much and remained suspicious of
them. Under Dr. Black, the hospital made few adjustments in treatment philosophy or organization in switching over from a select population of patients for training and research to a quite typical urban population. Staff and residents reacted badly in a way that belied their
professional values. They were outraged at the number of incontinent
old women and inarticulate poor blacks they had to treat. Dr. Black listened to these complaints and said, essentially, "Work it out." He
heard eloquent arguments as to why these patients were poor teaching
material and how chronic cases were piling up, and repeated, "Work it
out." This infuriated chiefs of service and other residents. In their
more thoughtful moments, they could not decide whether Dr. Black's
unelaborated policy was brilliant, by giving staff at all levels a major
challenge and responsibility, or lazy, by failing to lead the staff
through these problems.

That these problems were real (and they are only "problems"
from an elite, acute-oriented, psychoanalytic point of view), yet ignored by the administration, led the chiefs of service to initiate their
own survey of transfers to other hospitals for the academic year
1967–68. (At this point the hospital still retained the old privilege of
transferring chronic cases to other state hospitals to keep its wards
flowing with more "interesting" acute cases). They found that 33 percent of the patients were over sixty-five, whereas virtually none had
been so the year before. Another category that jumped was chronic
brain syndromes, up from a handful the year before to 35 percent of all
transfers. The staff judged 34 percent of these patients to be chronic
for life, and 85 percent of them were either single, widowed or
divorced.

Ten years later, a more systematic comparison of all inpatients for
1965 (before the hospital switched to serving the catchment area) and
1975 confirmed this early study at the same time that it suggested in-

compatibility between service to the area's residents and good training. The study found that during the decade, nonwhite patients rose from 3 to 21 percent of hospital population, and the percent with less than 7 years of education rose from 2 to 25 percent. Patients over 55 years old rose from 2.5 to 15 percent. The hospital went from being a select institution which drew patients from many areas to one which by 1975 received 86 percent of its patients from the immediate catchment area. The patients in 1975 were more likely to have been admitted several times before (implying chronic disorders), and their stay in the hospital was shorter than patients a decade ago, even though this hospital has always seen itself as a center for acute, short-term treatment. Finally, by 1975, one out of every four patients was leaving the hospital by escape or against medical advice, while a decade earlier only 7 percent did so.

To observe training during the first period, however, was to observe residents managing their patient loads to maximize their learning experience with psychotherapeutically interesting patients and ridiculing the intellectual paucity of their small weekly assignments and seminars in community psychiatry. In these and other ways, the training program reflected national trends. In a 1972 APA survey of the nation's psychiatric residencies, most programs offered didactic training plus clinical experience both in the hospital and at community agencies, though there was no measure of how much residents learned from these experiences.[30] Junior staff at other prestigious residencies which were located at psychiatric facilities responsible for a catchment area described to me a dozen ways in which new residents minimized their time doing community psychiatry and took every chance to work with supervisors who were analysts.[31] That these residents later took jobs in public institutions at the start of their career reflects more the expanding job market which the community mental health movement provided than good training in or commitment to community psychiatry.

The national survey identified twenty-eight programs in child psychiatry, ninety-eight programs in mental hospitals not affiliated with a medical school, ninety-seven that were so affiliated, and sixty-five located at free-standing clinics, general hospitals or other facilities. Like other medical school programs, the residency at University Psychiatric Center was larger than other types, in fact, one of the largest.[32] Like such residencies, it offered both a general residency and a special one in child psychiatry. Residents and staff used the prevailing kinds of treatment—individual psychotherapy, group therapy, psychotropic drugs, crisis intervention, electroconvulsive therapy, family therapy and, in a more marginal way, behavioral therapy and milieu therapy. Also like other medical school residencies, training was offered to medical students, interns, nurses, social workers and psychologists. Large numbers of behavioral scientists and other physicians populate the staff of residencies at medical schools, but this survey by the American Psychiatric Association concluded:

> In spite of the fairly large numbers of nonmedical personnel and of nonpsychiatrist physicians involved in psychiatric education, it appears that systematic preparation for, exposure to, and involvement in inter- disciplinary collaboration is quite minimal for many psychiatric resi- dents.[33]

Work with paraprofessionals was even more limited. ". . . program responses clearly indicated little, if any, systematic preparation of resi- dents for work with paraprofessionals. In fact, not one response could be interpreted as describing such preparation."[34]

In the area of social problems, the residency at University Psychi- atric Center was similar to others. It did make strong efforts to recruit minorities. While residents were "exposed to experiences with minor- ity group members in the course of everyday contact with patients and other staff,"[35] no special efforts were made to understand minority subcultures. Community psychiatry has been discussed; child ad- vocacy was not taught either nationally or at this program; racism and poverty were not a focus of training, and like psychiatrists in the na- tional survey, staff at University Psychiatric Center would probably question whether these were psychiatric issues. Training in administra- tion occurred only for residents who assumed administrative positions, and the regular training program did not teach program evaluation. The APA survey concludes that the growth in community psychiatry, the sharing of expertise with paraprofessionals and the decreased emphasis on hospital treatment are not reflected in the training of psychiatrists, as they were not at this program. Yet the structure of the program, being housed in a state hospital and community mental health center, affected the careers of its graduates more than they anticipated; for while most of them saw private patients after hours, a large percentage spent several years in public service.

The First Year

Following a common pattern, residents began their training on hospital patients and moved to the outpatient clinic in their second year. The director of psychiatry assigned the twenty-five new residents to four services, consisting of three inpatient wards and the Day Hospital, where patients whose families would help them came in for the day but went home at night. A "chief," who was a third-year resident, ran the ward in conjunction with a "superchief," who was a junior but licensed psychiatrist legally responsible for the ward. In addition, each service had about ten nurses, sixteen attendants (for three shifts), three social workers, three psychology interns, three rehabilitation workers, two ministerial interns and one occupational therapist, plus waves of student social workers, medical students, nurses, and others passing through.

The first-year residents were responsible (under supervision) for the diagnosis and treatment of patients in the hospital. Arriving on July 1, they assumed responsibility for many of the patients just left by the second-year residents, an awkward and often painful arrangement that the structure of training required. As new patients were admitted to the hospital, the residents acquired more patients and discharged others until their load reached about twelve. Around these patients centered most of the first-year activities—about thirty hours of therapy, supervision by several hand-picked psychiatrists plus the chief and superchief, morning conferences on patient treatment, daily case conferences in which residents present a patient to a senior psychiatrist, and several weekly conferences with different combinations of ward personnel. In addition, residents attended weekly conferences on neurology, somatic therapies, social psychiatry, diagnosis, and the development of modern psychiatry. For limited periods they also participated in administering shock therapy and drug therapy. "Shock" was done in the basement at 7:45 A.M. while everyone else was eating breakfast. Finally, residents attended a year-long sensitivity group run by a well-known psychoanalyst, which purported to teach the residents by example the nature of group process.

Each resident had seven supervisors with whom he was to meet once a week for about an hour. Compared to other residencies, this was an extraordinarily high number. Officially, one supervisor was designated for "individual psychotherapy case supervision," to follow the therapy of the only outpatient assigned to each first-year resident. This outpatient was carefully selected by the outpatient clinic as an "interesting, fairly well put-together neurotic." Almost every first-year resident found his "outpatient case" fascinating, and this patient helped to sustain faith in the psychotherapeutic ideal amidst psychotic, "untreatable" patients. Three supervisors were designated for "inpatient psychotherapy." One was the adolescent supervisor, and each resident was to have an adolescent case if possible. The resident also met with his service chief and superchief. These supervisions were usually more administrative and ward-oriented than would be possible with a supervisor who comes from outside the ward or hospital. However, the superchief tried to let the resident talk about whatever was bothering him and gave him a chance to let off steam.

Finally, each resident was the doctor-on-call one-twenty-sixth of the nights for the year. From 5:00 P.M. to 8:00 A.M. he was responsible for clinical, medical, and psychiatric care for the inpatient services. He slept at the hospital and was not to make any other appointments during that time.

If one had to characterize the rhythm, the routine of residency, it would be the weekly meeting. Numerous meetings and appointments were set up by the week, fewer by the month or twice a week. Least common were occasional meetings, despite the emergencies and chaos that characterized a hospital for acute problems. They kept intruding onto a resident's calendar, but at the sacrifice of breakfast, lunch or going home. Nevertheless, all residents found the hours lighter than during their internship.

The Second Year

The second year of residency was devoted primarily to working with outpatients at the walk-in clinic located at one end of the hospital. When they left their services, second-year residents continued with a selected number of patients from the first year. Some were still in the hospital, while others had been discharged but continued with the residents on an outpatient basis. If the latter needed readmission, the second-year resident would continue to treat him or her. From these patterns one can see the emphasis placed on long-term cases as the best way to learn psychotherapy, and the emphasis on continuity of care whenever possible. From the patient's point of view, these rules could assure long, excellent therapy or the experience of being stuck with a resident who was painfully mismatched. A patient could not switch residents. The system took no cognizance of research showing the importance of good matching for effective therapy; rather, it believed that each resident should learn how to work with all kinds of patients.

The diagnosis and disposition of outpatients was a new and (at first) challenging experience. The second-year residents thus decided who would be admitted to the hospital, and they took on a certain number of patients they screened for short-term and long-term psychotherapy as outpatients. They also assembled and led a group and worked more with adolescents and children. They attended weekly meetings on child psychiatry, neurology and other elective courses. Another new experience was consulting with medical staff at a city hospital about somatic treatments. Overall, second-year residents had greater autonomy, more elective time (ten hours vs. five in the first year), and a richer, more interesting range of patients. They continued to receive extensive supervision in short-term, long-term, adolescent, child, and adult psychotherapy.

The Third Year

In many ways, psychiatric residency is a two-year program, even though formally almost all residencies in the United States go for three years. Essentially, the third year is elective, a time to explore or to begin a specialized program in, for example, child or community psychiatry. As the official manual states,

> The two-year program in general psychiatry affords the resident basic training in clinical skills and provides him with the introduction to various subspecialty areas. In addition, the . . . Center and the Department . . . offer a number of programs of advanced training in various subspecialties of psychiatry.

Besides child and community psychiatry, residents could take a program in biological sciences, forensic psychiatry, psychopharmacology, social psychiatry, liaison psychiatry at a number of hospitals, or they could learn to do research by joining a number of projects. However, an important option was to become chief, either of one's old service or of the outpatient clinic. To be selected brought the stature of leadership and valuable administrative experience.

As we turn to the actual experience of residents in training, we should consider some basic challenges which the residents faced. One was the relation between the nurses, veteran sergeants of the services, and the green new residents. Residents had to learn from them, yet give them orders and explain what was happening to patients the likes of whom they had rarely seen before. A related struggle over power and status involved the tension between drugging a patient to make her/him more manageable and wanting to diagnose or treat the patient in a natural psychological state. Was one's goal to make patients manageable on the ward or to treat them? Or were management and somatic therapy a form of therapy?

In learning psychotherapy, residents began (under the influence of the program) to see how similar their patients' psychological problems and processes were to their own. They faced the danger of even identifying with certain patients, rather than empathizing with them. Empathizing required residents to get closer and closer to their own defenses, neuroses and fantasies. The more deeply they understood their own psyche, it was claimed, the better therapists they would be.

4.

Experiencing the First Year

The experience of becoming a psychiatrist is so intriguing, so alive, that one wants to avoid the common pitfall of the author interpreting the residents' story for them, with a few carefully chosen quotations inserted here and there. Not only is the richness of feeling and action lost, but readers too often get no sense on their own of what is happening so that they can judge the interpretations of the author. In order to accomplish this in a reasonable space, this chapter will focus on one group of residents and let them describe the critical first year, using largely their own words when they were talking to each other on the job rather than to an interviewer. The disadvantages of so limited a sampling will be compensated for in later chapters, where the particular experiences of these residents will be balanced by experiences and patterns observed in a variety of other resident groups.

This chapter centers on six young men whose fictitious last names all begin with R because they are residents: Ned Reich, Ken Reese, and Marc Raskin, Carl Rabinowitz, Jeff Roche, and Dave Reed. Although they represent all three types of residents, we will simplify a complex process by focusing on what they experienced as they grappled with basic issues of professional identity. Guiding them were Eric Saunders, the Superchief, and Adam Cohn, the Chief of Service I. Like many chiefs selected by the program, Adam was a therapeutic, family-doctor type of psychiatrist who was immersed in psychoanalysis.

The First Day of Residency

Saturday was an off day for the hospital; only one psychiatric resident "covered" the three inpatient wards of mental patients with the aid of a small crew of nurses and attendants. To the twenty-six strangers on the second floor, however, this Saturday, July 1, marked the beginning of a new career, a sharp departure from medicine, an unknown. These doctors, having completed medical school and a year of internship, were the new cohort of psychiatric residents.

For four months, they had been anticipated by staff and old residents as "the new residents," and would be so designated throughout the summer. Slowly this term would yield to "the first-year residents," but it would be heard less frequently as references become more personal or more ward-oriented—the residents on I."[1] Well-groomed and slightly overdressed in their suits and fresh shirts, they chatted as they moved into the hospital's small library. There they received their first orientation from Dr. Black, the director of the hospital, a man of national fame and local legend.

Black—for residents allude to senior officers by their last name only[2]—introduced himself, other important directors of services, and the heads of different clinics, wards, nursing, and social work. Then Black introduced Dr. Elvin Blumberg, clinical director of the hospital, and turned the meeting over to him. Blumberg, a portly man with a soft voice, gently asked each resident to "introduce yourself and tell us a little about yourself."

The first resident replied by giving his name, where he went to medical school, where he interned, and perhaps his interest in psychiatry. This cautious professional answer to so leading a question was picked up by each resident in turn. There is, of course, a rhythm to this process of introduction. About the fifteenth man had said who he was, where he went to school, that he interned at Children's Hospital, when Blumberg asked, "Do you like to play with children?"

The resident, who had stood up to take his turn, gaped, wordless, his eyes darting as if to find a quick escape. The tension of hushed silence mounted, and then he replied, "Yes." As the embarrassed resident sat down, a few snickers came forth. Then a wave of laughter. The residents next to me looked quickly at each other; some whispered. Blumberg eased the moment with a joke and asked the next resident to introduce himself.

During the rest of the day and the weeks to follow, a number of residents talked about this moment and puzzled. Was Blumberg making a psychiatric joke? Why put a resident on the spot? The victim thought Blumberg showed indiscretion. Later in the year, residents clearly knew what had happened; Blumberg had given a first, dramatic taste of psychoanalytic technique for exposing unconscious motives. What might have been taken as a quip in another setting was taken here to illustrate Blumberg's powers to disarm and to indicate that a psychiatrist's unconscious is a shared, professional concern.

The meeting broke for coffee, and the old friends chatted. "Did you know . . ." conversations took place among those who had gone to the same medical schools or had interned in the same cities. These remained the most common ties and subjects of conversation during the next few weeks, a search for the familiar in a new setting.

Near lunchtime, the residents went to their assigned wards, (called "services" here), where the chief of the service briefed them. The chief and head nurse emphasized the importance of controlling disruptive patients. They explained how to use drugs and restrictions to this end, and it was emphasized how one disturbed patient excites the entire ward, impeding the progress of other patients. The residents also met the superchief, Eric Saunders, introduced as "the big man." He was the only licensed psychiatrist on the service, the chief explained, and thus legally responsible for whatever occurred.

The chief gave out the assigned patients, two for each resident, and described what was wrong with each one. The strengths of the patients were not mentioned, and several times he warned that a certain patient would be "a very difficult, if not impossible case."[3] One patient "is thought to be psychopathic, but his MMPI's [psychological tests] show he is schizophrenic." Another never had "a real relation" with her therapist. "Perhaps you can get into business with her," the chief said. There is "a first-break schizophrenic" and a "paranoid psychotic." One patient is "an obsessive-compulsive," and the question is whether we should use "electroconvulsive treatment."[4] The new residents had full responsibility for the administration and therapy of these patients, except for two cases in which the resident would administrate on the ward, while another person would be the therapist. The danger, the chief warned, was that you would become a second therapist.[5]

After these assignments, the superchief told the residents how they would feel—*like running away*. The most common way to "work out your anxieties" is to read, he said. A little running was expected, but not too much. The superchief also discussed a second problem, that nonprofessional staff on the ward would know more than the residents about patient care. He urged them to listen to the nurses, who know so much, and to learn from them.

After the meeting, which was held in the chief's office, the residents walked out to the lounge to meet their patients. The ward was very still. The residents moved awkwardly, not quite knowing how to behave or how to find their two charges in a room of staring sick faces. Using formal address, each called out a name. "Mrs. Kelly?" A figure rose too quickly or with studied indifference, and the odd couple moved away toward the doctor's dim office, with beige walls, linoleum floor and old desk, to get acquainted.

The patients said in private that they were very anxious, and had been for several weeks, about whether they would get along with their new doctors. One pretty patient came back from her first meeting and said she hated her doctor. Another said, "Boy, have I got plans for him."[6]

Of his first encounter, a resident said, "He was really very nice, much more than I expected. Then at one point he said, 'I've got to say this. You're a dirty Jew.' I asked him if he had had a Jew before, and he said yes (his previous therapist). On the other hand, he was very eager when I came out to the dayroom for him. He zoomed out of his chair and stepped on someone's toe in trying to shake my hand."

One patient said anxiously, "They look so young."

Her friend replied, "They must be so nervous. Just think! Here they have been studying for years and this is their first real patient. God! That's really something."

Indeed it was. The residents' first day is appropriately couched in the language of an observer, because these young men were much too anxious then and couldn't express their feelings until much later.

The First Two Weeks

In the first two weeks, the residents established relations with the significant segments of the hospital and began to respond. Before arriving, most of them had been impressed with the graciousness and kindness of the senior staff. In conversations, they contrasted this tone to that of surgery, where men give orders with harshness and Prussian strictness. "Of course," said one, "much more is at stake in surgery." (July 11.) The chief of Service I, Adam Cohn, said to one of the residents, Carl Rabinowitz, "If you want, you might sometime go down and just spend a few minutes with EST [electroconvulsive therapy or shock treatments]." Carl noted the cautious, gentle tone, which he said changed by the third week to "I think it would be a good idea if you go and watch EST" (July 22).[7]

At the end of the first week Ken Reese concluded:

"Anxiety is encouraged here, if not forced, it is so heavy-handed. Everyone tells you you know nothing, that all your education is if anything an impediment. Actually we may know a good bit, and most residents here have had some experience before where they have been judged competent. Why else would they be here?

"But you come and get *two* patients! Last week I had a thousand I took care of at night and dozens in the day. (Also) you get seven supervisors. As an intern you had none or one.

"The staff treats you like strangers who are almost imposing on them. You get the message you don't belong. The staff also makes it clear you know nothing. If anything, this impedes your relationship with the patient, because of the anxiety and insecurity you feel, some of which is probably conveyed."

On the ward, residents had a difficult time. There was little effort by nurses, old staff and the chief to integrate them into the ward.[8] The first ward meeting began with the chief asking, "Do people miss having the old doctors around?" Patients responded in a spontaneous chorus of "Yes!" Dr. Cohn asked the new doctors to give their names. Ken Reese, Ned Reich, Marc Raskin, Carl Rabinowitz, Dave Reed and Jeff Roche. But the emphasis was on *loss,* and the chief guided the meeting in this direction according to the dictates of his psychoanalytic training. After the first ward meeting, Jeff Roche felt like an observer. Ned Reich didn't feel he could speak, didn't know what was appropriate. In the meeting it was a patient finally who said, "I think we should welcome the new doctors."

The residents did not confide much in anyone during this time (except for one). Their own efforts to belong to the ward seemed to consist of trying hard to do everything correctly, with a strained sensitivity and jumpiness which confirmed the old staff's feelings that they did not belong.

The nurses offered the greatest resistance. To summarize many pages of observations, nurses began to experience feelings of "termination" with their group of residents early in the spring, before other staff and patients did; they suffered the most of any group on the staff; they resented the new doctors the most, and they took longest to adjust to the new residents.

> A nurse came in the conference room to tell Rabinowitz he had a phone call and said, "Dr. Rabinowitz?" Looking around the room. She didn't know which one he was. I asked the nurse next to me, "Do you know the names of the new doctors?" She said, "Heavens no. I can't even look at them." (July 6.)

Social workers, the occupational therapist, attendants and other staff experienced the turnover in a similar but less intense way.

The nurses' resistance to accepting the new residents was reflected in how long it took the head nurse to learn which patients belonged to which resident. Watching her conduct Morning Report, I noted that it took her *three months* to learn this elementary information.

The felt hostility of the staff made the residents turn immediately to their patients, some of whom were eager to know them and all of whom had to work with them. They tried to know the patients as persons, but at the same time they were afraid the patients would go out of control. Recalling this period, Ned Reich said the first kind of uncertainty was one of being new and knowing nothing (March 2). Carl, who was quite hostile to me during this time, walked upstairs with me saying: "It's not you, I'm just bothered." And he still shut me out with his body as he went up the stairs. "What is it?" I asked. "Oh I'm just very worried about how to handle my patients," he replied. (July 13.)

And with reason. One of his patients told me how she asked him if she could go with a friend to the botanical gardens. He said that this hospital was no hotel. You're here to get into business. No. Later, she said to me that she was very pleased with his refusal. She said she didn't really want to go, that she was testing him to see if he cared. (July 13.) This example illustrates the complexities of human management which a resident faces.[9] Although Carl's reply turned out to be very competent, he was never sure of what he was doing or its consequences. He tried to carry out the constant instruction of his chief and nurses, to be in charge and to control the patient, but he never knew what he might be doing to his patient.

The elements of this period—silence feeding on itself and the psyche of the resident, groping to know one's patients, chronic tiredness, the sense of incompetence and estrangement—are beautifully portrayed in an intimate Saturday meeting of the residents, the chief, and the psychological intern. The first several minutes of the meeting included three long silences, one timed at two minutes.[10] Each time Jeff Roche broke the silence. The third time he asked about psychological tests. How are they done? What do they mean? He said he had heard that normal-appearing people can get crazy scores.

> *Adam Cohn:* Yes. You know people in analysis often give psychotic scores.
>
> *Jeff Roche:* People told me if I didn't go into psychiatry I'd go crazy. And now you say people in analysis get crazy scores.

For a half hour the psychologist talked about psychological testing.

> *Adam Cohn:* It seems to me we are avoiding our anxiety about being here. We're asking how can we know about our patients. We're looking for tests, like lab tests in medicine, which will tell us with reasonable reliability what is wrong, and we want to read all about the problems of our patients. (Jeff had previously asked for books to read.)
>
> *Dave Reed:* Yes, It's very hard to go from medical school where there are reasonable lab tests.
>
> *Jeff Roche:* We've talked among ourselves and we can't understand why we are so tired at night. We worked so much harder as interns.
>
>   . . . .
>
> *Marc Raskin* speaks of the negative aspects of the term "sick." He thinks it is a bad word. Reed defends it. It has connotations of doctors, of being cured, and being taken care of. That is good.
>
> *Ned Reich:* "University Psychiatric Center" is much better than the

old name, "Boston Psychopathic." Also, I don't like the word "crazy."

Mike (the psychologist): I'm not so sure that I don't have some of the same problems that the patients have.

Others picked up this theme and agreed with it. "The question," one resident said, "is where the doctor ends and the patient begins."

This meeting took place on July 8; the penetration of the old medical shell of habits and values begins quickly and is deep.

The First Month

Eric Saunders, the supervising psychiatrist on the service, began the second two weeks of July with a talk on control. The patient is more agitated than he shows, he said, and he wants control as little children do. He may not *say* he wants it, but in two days he will thank you for it—or if he doesn't you can tell that he is relieved from his non-verbal actions. Agitated patients agitate others, he continued. You will find you resent it when your colleague gives his upset patient less drugs than you would wish, because it hinders the progress of your patient. (July 13.)[11]

Later the same day, Ken Reese said that *he asked his patients* what their old doctors did to determine the right amount of restrictions. It seemed like a good way to the residents listening, and the next week at a staff meeting Dave Reed translated this practice into a continuing theme: "There is this question about responsibility, and we have tended to point to the staff and say they are responsible. I think that everyone, the patients too, must be responsible for their own actions." (July 20.) To the reader this may seem an odd theme to apply to psychotic patients who reach the hospital largely because they lack control in some manner, but it formed the second part of management. On one hand, "control the patient, even more than he says he wants." On the other hand, "The patient must manage himself." This paradox of management, barely formulated by residents in the first month, reflects the small but growing conflict between the ideology of administration and that of therapy. It marks the first annoyance at patient care which could be resolved by the policy: "I do therapy; you manage yourself."

The residents also began to devalue certain *kinds* of patients, but not individual patients they liked.[12] Sociopaths and psychopaths caused trouble, more so in the tolerant atmosphere of the hospital than outside. Chronics were "dead." A new category became explicit, "the catchment patient." In time it became clear that a catchment patient was one who offered no potential for psychotherapy. Often she was a woman, lower class, not very educated, old. Take Mrs. Ackerman, whom Dave Reed presented to a conference. (July 18.) He began:

> "Mrs. Ackerman is seventy-five and has slowly regressed since her husband died six years ago. Recently she was evicted from her home, which was a great blow. This is a classic case of catchment."
>
> Ten minutes into the conference, Ken whispered, "Obviously no one is taking the case seriously. You can sense it. Everyone sees her as depressed over losses, feeling attacked, demented. What can you do," he asked, "except send her to a nursing home?"
>
> "A local hospital sent her here to get our evaluation," Dave continued.
>
> The superchief said, "I think it was just a dump," and everyone laughed.

Not only did residents exhibit detachment from less desirable patients in the first month of training, but they also began to talk about their patients as case pathologies. After a ward meeting, Ned Reich remarked, "It's surprising when you get to know the patients a little and see how predictably they talk. . . . It's sort of scary to see how they find a grain of truth of seeing the world through their pathologies." (July 20.) Soon afterwards Carl said, "Each patient will see the ward according to his own pathology, and that is what you have to deal with." (July 22.) The psychiatric construction of reality was quickly absorbed.

Some said that the patients, moreover, were getting significant messages which we shouldn't ignore. One was that they wouldn't be believed. Carl responded by strongly arguing that the patients are in fact *not* to be believed, and he supported his case with examples of patients who had very erroneous ideas about him. Another message was that anger would not be tolerated. Ken summarized: anger which is expressed will not be tolerated and will be dealt with by discharging you or giving you great amounts of freedom.

At this point, the chief broke in and gave the psychiatric side of the management-therapy dichotomy. The message, he said, is that we treat each case *individually* and we do what we think is best for that patient at that time in that situation. If the patient thinks that we can't take anger, that is something to discuss with him in therapy. (July 22.)

The residents' initial discomfort about the ward and staff did not dissipate, and in the third week they expressed their wishes to get away or to detach themselves. Already they were talking about which holidays they wanted to take. Then they talked about vacations, and it emerged that each was planning when he would take the first of his four or five weeks. Adam Cohn, as noted before, had become more firmly directive and said: "You will find that the year really goes very fast, and that you won't want to leave your patients very long. [Murmurs.] There is so much going on and too much to learn. In any case, you cannot take a vacation before September 1." The residents responded by recounting how in internship they always squeezed the two weeks they had to the limit. Someone mentioned that as one gets more patients, it is harder to leave.

Meanwhile the residents were trying to master therapy, and they focused on specific techniques used in demonstration interviews between a senior psychiatrist and one of their patients. One technique which many residents talked about and tried was the look-into-your-heart approach. Here is the original model.

Patient: You can't see into a person's head here, can you?

Interviewer: Not really. And we can't really look into their hearts either. [Silence.]

Patient [who has been looking off, looks at him for the first time]: You mean the real heart?

Interviewer [smiles]: I think you know what I mean. (July 21.)

The residents thought that was great and constantly tried such techniques. But techniques have another, more subtle purpose in socializing the resident to his new profession. They show how a therapist's personal weaknesses can be seen as strengths, and that what they thought was incompetence in themselves can be seen as productive to therapy.

We talked about case conferences. Ken and Carl said they were very important. They tried out all kinds of things they saw in interviews, and they said they couldn't wait to try out others.

Ken said he tried the "body bit" (by the interviewing psychoanalyst above), asking the patient "where do you feel sad," etc. It works, he claimed. One girl pointed to her genitals. At the least it gets the patient to look at her feelings. Carl hadn't *dared* to try it, and he seemed very interested in Ken's account. Both had tried the look-into-your-heart business (also by the interviewer above). Jeff was silent, and I asked him if he had done any of these. He said he had not thought of it, but he realized from the discussion how techniques might be tried out.

Two of the residents tried to guess what the interviewers would say next or ask next. Carl said, "I've learned that if I ask a certain question at a certain time, the whole course of the interview changes later on. There is some sort of inner logic to the sequence of a session. It's very complex, and I'm trying to learn how to make the right decision of what to say at each point so the thrust of the session goes the right way."

Carl felt that often he doesn't know what to say. He has always taken this as a sign of weakness; a good man would know what to do. But he learned from one senior psychiatrist to shut up and think if you are not sure. That is what Fromm-Reichmann says too. Now he plans to have times of silence, and the patient knows that you really care and that you are thinking of what is best for him.

Jeff thought he had to keep the hour going full steam, and he was always trying to think what to say. (One resident remarked, "It's a tribute to the program's breadth that someone so unpsychological as Jeff is with us.")

Later, Carl talked about an interviewer who seemed quite angry at the patient. He emphasized how the man used his personality, his anger to therapeutic advantage, to get the patient to express anger. Ken could not separate the interviewer's personality from him as a model; so he rejected the man as a model altogether. (A few months later, he saw the man as Carl did.) (July 29.)

Carl's emphasis on technique became a major preoccupation with time. One can see how the complexity of deciding what to say when and of thinking that a session's entire thrust can be altered by what one says or does not say could preoccupy a therapist indefinitely.

These microtechniques also contribute to a diminished sense of cure. (If you are concerned with what to say next, the goal of curing the patient becomes remote.) Ned told me that he was pleased with his work with one patient. She came to sessions every time and stayed the full half hour, "which means she tolerates me." (She had run out on sessions before.) He interpreted as progress what may not have been:

"As she comes to trust me more, and she likes me a lot, I think, she also withdraws. She is trusting, but she is also pulling away, and doesn't want anyone to know that she is coming closer." (July 28.)

Ned's seeming comfort with his progress was not shared by others. At a group meeting, Ken Reese found sympathy when he complained about the paucity of milieu therapy.[13] "It seems that around here the ward is just a depository for the patients between therapy sessions, and that people believe that they have a special grip on the patient in therapy which overshadows whatever happens to the patient in the ward." (July 22.)

The residents did not relate their diminished sense of cure with their focus on technique, but the two occurred together throughout the year. In his review of the year many months later, Jeff Roche said: "I never dreamed we would be so excited and satisfied by so little. . . . I brought a tape measure this year, when I needed a millimeter rule." (June 4.)

In the second half of July, residents began to see the impact of their own personalities on their work. Adam Cohn helped them make these discoveries.

> Mike, the clinical psychologist training on the service, said that he was beginning to realize that he may not want to let his patients go.
>
> *Adam Cohn:* You find in the middle of your second year that the patients you still have or who are still in the hospitals are those who have the same problems you do.[14]
>
> *Mike:* I want to keep them dependent so I can be independent.
>
> *Adam Cohn:* You express your dependent side through them, which allows your independent side more freedom.[15]
>
> *Mike:* At the same time, you get gratification in curing your patients.
>
> Jeff looked bothered. He blurted, "That's a real dilemma. On the one hand you want to cure your patients and on the other you want to keep them." Jeff did not understand the idea of countertransference. "I don't understand. If you assume that we are reasonably normal [looks at the chief], and if we have some perspective on the matter and if we understand the doctor's role, then why can't we let the patient get better with no loss to us?"
>
> *Ken Reese:* "That's a lot of 'ifs'." Everyone except Jeff laughed. (July 15.)

In learning about professional success, the residents came to regard psychic weaknesses as assets.

The residents talked about the gigantic egos of Black and Blumberg. They claimed all top analysts had big egos. Jeff thought you were not supposed to be a good therapist unless you had some real neuroses yourself.

Ken agreed. Harry Stack Sullivan hallucinated at times. Carl added Sullivan's transcribed lectures really went all over the place at times. Ken said how human Sullivan was, and how the sick analysts are the humanitarians, *because they have been there*. They are the ones who argue for the idea of a continuum of illness from healthy to psychotic.

Carl insisted that there is a clear difference between some really ill people and the rest of us.[16] He added a bit later that X had a beautiful article of analysis as a game, that it was so set up that only the analyst could win, and you taught the patient the game.

I asked him if he thought that was what he was doing. "I hope I'm doing more than that, but there is more than a grain of truth to it. I am unsure." (July 28.)

By the end of the first month, residents have experienced one phase in the four great issues of psychiatric socialization. These are the tension between relating to the patient as a person or as a case: the conflict between management and psychotherapy; a primary focus on curing and progress versus preoccupation with therapeutic technique; and the tension between seeing a case in terms of a patient's illness or in terms of one's own neurosis. Throughout the rest of the year, the residents would move between these polarities several times, each oscillation longer and more refined than the last.

August and September

"... taking the risk of suicide is better than ... keeping therapy superficial." (August 5.)

In the second and third months of residency the staff still guided and taught residents on how to manage patients. For example, a resident told the staff that he was going to take one of his patients off thorazine "to see how he is." If he got more sick, he would be put back on thorazine.[17] Also, he wanted to let the patient off the ward. The chief interrupted, saying that you do not try two things at once, because it contaminates the data you want. Moreover, he might run away as he had done in the past. The resident said he had not found evidence of escape in the patient's record. The chief replied that the patient had run away twice before becoming an inpatient; so it was not in the record.[18] He suggested: "When you're making a major decision, especially regarding administration and restrictions, see the staff."

Despite such evidence that they had not mastered managerial skills, the residents talked about therapy instead of management. Therapy was "the real business," and while talk increased about the skills of therapy, with the constant effort to make general rules and derive guidelines, no comparable conversations were heard about the skills of management. Concern with therapy became even stronger in September, when all the supervisors returned from vacation and the full program commenced. By "therapy" residents usually meant individual psychotherapy, and within that realm they preoccupied themselves with technique in order to master their hour, their patient, and themselves.

I asked Carl if he had learned anything from one of his patients.

> In general, Carl thought he had learned things from this patient. He is here to learn from patients, and that is why he will reject this one if he "does nothing" in the next two months. First, he learned from this patient's pathology, which was new for him. Not the "passive aggressive" level, but the rest: the hate of self, the feeling of evil, feelings that the patient has of destroying females and is guilty about. Second, he learned from the maneuvers, which amount to trying to get a patient to work, to relate. He did not think these maneuvers interfered with his main work, which is *to understand*. (September 5.)

Carl's first statement, that he was here to learn and that he would not let patients get in his way, was the most important. Moreover, the *way* one looked at patients changed from psychiatric diagnosis to psychodynamics, such as the ones Carl mentioned—the hate, the sense of evil, a special sense of destroying. The resident now diagnosed a patient on two levels, dynamics and psychiatric categories. He quickly assimilated what his mentors told him, that the two kinds of diagnosis had little to do with one another. Carl's patient, for example, was a "schizophrenic" but one could not infer from that his personal sense of evil.

The residents were also preoccupied with that major feature of psychotherapy, talk. They wanted to learn how to talk well, and they looked constantly for good talk. "Good talk" was conceived of as either enjoyable or instructive. Once a patient "does nothing" and becomes tedious in therapy hours, the resident would try to see him less or get rid of him.

Residents also discussed psychiatrists who interview patients in conference according to how entertaining or instructive a man was. They continued to try out techniques of interviewing which would enable them to penetrate the defenses of their patients.

> I learned something about interviewing. I had thought I was direct and tough when I said, "Do you have any trouble with girls?" or the like. My patient would become very embarrassed and not answer.
>
> What Blumberg does (in a case conference) that is different is to *assume* the patient had these troubles. His questions took them for granted, which must have been a great relief for the patient, to meet a man who knows what's the matter and is not upset about it. I think I am a pretty good first-year resident, but when I see Blumberg I realize how far I have to go.
>
> The other thing that is great is the way Blumberg brushed off the patient's defenses. If you plot the statements of patients with Blumberg, they are pretty close, and if you plot Blumberg's questions, they stick to one area very tightly for a while and then shift to another area. If you plot a patient's sentences with a resident, they jump all over and that is because the patient is using different defenses to avoid talking about what is important. If you plot the resident's questions, you see him letting the [patient's] defenses work. (August 4.)

These were the complex skills which residents tried to acquire, and just as they found cure elusive, so they also found the mastery of the therapeutic hour difficult. They began to realize that psychotherapy would take years to learn well. When I asked Ned how he would learn not to give his patients "unconscious messages," he answered, "bit by bit." (August 14.)

All of these developments in the residents' lives are continuations of earlier themes. A new element was how the resident used himself as the measure for diagnosis and treatment. This self-orientation also reflected the primacy of learning; for everything one learned about psychiatry centered on the self. A resident and I were talking about how he knew when a patient was crazy.

> [The resident] emphasized that "crazy" is in terms of one's expectations. You have a crazy patient who will be always a crazy patient, in

terms of "normal" expectations. But with time, you begin to expect that patient's craziness to come in certain ways, and so on a short time span, you stop thinking that she is acting crazy; that's the way she is.

On the other hand, if a well-known patient suddenly starts to act *differently* than before, you say she is acting crazy, not in reference to general society, but in reference to your own expectations of her. (August 21.)

Concomitant with a focus on learning techniques and one's relation to it, the resident took on a more instrumental view of his patients.

. . . The question came up of a suicidal patient. What emerged was that some residents would rather see a patient kill himself than leave the hospital or leave therapy.

Jeff Roche assumed that you "have to go through the pain of understanding" (a common slogan here) to gain anything.

Ned Reich explained to Jeff that the patient may even get worse while you're sharing his pain, but that is a risk you have to take. In the conversation, it became clear that for him, Raskin, and Roche, taking the risk of suicide is better than no therapy at all, or having the patient quit therapy, or keeping therapy superficial.[19] (August 5.)

The new attitude which accompanied the greater distance residents took from their patients implied that patients were responsible for themselves in therapy. By the end of July, residents had begun to feel that patients must be responsible for their own actions in *management* on the ward. Now the same basic idea was extended to *therapy*. It was up to the *patient* whether he got well or not, whether he murdered or not, whether he committed suicide or not. In part, this psychiatric version of medical responsibility came from the tremendous pressure residents felt when they had a suicidal patient. They were told that patients can attempt suicide any time and that ultimately they cannot be stopped. For the therapist to feel responsible for his patient's life day and night becomes unbearable. As the resident experienced this pressure, he "realized" the patient must take care of his own well-being. Again three attitudes of training psychiatrists occurred simultaneously—a sense of diminished effectiveness, an emphasis on patient responsibility, and an interest in technique.

These acquisitions of professional psychiatry did not come easily, and the residents were too emotional not to feel some pain. Two months after the "sensible" discussion above about patient responsibility, the same residents talked again. In the interim, they had also acquired greater experience of failure, including suicide.

> Roche and Rabinowitz realized there were patients who could be put on drugs and gotten out, but claimed we minimize drugs in order to learn. "We learn more about the dynamics, but we don't get them out," they said. "And learning about the dynamics does not necessarily help either."
>
> Roche said, "What are we doing here anyway?"
>
> Another answered, "We are learning at the patient's expense." (Sept. 23.)

Guilt combined with a sense of helplessness, what one chief called, "the most dominant feeling of the first year."

> The residents expressed great skepticism about whether therapy helps at all. One recalled that after the guest interviewer on Friday said that the patient could go out if put on drugs, he had concluded, "So when you're through learning from him, get him out." The resident felt guilty about that cynical view.
>
> One resident defended this position, saying that the choice was between keeping the patient here and changing his character structure or sending him out and letting him function on drugs in his half-crippled way.
>
> Immediately, Ken and Carl retorted, "That is not the choice. How could you give that party line where there is no guarantee of character change? In fact, any basic change is unlikely. The real choice is getting him out or keeping him with some small changes over a long time."[20]

The growing sense of powerlessness was accentuated by two suicides in close succession on one service. At the end of a ward meeting following one of them, a resident said, "I feel sad, frightened, depressed. It is very hard to communicate feeling." A patient noted that throughout the meeting, no one had paid attention to the deceased patient's resident, who was sitting on the fringes of the group. (August 8.) Two weeks later, a resident on that service said that some residents were thinking of resigning. They felt everything was falling apart, and the senior staff was giving them no support. (August 17.)

The older residents considered these events and feelings as a routine stage in the first year. One chief said that the day after the first suicide on his ward, three of them came up smiling and asked, "Well, how are things going?" "The bastards," he said. "It's like initiation, going through what makes a psychiatrist. The *rites de passage* are a suicide, a patient who won't get better, or one who escapes.''

In sum, as the residents eagerly moved toward learning technique they experienced a complementary oscillation toward wanting to cure patients which left them guilty and feeling helpless. The most important support came from each other, that they were going through this together.

Not sure they could do any good, frightened and depressed by what they saw around them, the residents, not surprisingly, began to talk more than before about countertransference issues, unconscious and characterological feelings they had toward their patients which interfered with their work.

> Ned had learned a lot from the interview today. The biggest thing was, "how I am giving [my patient] the message that I don't want to see him." He said it "ties in with my wanting to leave the hospital now." (August 4.)
>
> I asked Ned if he had figured out whether he was giving [the same patient] negative signals or not.
>
> "I haven't thought much about that, frankly."
>
> "Why not?" I asked.
>
> "It gets pretty frightening when you think that not only might you want to get rid of a patient, but that unconsciously you might be doing something you don't even know about. Wanting the patient gone is not very far from wanting him dead!" (August 14.)

Uncontrolled messages of anger again preoccupied residents, but Ned's last remark illustrates a new development—that fantasies and extreme extentions of one's thoughts were encouraged. If such a thing is possible, neurosis was encouraged. When, for example, some residents admired a famous analyst for her gentle, positive style, their chief said, "Perhaps you like her because you want to avoid your feelings of despair." (August 17.)

It is at this time that residents began to accept the staff's view of their patients as extensions of themselves. The line between patient's and resident's psyche became blurred in the resident's mind. One common saying among all personnel was that you cannot really understand a patient unless you have gone through the experience yourself. Once again, one's own neurotic traits seemed an asset, but a troubled one.

The First Half Year

In the fourth to sixth months, October to Christmas, the residents felt the conflict between management and therapy sharpen. Up to this point, the residents had tried to be as therapeutic as they knew how. For example, although they were doctors by training, they had been reluctant to administer drugs. "It changes your ideas," said a young psychiatric resident, "when you realize you have to give drugs, and the drugs get the patient better." (September 28.)

By the winter, residents became better, more realistic managers of inpatients, but their main focus remained on therapy. Having concluded that therapy was difficult in the first year with inpatients, they looked to the outpatients they would have in the second year of residency. The important socialization process was that they learned not that psychotherapy does not work but that it fails in the circumstances in which they practiced it, circumstances which would change by the second year.

In October, the issues of management versus therapy were accentuated by two executive orders. One, from the director, Dr. Black, stated that patients who had been in the hospital over ninety days should be discharged or their continued presence should be explained in a note to him personally. Attached was a list of the thirty-four patients who had been in the hospital for more than ninety days. Dr. Black also indicated that psychopaths and sociopaths should not be kept in the hospital, because they did not benefit from therapy. A number of these patients were suicidal, which was seen by Black and some chiefs as a manipulative device which the hospital could not tolerate indefinitely.

The residents' main response to Black's edict was that they did not want to take the responsibility for sending their patients of long duration "out on the street." The six residents on Service I discussed this order, and all but Marc Raskin felt uneasy. Since the beginning of the year, he had taken an attitude which represented the values of a fully-socialized resident psychiatrist. For example, in discussions about suicide he displayed calm assurance that the doctor was not responsible for the patient's life. The others, who were constantly anxious about this antimedical position, always became angry at him for his "irresponsible'' attitude. Responding to the executive order, Marc told the residents that Black was right:

> Nobody benefits psychiatrically from being in the hospital, Marc said. The only reason for being in is because society cannot tolerate you or because you need a rest from pressures. But neither reason helps therapy. *The hospital impedes therapy.*[21]
>
> Specifically, Marc told Carl that he had kept a suicidal patient in and she had regressed. ''That's the whole point; you s̄hould have kicked her out long ago.''
>
> Carl replied that she used to manipulate, but he was sure she would kill herself if she was discharged.
>
> Marc persisted, ''She can manipulate anyone. What she needs is to find someone she *cannot* manipulate whom she can trust and get into business with.''
>
> Ned said, ''We can't tell who is really asking for help and who is not.''
>
> Marc replied, ''But they're *all* asking for help. The question is what is the best form.'' The chief agreed. (October 7.)

In contrast to Black's promanagement edict, the clinical director, Dr. Blumberg, issued an antimanagement order stating that hypnotic drugs were not to be used unless cleared with the chief *and* superchief of the service. (Hypnotics are mainly used to help patients sleep at night.) In the classic psychoanalytic tradition, Dr. Blumberg argued that drugs impede therapy. You cannot do therapy with a drugged, dopey patient. In response, the chiefs felt this order showed that they were not trusted, and the residents said the order deprived them of their doctorhood. They also thought the policy unreasonable.

> *Dave Reed:* If the higher-ups are going to make drug policy, they should back it up with some data. A lot of things being said are just not true. It isn't true that a half grain of chlorohydrate gets between you and the patient in therapy. . . . When a patient is tossing in bed and can't sleep, he is no good for therapy in the morning. (October 14.)

These two edicts and the tenor of the times reflect the deep ambivalence residents experienced about their identity and their relations to patients. When their medical license was challenged, they defended their doctorhood and the use of drugs which they saw work. Yet they had committed their doctorhood to psychotherapy without knowing how well it worked.

Only Marc, who had come to terms with the nature of psycho-therapy before he arrived, supported Dr. Blumberg's edict (as residents called it). It made clear what the real work was; it separated administrative actions from real depth therapy.

> *Carl Rabinowitz to Marc Raskin:* Don't you feel a little bit like making the lame walk and the blind see?
> *Marc Raskin:* No.
> *Carl Rabinowitz:* You're lucky.
> *Ken Reese:* On the contrary, it's tragic. (November 4.)

Yet Ken was finding that despite his best efforts, he had little impact on his patients. Everyone except Marc felt ineffective. Although patients got better, many residents said that they could not credit themselves with the successes. Patients improved at the "wrong" time or for the "wrong" reasons. Psychoanalysis came in for harsh criticism. After a bad case conference conducted by a member of the Psychoanalytic Institute, two residents said, "Well, that's three strikes against the institute." On the same day, a chief said, "Blumberg is useless." (October 19.) Also the same day, another chief told me, "Now analysis is out, not only out but being challenged. The new things are community psychiatry and biochemistry." Carl summarized the general feeling.

> *Carl Rabinowitz to psychological intern:* At the start of the year, you felt that you were powerless, that all you were supposed to do was "understand," while we doctors could prescribe drugs and administrate.
> But now we are feeling the same things, because of the edicts, and we are told that all we have is our personality and that we are to understand. (October 28.)

Nothing works. The residents felt stripped bare. Looking at treatment from a psychotherapeutic perspective, they complained against the hospital.

> *Carl Rabinowitz:* We've become a traffic station. We just ship people here and there. People come in from the courts and we send them out.
> *Ned Reich:* People are admitted when it is not necessary. No point in evaluating a patient who goes immediately to a state hospital. [Evaluation here takes over one week of work.] We can evaluate him at the door.

> *Ken Reese:* I have fallen into the practice here of not doing what is best for the patients. Taking a throat culture is such a nuisance here, you don't bother. No one here has ever heard of blood cultures.Last year [as an intern] I would have been in charge. I would have done a lot more. I like the medical model. It embodies great care and concern for your patient. Here, everything gets sloppy. We don't take patients seriously. (November 2.)

From this nadir of frustration and futility, residents began to work out a definition of their work on which they built a new professional identity. A critical event for this group was the talk given by a visiting analyst at one case conference. Hearing them, before the conference, complain about the pressure they felt from the patient's demands for cure, the interviewer talked to the residents about coming to grips with what you can and cannot do. "You have to learn ways of looking at your work and at patients so you are not disappointed when you can't give what is demanded; so you aren't too upset, but can roll with the punches. We must learn what our powers are."

The interviewer then held the conference, and afterwards the residents talked a great deal about her brilliant interview and technique. The guest seemed like a prophet who had come at a time of despair and lost faith in curative models and had told the lost tribe what they must do. Then she had shown them wherein their new powers lay by displaying the power and mastery of a superb interview. (November 4.)

The analyst had advised the residents to find a new and liveable perspective on their work. This happened over the next several weeks. More and more of them began to realize that desires to get patients better as they had in medicine were indeed "rescue fantasies," and they would be less miserable if they stopped trying so hard to cure the patient. Second, their mentors emphasized in supervision and conferences the fine points of the therapeutic process. Thus mastering the therapeutic hour supplanted cure as the primary goal. Paradoxically, then, residents found their salvation by immersing themselves more deeply in what had been destroying them—therapy with their patients.

> *Ken Reese:* This week I have been involved in my patients like never before. Qualitatively it's been different. Very deep. And it has made me angry.
>
> *Marc Raskin:* My patients have made me very sad.
>
> *Jeff Roche:* I can imagine that [Raskin's patient] made you very sad.

Marc Raskin: [Nods.]

Adam Cohn: And the two patients Marc's been working hardest on have gotten worse.

Jeff Roche: Yeah. You weren't exactly enthusiatic about giving her EST.

Marc Raskin: [Nods.]

Carl Rabinowitz: Well, my patients have made me sad and angry. Mrs.—— makes me so sad that it takes me an hour to recover from being a half-hour with her. And Mrs. —— makes me mad. She has a talent for assailing my narcissim. (November 18).

Ken Reese told about a dream in which his patients were corpses floating in a solution in a basement autopsy room at his old medical school. He approached one vat, and a patient suddenly kicked, splashing solution on him. Ken continued:

Yesterday I had a beautiful session with Mr.——. We shared a very touching experience in his past, when he was an altar boy, and as he left I thought, perhaps someday he will be a cardinal.

Can you imagine! Having both of these experiences together? You get tossed so high and then sink so low.

Dave: What is so interesting is that we spend so much time over what to do when there is no evidence that any of the alternatives do much, outside of drugs.

Really what we do is look for a style that suits us. (November 18.)

In the week of December 4, three of the six residents on Service I said that for the first time they felt like real psychiatrists. Much later in the year, the psychological intern, Mike, explained what was a basic cultural force which pushed residents through depressions and involved them more than ever: "I felt great pressure when I came here to identify with my work, and *that* takes a lot of energy."

Now when residents criticized Blumberg as the supreme psychoanalyst, it served a different purpose than a few weeks earlier.

Jeff Roche: Well, I always thought how poor I was and thought if I were Blumberg she would move. But yesterday he didn't get anywhere with her, not at all, and I felt a whole lot better. (November 18.)

No longer were residents challenging the psychoanalytic model but they were rather measuring their worth as junior analysts. An alternative was Dr. Black's administrative approach to patient care, which some embraced but most rejected.

Ned Reich: And Blumberg never talks about getting the patient out of the hospital. On the other hand, others are telling me the patient is very sick, and Black is asking why is the patient still here. It's very hard being tossed between these totally different views about a patient.

I'm still sticking with Blumberg. You see, I'm here to learn psychotherapy for patients who don't even exist here. It is harder his way, but I'm here to learn it. *It's too easy to use drugs.* (November 18.)

Residents wanted to treat patients who didn't even exist here. Dr. Black's approach made sense to the residents for inpatients, but they had learned that hospital administration lacks professional lustre. Moreover, Black was a psychoanalyst as well as an administrator and would probably not be director unless he were. Thus long-term therapy became the goal. While they tried to do it as much as they could with their inpatients, their new perspective emphasized outpatients and the second year.

Ned Reich: This week has been the high point for me as a psychiatrist. Mr.——, the first patient I have discharged who is not a court case or did not sign a three-day paper, returned for his first outpatient session. [Laughter.]

Of course he was drunk. [Laughter.]

And he was ten minutes late. [Laughter.]

Ned Reich: But he came! This is what I came here to do. To give psychotherapy to outpatients, and now I'm doing it. (December 2.)

The end of the first six months brought the residents full circle. Just as on the day they arrived, they felt helpless, only more so because they now had tried the tricks of the trade. December felt like the end of the year, and it was hard to imagine what the next six months could bring.

Ned Reich: For most patients, [Christmas] is a time when families usually gather. And also it is the beginning of a new year, and they wonder where it's gone.

Someone: That's it.

Another: I'm ready for my second year.

Another: Yeah, six months of this is enough. [Nods.]

Ned Reich: I don't know. I'm very glad to have this year, where I've gotten experiences I won't get in the future.

Carl Rabinowitz [disgusted]: Like what?

Ned Reich: Oh, I have seen patients I won't see again, many kinds that are very interesting.

Carl Rabinowitz: You know I was thinking what I did for Christmas last year and what I will do this year and the year after that, then the one after that.

Adam Cohn: All this week I've been running around making plans for next year [*smiles to self*].

Ken Reese: I was thinking, not to be Oedipal, who will be in your chair next year.

We'll blink twice and the two years will be over.

Adam Cohn: Blink twice and you'll be on Medicare.

Carl Rabinowitz: Blink again and you'll be dead.

Dave Reed: Exactly.

Ken Reese: The question is whether there is life before death. . . . [*Great, continuous laughter.*] What are we getting? For these years? Who will repay us for all these precious years spent?[22] (December 16.)

Through the Winter

"My fantasy is that some day I'll be so competent that I'll have no feelings about the case." (Jeff Roche, March 2.)

By the end of the calendar year, the residents wanted the second year to begin. Six months remained, however, and during that time they solidified basic attitudes toward work and the profession, intermingled with cycles of hope and depression.

After Christmas, residents still tried to escape from their work, in mind if not in body. Carl said that some of them were talking about academic appointments, and that his dream would be the University of Hawaii. (January 6.) Several mentioned they had been thinking about their third year. Even the chief, Adam Cohn, felt worn out, and he could not wait for his winter vacation. (January 18.) He said he felt guilty about his extravagant trip, but not about leaving his ward. Slowly, resignation to reality replaced escape, a realization that nothing would change for many months. Ken Reese said, "The day is so long now that you go home and get up, and it feels like the same day still going on. There is no relief." (January 18.) When Carl had similar feelings, Adam gave them his usual interpretation: "You're beginning to feel their pain, how they [the patients] must feel all the time." (January 20.)

Soon after the holidays, one conversation among these residents unveiled the themes of the winter months ahead.

Jeff Roche: Last year was so clear-cut. [*Whining voice*] I always had a clear conscience. I always knew I had done everything possible.

Ken Reese: Last week was the worst of the year for me. I went around gloomy, not really here. This week was better. . . .

Jeff Roche: Why should I see my patients twice a week, that's what I'm wondering?

Ken Reese: Why should you see them once a week? What do we think we are that we can do much by seeing a patient one, two hours, even four hours a week?

Carl Rabinowitz: Marc, how do you feel?

Marc Raskin: I am enraged at what goes on here [at the residency] . . . but I am able to stay for the piece of paper.

Marc, Ned, and Carl all say in sequence that they are learning a lot, "a tremendous amount."

Ned Reich: I escape some of the pain you mention by thinking of the healthier neurotics I will treat and by having less hope for these patients.

Jeff Roche: I'm beginning to think there are no neurotics in the world.

Ned Reich: Don't worry. You're sitting next to one. [*Everyone laughs.*]

Adam Cohn: Two days ago, I threw a glass against the wall at home and smashed it to smithereens.

Jeff Roche: I'm kind of sickened to hear you say that. I think of you as very peaceful and controlled.

After the meeting, two residents talked about the medical problems of a patient. They really talked shop, using many medical terms in telegraphic sentences. (January 27.)

Feelings of therapy being ineffective yet of learning a lot, of looking to work with neurotic outpatients for hope, of thinking about one's own neuroses, and of bottled-up frustration with the hospital characterized this passage to springtime.

Marc's views of patient care and the hospital, once considered irresponsible, gained favor. About this time he gave a talk elaborating his views, and the residents liked it, though some said he overstated the case. At University Psychiatric Center, he said, everyone is labeled—doctor, nurse, patient—and everyone introduces himself that way. Status is very strong, and everyone on the staff knows anything he wishes about a patient, but not the reverse. More striking, he said, the patients are kept from information we have about *them*.[23] Thus status is confirmed by the system, which claims that we know more about them than they know about themselves.

In treating patients, Marc continued, we normalize them. If they offend us with their behavior, we tell them to shape up or ship out. We use denial a lot, denying a man's feelings by passing over them. Recently, a patient greeted a resident, "Hello, shithead." The doctor replied, "Hello, Mr.——."

We also objectify patients by putting their feelings into theoretical classifications, Marc said. There is a demand for a lot of personal material from the patient. If he gives it, he gets more attention, is a more "interesting case." If he only acts on his feelings instead, he is not tolerated. (January 18.)

In part the residents responded to these features of psychiatric work by withdrawing from the ward as much as they could from a place where they worked every day. While before the residents had attacked the hospital and struggled with problems of management, now they minimized efforts on these matters and ignored the nurses. Ironically, they could now ignore the nurses because they had learned what the nurses had taught them.

> *Adam Cohn:* I think they [the nurses] want a party, because they want some expression of unity and caring from you [the residents]. More recently, you have not been consulting the nurses or staff, and you work on your own more. (January 6.)

A week later.

> *Jeff Roche:* I think of a party as meeting other *residents,* with a word or two to keep the nurses happy.
>
> *Marc Raskin:* I fear not knowing all the names.
>
> Cohn talked about how the nurses don't feel consulted, not even in case conferences or staff planning conferences.
>
> *Carl Rabinowitz:* I feel in those meetings I'm just telling the other residents about my patients. (January 13.)

The nurses, recently an object of uneasy respect, received more and more criticism from this group of residents.

Ken Reese: The nurses are really dumb and rigid. They are the most rigid group. For example, I have a patient who is upset, but I want her to have as much freedom to move around as possible. The nurse said, "How can you do that? She [the patient] obviously is not ready for those privileges. She will show she is ready, when she stops getting upset each night." [24]

One big difference between the medical team, which is all doctors, and the psychiatric team, is that the rest of the team is far below your level of skill and brains. Except for some attendants. (March 16.)

This last opinion marked a change in confidence as professionals. Through the winter the earlier feelings of futility were supplanted by a growing sense of mastery. This first happened in management, by learning rules of procedure. Many residents disagreed with my emphasis here on rules, but their examples always turned out to involve them. Here are my notes on what happened when I asked one of many residents if he had learned rules of management.

He said no. You learn like you learn a foreign language by living with a family. Someone asks you how you make plurals, and you say by adding s, but you know the exceptions too.

I asked for an example.

He thought for a while (it was hard) and then said a patient had come up to him in the hall and started on something. He said to her she should bring it up in therapy. She continued, and he persisted.

He said in July he might have done a number of things. He might have gotten concerned and taken it up there. He might have invited the patient into his office to talk about it. He might have gone to the head nurse to talk about it. But now he always knew what to do.

I said that sounds like a rule to me.

He said yes, and he could not think of something analogous to the plural of goose.(!) It bothered him that he could not, and he said he would tell me later. (He did not.) (January 9.)

A month or two later feelings of confidence as a therapist emerged. Two important dimensions were *sustained focus* and *comfort.*

I asked Ned Reich what he had learned in therapy. He thought a while. No quick answer.

Finally he said that he had learned to get to what's on the patient's mind, and that was central. He had learned how not to distract the patient's thoughts, divert him, or sidetrack him. (I think that really means learning how to shut up and not interrupt.) What this means is to understand his defenses better so that you don't get caught up in them.

He gave an example. A patient came into therapy, having missed the previous week's appointment. He said he missed the hour because he was afraid the therapist would stop therapy, or make him stop seeing his friend, or stop wearing red.

"Red," Ned asked, "why red?"

"Oh," said the patient, "it could have been anything."

"No," insisted Ned, "you are responsible for what you say. Why red?"

"Well, I didn't get it from this Marlboro pack [*on the desk*]."

"Where did you get it?" the resident asked.

"Well, this is silly," said the patient, "from my jacket [red, green, and black checks]. I was in New York last week and my friend gave it to me."

Ned was very satisfied with this success. The patient wore that jacket, he said, almost as a symbol of why he was not at therapy the last time; he had chosen his friend over the resident. That is what underlay "red."

The lesson is to stick to something, said Ned. That's what you learn from Blumberg. He never lets go.

"But how does he know he's not on a sidetrack?" I asked.

"Well, there are certain basic things all people here are concerned with. Anger, loss, sex."

"Freud," Ned concluded, "reduced them to two. *Lieben* and *arbeiten*." (March 2.)

Here is an example of comfort.

Ken Reese told me that the therapy with his patients is better than ever. He feels he knows them better as people, that the sessions go quickly, so that you want to see the patient more, rather than their being a drag.

"Why is that?" I asked.

"Well, he answered, "I think I am more skillful now than before."

"What are the new skills you have?"

"Well, much of it is feeling comfortable with the patients. I have less anxiety. I can tolerate the patient getting angry at me more than before. Before, if the patient would complain about nurse's group, I would sympathize and see what could be done. But this is a way of covering over the anger with kindness 'You kill me with kindness.' Now I am more likely to ask the patient why she is so angry, and to see why she is angry at me.''

"Is she?'' I asked.

"Well, you know that all hypotheses go. She may be angry at her mother too, but I can deal directly with her anger at me. The point is that if you guess she is angry at you, and she gives clear signs that she is, then your hypothesis is right. But had you suggested she is angry at her mother, that would be right too. They're all right.'' (March 30.)

Thus, even though Ken saw that a given interpretation is arbitrary and self-confirming, he was sure that his old, indulgent manner covered over the patient's anger. Less logical but more real, he exchanged the patient's comfort for his own. As residents moved away from the hospital and a curative orientation, they became increasingly concerned with technique and feeling comfortable. Most gains in comfort, like this one, were seen by the resident as therapeutic for the *patient*, not for himself.

Earlier, Ken Reese had suggested how I might study the professionalization of residents. I could use a questionnaire, he said, asking the resident what he would do if a patient said he was going to kill himself, or if a patient came up to you in the hall with a complaint about other patients, or if a patient embarrassed you and you blushed and he noticed, or if a patient refused to come into the office or left the office prematurely? His questionnaire, I thought, saw professionalization as learning how to handle embarrassment and how to become comfortable. (January 9.)[25]

A final dimension of professional confidence is diagnosis.

Ned Reich and I talked about what he has learned since July. Ned replied that he could diagnose patients much faster than before. He said there were three elements, delusions, hallucinations, and loose thought patterns. The first two are gross schizophrenia, and they are easy to detect. He had learned to do better with them. Now, if he hears that a new patient thinks that his body is changing from a man's to a woman's, he thinks it can hardly be anything else but schizophrenia.

But some schizophrenics, he said, have "a thought disorder.'' That is more subtle. They say coherent sentences, but the sentences "somehow don't hang together.''[26]

I said we all do that at times.

He said, "but with them you sense that they are trying to escape feelings. No, not feelings; none of us want to face those. But you sense that the looseness is 'bizarre.' "

"What's that?" I asked. He could not explain.

After talking about schizophrenics for twenty minutes, he mentioned that he only worked with two cases like it. So he was talking mainly on the basis of watching and being told stories in conference and in supervision. (March 2.)

Although the residents felt like true professionals for the first time, the complexities and disappointments of therapy constantly set them back. Early in the winter, Ken said:

"We are all gigolos, stabilizing patients by love. For a few bucks an hour they can come to us and get reliable, concerned involvement without giving anything of themselves. And they can meet probably the most solid, perceptive person they have ever known. And they don't even have to go through the sex mess, which most of them don't want.

"I just feel they are so narcissistic, so demanding, just sucking on me all the time." (January 6.)

Not only did many residents feel they were not doing therapy, they felt they were hurting patients. In part, the harm came through the hospital, as described before. In part, they themselves felt responsible.

I'm looking after Mr.———, and his treatment has been a real mistake. His spirit is broken . . . I don't think any one of us could stand the humiliation of what he's gone through. (February 3.)

Yet despite their "working with the wrong type of patients," residents got more involved in therapy. Near the end of January, Carl Rabinowitz said that it took him two hours to get over one therapy hour, not just with his closest patient, but with all of them. Other residents seemed more even, emphasizing neither detachment nor involvement.[27] But those residents who talked of their diminished involvement soon complained of the pains of overinvolvement. Much talk was devoted to allowing the patient to express his rage and sadness without its destroying you as a therapist. A psychoanalyst might interpret this as the resident letting the patient speak for him. When Jeff Roche said, "My fantasy is that someday I'll be so competent that I'll have no feelings about the case," other residents agreed.

Marc Raskin: I feel I know more about ———'s dynamics now, but I'm not sure it makes any difference.

Ned Reich [*soberly*]: My fantasy comes from meeting Theodore Reich, who said that with the right patient at the right time, the analyst's tool is as precise as the surgeon's.

Marc Raskin: So?

Ned Reich: So you can cut out the disease and cure the patient.

Carl Rabinowitz [*sarcastically*]: Are you interested in cutting or sewing.

Ned Reich: Cutting. [*Carl smiles.*] (March 9.)

The tremendous pressure of therapy and of their dreams also led the residents to greater self-consciousness.

I asked Jeff if he still thought people who go into psychiatry may go crazy.

No, he answered, he felt more relaxed than ever before. . . . He said he has been thinking about analysis, because "everything I read or hear seems to say the same thing—that regardless how well put together you are, your unconscious enters into your therapy so much that you can't really be good until you know it."

But he said he would never go into analysis for personal reasons. "Why should I? I do just fine."

. . . .

"I told my brother that I think I ought to get married before I get analyzed so that I decide who I'll marry on a sound, irrational basis." (January 4.)

The awareness of the unconscious and its role in therapy was for many the most important discovery of the year.

Marc Raskin: This week, no one has gotten in the way of the progress of my patients, except themselves.

Ned Reich: How about yourself? Countertransference?

Marc Raskin: I work very hard not to interfere.

Ned Reich: I don't know how hard I try.

Mike (*the psychologist*): In the last three months, all my supervision has been on countertransference.

Marc Raskin: I should think so, since you only have one or two patients. . . .[28]

I've seen [a patient] six times a week since he came, a half hour each.

Ned Reich: Wow!

Mike (*the psychologist*): No wonder he's running around!

Marc Raskin: It's the first time I've really become aware of coun-tertransference. It's been the greatest teaching experience of the year. (February 24.)

By March, five of the six residents and the chief were thinking of applying to the Psychoanalytic Institute.

I told Ken I felt full of energy today, and he said he did too, but now he thinks of it as "manic," with the implication that depression will fol-low. We joked about how this was a self-fulfilling prophecy.

Before coming into psychiatry, he said, he was often full of life, but he didn't think of it in the same, self-conscious way, suspicious of his mood and nature. Before, he also got depressed. "Depression is my next-door neighbor, but it didn't follow exalted states."

"This is the dangerous thing about this business," he concluded. *"You can't be happy so easily. You suspect yourself."* (March 23.)

To summarize, the first three months of the calendar year found the residents again in cycles of exhaustion and anxiety. Chiefs and supervisors interpreted these as learning to feel the pain of the patient, to work through the rescue fantasies of curing patients, and to face "termination" or the end of the first year.

Desires and small efforts to come closer together accompanied this time of trial. But as Ken noted, "We're not a getting-together group like Adam's was, where the residents met every weekend, even more, to talk and do things." (January 13.)

Adam summarized the meeting by saying: "You guys have been using many images in our conversation this morning of physical contact with each other, touch football, skating, having dinner."

A resident: You mean there's homococktis going around? [*Peals of laughter.*]

Another: Adam, you have a dirty mind. You should be an analyst! (January 13.)

Renewed efforts were made in March.

Ned Reich: On Wednesday, let's have a half-hour open, for coffee and talk. This meeting here is great, but during the week we hardly have time to talk to one another. At [another school] they had a coffee hour, and it was a great way to see the staff.

. . . .

Adam Cohn: I think we're trying to get away from the hospital. [*Laughs, then silence.*]

Carl Rabinowitz: You can tell when Adam makes an interpretation, because there is five minutes of silence after.[29] (March 16.)

This group's inability to succeed in becoming comrades did not represent residents generally. Some first-year groups, both in this year and in others, had warm, close comradeship. Despite such variety, the psychiatric culture rendered a uniform interpretation on all of these group experiences. If the group was close, its members, after a year's distance from the experience, invariably said that they never expressed the considerable anger they had for each other. If, like this group, they never got close, members came to see how much warmth existed which was never quite expressed.

Getting Comfortable

The chief [*instructing*]: Here we sit and listen.
Ken and Carl: But that's all. We don't learn. Here, we get the *Reader's Digest* version of the analytic tradition. (May 18.)

Spring found the residents more competent, yet less happy with the residency.

Carl Rabinowitz: Some time ago I passed that point of diminishing returns here, and I'm just pushing through now. I'm getting very little out of here.
Marc Raskin: If what were implicit here had been made explicit in the contract, I would never have signed it.
Ned Reich: Like what?
Marc Raskin: Like the infantilization all over. The requirements, especially the case conferences.
Ned Reich: I sympathize. I like to be infantilized; so it's not so hard for me. But I don't think all the conferences are necessary.
Ken Reese: What is worse is that this place is so intellectually vacuous. People are dull and picky. Like the restrictions on lithium. . . . It's absurd, like Gilbert and Sullivan. Remember the community psychiatrist at conference? She went on [*sings*]
Oh the social worker is very nice, very nice, very nice.'
Then the social worker dances on stage [*sings*]
And you are toooooooo.

Then we have the chorus

We all like community psychiatry, community psychiatry!
It can do so much for us.

[*Peals of laughter.*]

And with Sally, the head nurse. You know, when you go in the office, if you say "Yes," she will take her cue and sing

NO! No, no, no, no.

You sing back, *"I really think so. I do, I do, I do."*
She insists, *"No, no, no, NO!"*
You sing, *"And tha-a-at is the way, it will be."* She grows red and runs off stage. Act II, Scene I. You play it over and over. There's no intellectual stimulus. (March 30.)

Such widely felt despondency as documented in these pages could not last forever. The most impressive fact of April and May was how residents pushed through. The sheer weight of work and patients kept them going at a time when some might quit. Feeling dumb, stupid, numb, emptied (to use their self-descriptions), they went on seeing patients and handling ward routine "better" than ever. The communal responsibility for the ward and the comradeship among each other also kept them going. During this period, their desperation for action turned a minor accomplishment into a feeling of triumph. One instance stood out because it never happened (but could have) before or after.

In ward meetings, the patients often complained about the stark facilities for living; for example, the women's dormitory had no curtains, so that the sun woke them early in the morning. (They also had to hide from the window when dressing.) Residents, by example of the chief, learned to respond to such complaints by psychologizing them. In this instance: "It seems to me, Mrs.—— is saying it's hard to wake up and face that we're still here."

In April, the patients complained that they could not go out of doors or off the ward easily, because staff who might accompany them were too busy. Immediately, the residents responded with a suggested buddy-system, where patients with more privileges could accompany more restricted patients on prescribed outings. After the meeting, the residents were elated by the idea of having solved a *real* problem. A senior psychiatrist might have seen this action as a relapse into rescue fantasies, but the residents did not choose to consider it that way. Jeff Roche said, "We actually decided something! It was great!" Carl Rabinowitz added, "This is the first time we have been able to *act*."

Ken Reese told me there was a real change in mood. Even Carl reversed the general ideology of ward meetings, that feelings should be shared and that action is an escape from feelings:

> This showed what group meetings can and cannot deal with. They can be used to make community decisions, but when —— brought up his homosexual feelings, everyone shut him off. That stuff belongs with his therapist, not weekly meetings. (April 11.)

This one communal decision became implemented. It seemed to satisfy the needs of residents to *do* something, and perhaps to want to get out of the hospital. Residents said they sympathized with the patients, and at their next private meeting, the residents decided for the first time to meet outdoors rather than in the chief's office on the ward. In the subsequent two weeks, more than a usual number of residents said they wanted to do something for blacks or for peace in Vietnam.

Despite these efforts to do good for someone, the residents continued throughout the period to feel "chronically tired." They felt they too had become like the program.

> *Carl Rabinowitz:* I have been surprised at the dullness here, because when I came to visit, this place impressed me as having the most stimulating residents.
>
> *Ken Reese* [*smiles*]: It's the way we *become*. We lose our enthusiasm, fun, and critical faculties. At [another hospital] the atmosphere is so different. People joke, and they run around looking things up. . . . (March 30.)
>
> Carl felt he had been emptied out. The feeling persisted into May. Ken mentioned how terribly exhausted he was, although he had more free time than ever before. "It's from wanting to get out of that hospital all day." The height of his day, he said, was lunch. "I think about having it all morning and I think about how great it was all afternoon!"

Residents also adjusted and pushed through by doing their business more coolly and efficiently. By this time of year they accepted and treated most patients as cases for management, not therapy. therefore they saw fewer patients fewer hours, giving themselves more leisure time than ever before. The kind of patient who would have received two hours of therapy a week in July now got twenty minutes. (May 24.) Silent patients, once fascinating and attractive to new residents, were now given drugs. Once silence was good talk, intriguing. Now no talk was bad talk.

The only resident who did not show signs of depression was Marc Raskin. He said his patients were coming along fine. Commenting on the depression of a more typical colleague, he said the man had unrealistic expectations. In contrast, he said he never expected to accomplish much with these patients from the start. "You have to sit there for hours and hours chipping away at the defenses." Slowly, one saw the other residents learn this basic lesson, that much of their misery came from their rescue fantasies, i.e., their desire to cure patients. This lesson led to a major professional adjustment. Residents began to *care* for patients, aside from cure.[30]

> *Dave Reed:* OK, but does therapy work? Do patients get cured?
>
> *Ken Reese:* Yes. You help the patient by caring for her and expressing interest.
>
> *Dave Reed:* You need no training for that; anyone who is concerned can do it.
>
> *Ken Reese:* But that's learning to *care*. We care by trying to see what the patient really means and needs and wants. (April 6.)

At the end of the year, Carl summarized his experience.[31]

> He could not think of one instance where knowing the dynamics had made any difference for a patient, or where working through an issue in therapy had been completed. People just don't get mourning out of their system. They rarely get over a big issue.
>
> Nor does he think as manager he had really helped someone get better. So the only way he sees that he made a difference was that with some patients it was important that there be someone who is trustworthy, who cares, and who is willing to help. (June 27.)

Caring for patients was a selective process of getting comfortable. One could only care for someone one cared for, that is, someone one liked. Marc Raskin (a bachelor) said that he thought you saw patients intensively whom you liked, either because they were attractive or because you and they shared some problem. All five of his long-term patients were under thirty; three were attractive women, "marriageable," as he put it. Both men had homosexual problems. He thought that perhaps this was the way he expressed the homosexual in him, through treating them. (May 24.) Analogous situations abounded. Since the first month, residents had been selecting patients for long-term therapy and abandoning the medical edict that one treats anyone in need.

Increasingly, references were made to finding self-satisfaction in one's work. Ken said that therapy with his patients was better than ever. I asked him what he meant, and he replied that he felt he knew them better as *people,* and that the sessions go quickly so that you want to see the patient. He felt he interviews better. Thus, it seemed to me, how well therapy was going depended on the experience the *therapist* had in therapy. Another resident told about a puzzle he solved, calling it "a good piece of work." His patient would say no ill of his half-brother and the resident wondered why. He got the patient to recall that when he was six, his mother had threatened him should he ever speak against his brother. Another part of getting comfortable was fully realizing how powerful you were, even though you might feel ineffective.

> In the discussion, two residents said that they gave nothing to some patients and the patients loved them for it! "We are the greatest thing for those patients, even when we are cruel to them." (April 13.)

At a ward meeting, some patients spoke.

> *Patient No. 1:* Sometimes I think my doctor is God. I mean I put all my faith in him.
> *Patient No. 2:* He has to be. There's no one else.
> *Patient No. 3:* Or he tries to be. Doctors always act that way, they think they are right.
> *Patient No. 2:* They are paternalistic.
> *Patient No. 3:* But not mine.
> *Patient No. 2:* You only think the therapist is God because he acts that way.
> *Patient No. 1:* No. You feel desperate. You grasp at straws like a drowning man.
> *Patient No. 2:* Switching doctors is the most terrifying thing in the world. (May 16.)

Finally, residents became more preoccupied with their own therapy.

> *Jeff Roche:* I think we learn. A crazy patient came in when I was an intern, and I was petrified! Now we're very comfortable with crazy people. [Note the phrase.]
> *Dave Reed:* I feel better about my own analysis. You get something personal out of your own. Also, you learn techniques and have better

tools, and if this is going to be your profession, you might as well be as good as you can. Also, I feel you can do more about neurotics.

Ken Reese: You wouldn't want to sell false products. . . .

Dave Reed: It depends on how you sell them.

Marc Raskin: I'm glad we're no longer hung up on the medical model. What we've done is become good patients! (April 6.)

Increasingly the residents were immersed in seeking a more perfect self, despite the dangers.

Jeff Roche: Let me throw out several negative things I've heard about analysts. If an analyst wants to have his patient get better in some way, the analytic tradition sees that as a problem the analyst has not overcome.

Carl Rabinowitz: I'll give you one view, that the tradition would not be so concerned about that if analysis were not ineffective. [*Laughter.*]

Reese and Raskin then said that they are thinking of going into analysis.

Mike (the psychologist): In analysis, you are broken into a thousand pieces, dissected.

The conversation continued with stories about famous analysts who never succeeded in putting themselves together. (May 18.)

June: The End of the Year

"This has been a year of learning how to be passive, after having been active for so many years (from Jeff Roche's Review of the Year).

Although many residents felt in January that there was nothing more to learn, June brought a feeling for some that they were not yet ready for the second year. Ned Reich said, "Well, isn't it June first?"

Jeff Roche: I have one more day as DOC,[32] and then I wonder if I'll ever use that little black bag again.

Ned Reich: Well, being a medical doctor has never been my problem. . . . I'm angry, because I don't feel prepared for the huge change in June. I've had no time to adjust to being off the ward. I have almost no time to prepare myself, but I know I've arranged it by ignoring May.

Jeff Roche: This year is the first time I've drunk coffee, and every time I do, I think of this group.

Ned Reich: You'll be drinking coffee for a long time.

Ken Reese: I have feelings for the group, but I'm skeptical about this "community" having been formed this year. We're artificial as a group. . . . I doubt if a community is possible here, but I'm sentimental and sad there wasn't more community this year. (June 1.)

For the first time in a long while, the feeling of exhaustion lifted. By June, the residents had considerably lightened their patient load and had begun to indulge themselves by leaving before five o'clock. Ken Reese, for example, reduced his therapy hours with some old patients and saw new patients much less. The end of the year, he reflected, was very different from internship, where you would work all night the last day, if necessary, on a new patient. Nor were there all these sentiments about "termination" in internship. But here, any patient who comes in after April gets the short end, and we talk of nothing but "termination." (May 7.)

The residents cut therapy hours in several ways. Perhaps most important was that they learned to *see* how few patients were "therapy patients," and therefore they did not invest time in them as they had indiscriminately at the beginning of the first year. Although residents still spent more time with new patients during the first weeks of evaluation, many reported that evaluation now took them much less time. Therefore, with new patients, residents saw them intensively for a shorter time to evaluate them, were much less likely to accept them for psychotherapy, and if they did, saw them less.[33] As for the quality of the work, some residents thought it had slipped, while others did not.

Few residents had simple feelings about leaving the first year. Some looked forward to it; the rest clung to the ward and the community it provided. Ken Reese said, "I am, frankly, happy to leave." (June 27.) A good cross-section of responses came out in the last meeting of the Group Dynamics Seminar, known as "Group," composed of residents from all wards.

Resident No. 1: I find I'm hanging onto the first year. I am way behind in my anamneses; I don't want to sum up those patients. But I pulled out the files of the patients in my group for next year.

Resident No. 2: I find I am making a hypermanic flight into the second year.

Resident No. 3: I am making a furious, fifteen-hour-day drive to get done with the first year.

Resident No. 4: Knowing now that I really have an office makes the second year much more concrete. (New offices were not assigned until the last week of the year, much to the residents' annoyance.)

Resident No. 3: Every time I tell someone about how this year was, I end up saying, "Well, that's another year shot." I don't know. Somehow I feel that way even though I feel I've learned a lot. (June 27.)

Although some residents clung to signs of their first year, when the change actually occurred, almost all residents reported relief that the first year was over. However, for some the process was difficult. Ken Reese, just cited as looking forward to ending the first year, said he found it very hard to leave the service (July 3).

During June, disengagement continued, and the attacks on the program or on psychiatry dwindled. Residents skipped supervision. They reported that the senior staff removed itself too. On the ward, the nurses reported that residents had become slack, which hurt the nurses sorely; for by anyone's account they were most upset by the end of the year. Every July they lose the men they have come to respect, and they have to start from the beginning with new residents. On some services, the nurses take seven to nine months to work harmoniously with a new group of residents!

The residents created informal, comfortable distances from each other. The short strained effort to get quite close in the spring never succeeded. Now, at Feelings meetings,[34] almost everyone read the newspaper before the hour began. The entire meeting of June 15 was filled with light stories and jokes, and aside from the content, the atmosphere felt relaxed.

Nurse [*anxiously*]*:* The ward is very tight. We have three colored women doing crazy things. [*She mentions a patient.*]

Mike (*the psychologist*)*:* They took care of her in conference by diagnosing her "psychotic character" [*laughter*].[35]

The first ten minutes went to stories, like the following: there was a girl who came in with a football helmet under one arm and a bunch of flowers under the other [*laughter*]. We had nothing to do that night, so she put on a real show for the medical students on night duty.

(All the stories were about the crazy things patients do.)

More stories. Among them, Carl recalled a patient who came in here with a loaded gun.

> *Dave Reed:* Well, last year in the country four psychiatrists were killed by their patients.
>
> Lots of talk on how to kill the patient who has a gun, before he gets you. Boisterous talk about how you could have machine guns built into the ceiling and walls of your office. (June 15.)

During this meeting and others in the late spring, the residents made no interpretations about what they were saying, such as how to kill your patient before he kills you. No introspective discussion occurred. For example, in the same meeting the residents discussed how one of them had no birth certificate and how easy it was for anyone to get anyone else's birth certificate, how anyone could become *you*. They also mused about how nice Stillman Infirmary was if you ever got sick and how nice another hospital was, because you could walk in any time and talk with someone. Finally, they talked about arrangements for using their old offices on the ward when they were seeing inpatients, even though new residents would occupy them. Despite such rich material about being lost and lonely, residents' talk remained completely unanalyzed.

To understand the residents' efforts to get close and then become comfortably humorous, one must see them in their culture. The last Feelings meeting ended this way:

> *Ken Reese:* This meeting is something I will miss. It is the most valuable scheduled event we have. It's better than Group.[36]
>
> *Jeff Roche:* I'm surprised to hear you say that after all your criticisms about our not getting close. But I agree. I thought you wanted therapy here.
>
> *Ken Reese:* No.
>
> *Ned Reich [to Jeff]:* You assume that to be personal is to have therapy. That's the general assumption in this profession, but it's just not true.
>
> *Jeff Roche:* That's what [a senior figure] says. When the group becomes therapy, it gets more personal. (June 29.)

To be in therapy may be to get more personal, but the inverse was also assumed in psychiatric culture, as it is not among laymen. This was one of the socially inhibiting forces in the culture, that getting close to your colleagues may turn you into a patient.

At a case conference, the chief said that we were given the sickest patients first, so that we could tell ourselves from the patients. The residents laughed.

> *Chief:* No, I'm serious.
>
> *Marc Raskin:* Why do you want to do that?
>
> *Chief* [*missing the point*]: So you know who is the doctor.
>
> *Carl Rabinowitz:* But why would you want to know *that?*
>
> The chief looked blankly at the residents. (June 26.)

What the chief did not recognize was that Marc and Carl had long since gotten over the shock of seeing themselves in their patients and now considered themselves so much *as* patients that they saw no use in distinguishing between patient and doctor.[37] Is there any other profession where this could happen?

Because of these feelings and their sense of inadequacy as skilled professionals, residents turned to psychoanalysis. They continued to talk about their poor "tools." The sequence several times went like this: our tools are lousy; but *we* are the "tools"; so we'd better get into analysis to improve ourselves as psychiatrists. These ideas were encompassed in the central belief that "*you can only treat a patient when you can go with him, when you've been there yourself.* This is the point of analysis, to get in touch with your sadness and rage, so you can mobilize them with the patient." (June 22.)

Only one case made the residents feel that this principle of "therapy through empathy" might not work. It deeply disturbed the residents and scared them as therapists. This patient so repelled them that they could not talk about him rationally or professionally. In fact, they did not (or could not) talk about him openly or at length until the end of the year. Joe, the patient, was a murderer.

> *Dave Reed:* When he said he was angry, I could image his rage. . . .
>
> *Carl Rabinowitz:* Yes. I have never been able to talk to Joe either.
>
> *Dave Reed:* All year I have not been able to talk to that man. Every time I try, what he did just wells up in my mind and blocks out all other feelings.
>
> *Jeff Roche:* I felt quite differently. I didn't feel like a doctor but very much like a member of a mourning community. I couldn't evaluate.
>
> *Ned Reich:* That's how I felt too.
>
> *Mike (the psychologist):* You somehow feel violent. All I could think of was images of violence. You feel that the best in you can't come out and the worst is brought to the surface. (After a ward meeting, June 6.)

Joe's therapist talked to the residents about working with him. He said that when his supervisor told him to "get at the affect," he realized that as therapist he must take the patient back to the scene of pain, that the patient can go back only as far as the therapist takes him. "With Joe," he said, "I would begin to cry as he described the crime, and Joe would say, 'Oh, if it bothers you I won't go on.' "

> *Carl Rabinowitz:* I couldn't treat him. [*Sternly moralistic.*] He must serve sentence for what he has done. How else can he live? To plead insanity is to double his burden of guilt, for what he did and for not owning up to it.
>
> *Therapist:* Yes. I sometimes see my job as setting up tasks for him to do to pay.
>
> *Carl Rabinowitz:* I could treat him if he were in jail.
>
> *Ken Reese:* I can't agree. You're saying in essence that sociopathy is not to be studied, because of the moral horror. But why can't you study it as a disorder, like others?
>
> *Jeff Roche:* Yes.
>
> *Mike (the psychologist):* No. Treatment only comes with empathy, and how can you empathize with a case like this?
>
> *Ken Reese:* Is empathy necessary?
>
> *Carl Rabinowitz:* I'm not saying he *can't* be treated. But *I* couldn't pay the price.[38] (June 22.)

These discussions were among the few when a sharp distinction was made, at least implicitly, between action and feeling. In this case, one might have had murderous ideas or dreams, but to actually confront someone who had *done* it exceeded the fantasy so much that many residents could not face it. Aside from these rare exceptions, psychiatric culture treated feelings as action. After the meeting, Ken Reese pursued his point, saying that we face this discrepancy with every patient, that to know sadness or to sense psychotic rage inside you does not make you like someone who had actually gone crazy. He also challenged the unexamined assumption that such empathy was necessary for treatment. The other residents listening replied by emotionally returning to their feelings about Joe. Ken gave up. Afterwards he told me that throughout the program we do not examine our feelings with any acuity but simply send out "feelies" at the appropriate times.

Despite some success at gaining mastery, many residents felt unsure, if not angry, at their work. Intellectually, they craved tough discussion of what they were doing. In June, a senior analyst, whom most residents regarded as the best intellectual in the program, gave a series of seminars which two-thirds of the first-year residents attended. The residents found him inspiring, and coming at this time, just before the second year, he wrestled with all the doubts and wishes the residents had accumulated over the year. In his conversation he showed sympathy and, using a dramatic whisper, criticized other approaches, so that implicitly analytic psychiatry remained as the most substantial pursuit for future growth.

Resident No. 1: All the words and theory I've learned this year seem useless, not effective.[39]

Analyst: So the relationship itself and being with the patient is more than enough, or rather the core of the matter.

Resident No. 1: Yes.

Analyst: What's that called? [*No takers.*] When you come down to the bare experience and clear away all the intellectual framework, it's *phenomenological reduction.*

Resident No. 2: I would call it empathy.

Analyst: Yes, and what you end up with is *just* empathy. Phenomenology wants to enter into a person's mind, but this is hard. Often, it merges with existentialism or existential psychiatry. You've given up the analytic model thoroughly; you're really in existential psychiatry.

Working through the transference is very similar to existential encounter. It is a difference of rhetoric.

Resident No. 3: We assume here that the doctor is healthier than the patient.

Analyst: Given how much more treatment we get, it's a questionable assumption. [*Laughter.*]

Resident No. 3: But there is an inseparable world between me and a schizophrenic, and I don't understand those who say you have to live in their world to understand them. If that's so, no existential encounter is possible. So there is nothing to do. . . .

Analyst: Right. The patient's biases are regarded as pathological, while yours are called "knowledge." It's hard to get together under those circumstances.

. . . .

Analyst: Martin Buber says growth comes from conflict, when we can stand wholly in relation to each other.

You'll be comfortable putting it in analytic terms, I think. What is that called? [No response!] It's *genitality*.

Resident No. 4: Such words to me are vague. I don't see how putting things in those terms helps.

Analyst: To the extent you reflect on the patient, think he is a schizophrenic, you objectify him, right? The goal is spontaneous, unselfconscious encounters. You act in such a way that you don't know what you are doing, because to know is to reflect. . . . [But] existentialism says you can't get someone over schizophrenia until you stop looking at him as a schizophrenic. This is largely tautological. (June 10.)

From this critique of the residents' inclination to abandon theory for caring, the analyst showed that love is not enough and that psychoanalysis enables one to transcend the tautology and thus to pull the patient out of his pathology.

5.

A Sociological Calendar of Psychiatric Socialization

A perennial problem of field work is the paucity of analytic tools. Although field work continues to appeal to young researchers, and although it has distinct advantages over other methods such as observing changes over time, it has no way to report or analyze observations except in thousands of words. Simple tables can be constructed for calculating the proportion of respondents who act or feel a certain way,[1] but no comparable tool takes advantage of the developments through time which field work documents so well. The sociological calendar is designed to fill this need.[2]

Any observer of social life wants to discover the natural units of time latent in people's actions, fitting the hours, days, and weeks of Julian time to the social events observed. Thus a sociological calendar divides off *socially* equal units of time, even though they vary in length from those measured by the Julian calendar.

Besides marking off time, any calendar of events marks them against time. An academic calendar notes when classes begin and when midterm examinations are given. A racing calendar marks the starting time of different races. But the sociological calendar is more complex, because it marks off the interconnected phases of a social process. Thus, forming such a calendar requires one to identify the dimensions of a social process like experiencing the first year of psychiatry, and to discover the rhythm of the process. As I did this for each of the dimensions or themes of professional socialization, the calendar enabled me to see more clearly relations between what was happening to the residents in one area and their experiences in another. Much like a contingency table in survey research, the sociological calendar requires one to code the data and then enables one to see patterns of relationship that were difficult to discern in the raw data.

The Sociological Calendar for Psychiatric Residency

When the research materials reflected in the last chapter are analyzed together with observations and interviews in the second and third years of residency, six major levels of experience emerge. First, what was the residents' primary focus of energy? What did they most talk about, worry about, struggle with? In the beginning, it was *management,* the effort to "learn the ropes" of administration on the ward.[3] The variety of restrictions, drugs, use of nurses and attendants, must be mastered before anything else. The staff emphasized this as well. The residents' first patients were described in the most pathological way possible, and the superchief as well as the nurses emphasized control. Moreover, as Eric Saunders said, the patient wants control whether he appears to or not.

Although the problems of management challenged the residents for many months, the preoccupation with *psychotherapy* soon took over. This was the heart of psychiatric residency as they experienced it, and while the half-dozen types of restrictions could be learned in a day, the techniques of interviewing a patient could not. At first the style of approaching psychotherapy had an external quality; residents tried to pick up tips from senior interviewers or to imitate the style of someone they though was effective. But unlike medicine, they soon learned that this was not enough; the microtechniques did not make much difference in their patients. And from all quarters they learned that it was their personalities that were the heart of the matter. The primary focus became *countertransference.*

The idea of an unconscious is central to countertransference. One can be struck with examples of projection and denial from one's own therapy without really focusing heavily on the unconscious. Psychoanalytically oriented residents naturally became preoccupied with the un-

A Sociological Calendar of Psychiatric Socialization

	1 Month (July)	2 Months (Aug–Sept)	5 Months (Oct–Feb)	9 Months (Mar–Nov)	20 Months (Dec–June)
Primary Focus of Resident's Energy	Managing patients	Doing therapy	Countertransference	Knowing the unconscious	Individual style
MAJOR ISSUES					
1. Efficacy:	Get patients better	.... Nothing works	..... Care for the patient (I can make a difference)		
		(Learning not to cure ...)	(Learning to understand		Apply to Psychoanalytic Institute ...
2. Focus of Therapy:	Microtechniques	....	Whole models of therapy	Therapeutic models for self	
				..... Turn to technique	
3. Doctor-Patient Relationships:	Patient is a crazy person	.... A pathological case		.... Getting comfortable	
	—And I am neurotic too			.... I enter analysis (or therapy)	
4. Responsibility:	Responsible for patient's life			Patient responsible for own life and work in therapy	
		Patient responsible for own management			
5. Relation to nonmedical staff:	Learn to respect staff	....	Work with staff	.... Ignore staff	
	Fight with staff				

Choose electives for 2nd year ....
for third year ....

FIRST YEAR   SECOND YEAR   THIRD YEAR

conscious early, but by the spring of the first year, even managerial residents had sunk deeply into the matter of their own *unconscious*. This remained a focal point through at least the second year and often much longer. One's own long-term therapy, or personal analysis, or professional analysis at the Psychoanalytic Institute, was the most important thing in one's life. But as residents got into their electives during the second year and mapped out their special interests thereafter, less uniformity was apparent. Thus, *individual mixtures* arose, with one resident committed to administrative work but also a candidate at the Psychoanalytic Institute, another excited about group therapy with no involvement in psychoanalysis, still another active in community psychiatry, and most taking on a mix of all of these. As mentioned in the first chapter, the smorgasbord career made up of some private patients, a day at a mental health center, a little research on the side, some part-time administrative work, and, if possible, supervision of a new generation is an ideal many psychiatrists pursue.

The five phases of the residents' socialization indicate the discontinuity they experienced in the transition from medicine to psychiatry. It was not until the second year, in the crucial fourth phase, that many of these residents had defined for themselves a new professional identity that felt comfortable. The major issues in the struggle for a new professional identity constitute the five remaining rows of the calendar. The first reflects the residents' concern with *efficacy*, with helping patients get better. *What am I trying to do and how well am I doing it?* The second captures the more specific set of concerns about doing psychotherapy. The resident asks himself, *"How do I make therapy work?"* Third, residents constantly thought about their relation with their patients in terms of *who is really sick?* A fourth dimension of resident socialization concerns responsibility: *who is responsible for what?* Finally, the residents' *relation to the nonphysician staff* is a level of professional socialization that reflects the residents' struggle to define themselves as somehow professionally superior to other therapeutic agents. In the process of coming to ignore or minimize their involvement with the staff, they regained an earlier sense of doctorhood.

Now let us consider the interwoven dimensions and phases of socialization into psychiatry and see the discontinuities through time and their resolution, as well as the continuities between dimensions of the training experience. During the period of management, for example, residents focused on getting their patients better despite the staff's effort to eliminate desires for cure, which they called "rescue fantasies." In order to get the patients better, residents searched for little techniques, that is, for skills analogous to medical ones which specifically applied to a specific problem. This search is sociologically important, for it gave them the temporary security of acting like doctors while it shrank their expectations. They felt responsible for the patient's affairs, and they quickly realized that the nonprofessional staff knew more about managing these patients than anyone else. Although it threatened their already-assailed standing as physicians to defer to nurses and social workers, the residents learned to do it, resisting all the time.

In the second phase, the residents' primary focus turned to therapy. Now a workable competence in ward administration allowed them to refocus their energies. The calendar indicates that only one major change accompanied this quiet shift, the view that the patient is responsible for his own management. This, of course, oversimplifies the case. Psychiatrists in fact continued to manifest their doctorhood by giving orders not only throughout the first year, but in later years of practice. However, residents increasingly demanded that patients be responsible for themselves, as Dave Reed did on July 20th (chapter 4).

As the training program came into full force during the fall, major changes occurred in almost every dimension of socialization. However, this third period could not have occurred had it not been preceded by the two before it. For example, the residents had been trying in vain to cure their patients throughout the summer. Their experiments with microtechniques, picked up from watching senior staff interview patients in case conferences, had also proved uneven, and this left the resident with no effective tools, no basis for self-esteem as a physician. It was not merely that patients failed to recover; a number of them did. But even in those cases the resident realized that his ministrations had as little to do with those who improved as with those who stayed the same or got worse.

"Nothing works," as the calendar says. Yet each resident perceived that a few supervisors and guest psychiatrists seemed to understand difficult cases with great mastery. Residents abandoned the search for particular techniques and began to emulate one or two of these men as models for therapy. At the same time, supervisors continually pointed out how the young therapist's unconscious interfered with effective therapy. "Suddenly you realize," said one resident, "that it's not what you *know* that counts, but who you *are*." This fits closely with the emulation of great therapists—if only one could be a better, more mature *person,* one could do better therapy. Along with these changes, the lesson that had been pressed since the first day—to understand the patient rather than cure him—began to make sense amidst such discouraging results with patients.[4] Slowly the resident learned that his sense of failure was proportional to his "rescue fantasies." Likewise, what impressed the resident about his idols was not that they could cut and sew like a surgeon but that they understood so much.

Once the resident identified strongly with one or two favorite therapists, most of whom subscribed to psychoanalysis, and once he "discovered" that his personal neuroses impeded his work as a therapist, the rest of the socialization process was only a matter of time. By that discovery he submitted his personality to his mentors. Although the resident might choose alternative resolutions, the program discouraged him. Behavioral therapy represented "escape from personal involvement with your patients," and community psychiatry was "acting out."

The fourth period of socialization extends the concern with countertransference to a focus on the unconscious. Such a focus is narcissistic, as can be seen in the calendar. In therapy, residents turned to technique as a resolution to failure. This is not to be confused with the early search for microtechniques as a way to get patients better, for here the residents considered technique an end in itself. Having learned that their ideal of getting patients better only brought misery to themselves and their patients, the residents resocialized themselves toward this new model of core work. The goal was to become master of the therapeutic hour, an aesthetic and somewhat manipulatory pursuit.[5] Residents who, a month earlier, had talked about therapy in terms of a certain patient as improving or slipping back now described a "beautiful hour" and how they "elicited some great material." When one of the most sensitive residents talked this way about a patient whom we both cared for I asked him why. He said, "You have to believe in something to survive here." This account does not deny that such mastery of technique may contribute to the resident becoming a more effective therapist, but such is not its function in socialization.

This change toward mastering the fifty-minute hour means that the resident had abandoned therapy as the major source of efficacy, and he increasingly talked about the senior staff he admired not in terms of therapy with patients but as models for himself. He was getting comfortable. Already some residents had entered personal analysis, and the number increased through the fourth period. They also applied to the local Psychoanalytic Institute from this period through the third year.

The dimension of professional responsibility also reflects this basic change. Earlier, when therapy became the primary focus, the residents had increasingly tried to make patients responsible for managing themselves. In the third and fourth periods (and thereafter through the second year) residents more often came to regard the patient as responsible for working in therapy as well. A therapist would say that a patient is "not working hard enough" or that a difficult case "will not open up"[6] The astute reader realizes that *each of these shifts in responsibility implied a different kind of patient,* the final ideal in the second year being someone who could take care of himself and who was motivated to work hard in therapy.

Staff relations improved as residents became equally competent with nurses and social workers. There was a time in the third period when, out of despair with failures, residents were most likely to form therapeutic teams with a nurse, an attendant, and a social worker. All levels of personnel came together to help the patient. But as residents became increasingly preoccupied with long-term psychotherapy both for themselves and for their patients, therapeutic teams diminished. In fact, the residents became so competent on the ward that they could and did reduce their time with the staff to a minimum. Nurses complained about not seeing residents enough, and residents made half-hearted efforts to "be nice to the nurses," but the pattern was clear. In-depth psychotherapy was the wellspring of prestige, and by concentrating on it, residents regained a sense of being master professionals. Yet in private moments many of them recognized that were nurses and social workers—and even some attendants—allowed to do long-term psychotherapy, they would be just as effective. In short, it is the social organization of mental health services which generates and sustains the hierarchy of professional expertise, not the other way around.

Varieties of Experience

Depending on temperament and professional work style, residents experienced these stages of psychiatric socialization with differing intensity, and they found different dimensions of the process more or less important to them. The whole experience is probably clearest in Jeff Roche, for besides having a therapeutic work style, he was extraordinarily naive in matters psychological or psychoanalytic. His great strength was an intuitive sensibility, the way Benjamin Spock or Paul Dudley White might have been in their green years. But he did not start as psychologically attuned, and this is what a resident meant when he said without sarcasm, "It's a tribute to the program's breadth that someone so unpsychological as Jeff is with us."

Thus, countertransference and the subtle dilemmas of psychotherapy were true revelations to Jeff, as when he blurted out what everyone else in the room already recognized to be the underpinning of the conversation, "That's a real dilemma. On the one hand you want to cure your patients and on the other you want to keep them." His basic assumptions were those we all have about medicine:

> I don't understand. If you assume that we are reasonably normal . . . [*looks at the chief*], and if we have some perspective on the matter, and if we understand the doctor's role, then why can't we let the patient get better with no loss to us? (July 25.)

Everyone but Jeff had a good laugh.

Jeff was deeply puzzled. Not only did he fail to see anything funny in what he said, but as time passed he became exasperated that his Boy Scout approach to getting patients better did not work. (January 27.) By this time he knew about the unconscious but it was not real to him; intellectually he was persuaded that he should go into psychoanalysis, but he trusted his gut feelings more than some complex set of "insights" which psychoanalysis was supposed to offer. "I think I ought to get married before I get analyzed so I decide who I'll marry on a sound, irrational basis." (January 4.) Finally, Jeff loved being a doctor, being responsible, working with a medical staff, and getting people better. By the middle of his second year he had not so much abandoned these aspects of his work style as drastically altered them to fit the limitations of psychotherapy.

A much more sophisticated version of the therapeutic type of resident was Ken Reese. He combined a good intuitive sense of people's needs with intelligence and wide reading in psychology. Although he approached any work intellectually, his primary motivation was always to get the patients better. As he said, he was here "to relieve the pain." He did not speak of or treat patients as "cases." With much more awareness than Jeff, he went through the same discomfort when patients did not respond to his efforts. His desire to cure was finally reduced to compassion: "You help the patient by caring for her and expressing interest," he said when I asked him after six months how he could help a patient. By the third year, however, like most therapeutic residents, Ken felt once again that he was effective. This recapturing of effectiveness comes from a combination of having diminished one's expectations, treating healthier and more responsive patients, and *accumulating over time a selective set of success stories* which persuades you and your listener that in fact therapeutic intervention can profoundly alter pathological behavior.

Dave Reed exemplified the managerial type of resident. This is hard to capture in the text of chapter 4, but it came through in expressions of blunt realism. "If the higher-ups are going to make drug policy, they should back it up with some data." (October 14.) "What is so interesting is that we spend so much time over what to do when there is no evidence that any of the alternatives do much, outside of drugs." (November 18.) On caring for the patient: "You need no training for that; anyone who is concerned can do it." (April 6.) Almost never did he bungle an administrative matter, and his relation with patients was very businesslike. In his third year he was selected to be chief of a service.

In terms of socialization, administrative residents became upset with how ineffective they were, but they resolved it by focusing on management. The best you could do with inpatients, they argued, was to arrange their life at the hospital so that they gained increasing confidence and competence, until they could be discharged. More than the other two types, these residents continued to feel responsible for both the management and therapy of their patients. They also worked well with the staff and tended less to ignore them or to immerse themselves almost exclusively in their own analysis. This does not mean, however, that they ignored psychoanalysis. As Dave said, characteristically, when he applied to the institute, "it's obviously the right thing to do."

The intellectual type of resident is not necessarily bright but rather approaches his patients less to cure them than to analyze them as examples of psychic behavior. In this program, most such residents were psychoanalytically oriented, and Marc Raskin illustrates this perspective. Such residents were least affected by the change from medicine to psychiatry. Usually they disliked medicine, and even if they had absorbed the active, intervening style of medical practice through sheer exposure, they knew that trying to cure the patient was not the object of psychiatry. This made other residents uncomfortable and angry. For example, when Carl asked Marc if he didn't want to make the lame walk and the blind see, Marc said "No." Feeling his own extreme discomfort at how little good he was doing, Carl said, "You're lucky." Truer to his principles, Ken added, "On the contrary, it's tragic." (November 4.)

Thus, Marc reacted to the first year by declaring it a disaster. He believed that the residents were being forced to do more harm than good, and that the hospital impeded therapy. He hated having to give his patients shock treatments. (November 18.) On the other hand, he seemed unusually comfortable talking about his unconscious and its impact on his patients through countertransference. (May 24.) By the spring of the first year, most of the residents had changed their earlier opinions about Marc; he had only been ahead of the rest. Thus, for psychoanalytically oriented residents, the first year is not a time of transformation but a burden to be tolerated on the way to the second year. They had arrived before they began.

Socialization Beyond the First Year

Although extensive interviews and observations were made of residents in their second and third years, the shape of residency experience indicates that the major phases of socialization occur in the first year. Moreover, in the first year, residents must choose how to use their elective time for the second year, choices which most openly reflect what they have learned to value during the first year. In this way and others, the second year is designed as an outgrowth of the first. By centering around neurotic outpatients, the second-year program smoothly builds on the final phase of socialization in the first year.

Beyond this sociological argument, evidence indicates that residents learn little psychiatrically after their first year. In carefully designed tests, the Menninger research team found that, except for "psychodynamics," older residents did not score higher than residents ending their first year in clinical judgment, history-taking, psychopathology, psychotherapy, neurology, questions of fact, and ward management.[7] In fact, senior psychiatrists at the Menninger Foundation who were diplomats of the American Board of Psychiatry scored no higher than residents ending their first year in four areas—clinical judgement, psychopathology, psychotherapy, and ward management—on this examination "intentionally limited to the basic psychiatric subjects, such as psychopathology, hospital treatment, and psychotherapy, that are introduced to first year residents."[8]

This is not to say that residents do not experience significant growth after the first year. Rather, they turn to improving techniques which lead to what Rue Bucher calls "mastery statements," a growing sense of competence.[9] "I feel much more capable now," said a resident entering his third year. "I can handle a greater variety of cases," said another. With this overview in mind, let us look briefly at the second and third years.

The basic change which second-year residents described was one of increased freedom and autonomy. No longer did residents work on the ward, but instead they had offices of their own in other parts of the hospital. Residents uniformly found this a pleasant change; even those who liked the ward's atmosphere soon began to avoid going to see their inpatients any more than necessary. Often, the nurses greeted them like sergeants greeting captains returning to see how the second lieutenants (i.e., first-year residents) were doing. Yet returning to find a new resident occupying one's old office on the ward is not a comfortable experience.

Predominantly, the second-year residents worked with outpatients and nonpatients. They ran the Walk-In Clinic, which screened anyone who came off the street or who was referred to the hospital. Therefore, while they decided, in conjunction with Walk-In supervisors and a Walk-In chief, who should be admitted as an inpatient, most of the people they saw either became outpatients or did not return. Very little time, then, was spent managing patients with drugs and restrictions. Treating outpatients reinforced a lesson of the first year, that professional power and control comes not from management but from psychological interpretation and mastery of the person's problems.

At the same time, the inpatient experience left an important residue. Residents in the second year were likely to assume a patient with a problem sufficient to bring him to the Walk-In Clinic was "sick" in some sense. In therapy with outpatients, the residents tried to uncover the layers of defenses they saw which separated the surface personality from the basic, primitive feelings assumed to be there, the same ones seen in hospitalized patients the previous year.

Residents in the second year claimed they were treated differently. Even the same men who supervised them in June as if they were novices considered them as junior colleagues who could handle themselves by July. This was even experienced by a second-year resident in the attitude of a supervisor who had told me that the resident was the worst of last year's crop. In the second year the residents really begin to feel like psychiatrists.

When they began the second year, residents had been looking forward to treating outpatients for half a year. By the fall of their second year, several residents who had been skeptical about whether psychotherapy could do any good for the patient said that they felt they helped some patients get better. When asked for examples, they usually chose a long-term case (over a year of therapy) in which the patient talked about a problem and soon afterwards was able to overcome it. For example, a patient might have trouble working effectively. In therapy, the resident said, he and the patient discovered that the patient felt he was competing with his father's expectations all the time. Soon after, the patient improved markedly in his work and got a promotion. Often, the examples chosen illustrated worldly success or achievement.

Case conferences, diagnostics, and supervision continued as they had before, but no second-year resident continued with a first-year supervisor. The official reason was that "we don't want you to get too attached, and we want you to be your own man." While some residents began analysis in the first year, more began it in the second. For the past several years, about 60 percent of each class went into analysis.

The second year also permitted residents to apply to the Psychoanalytic Institute. Percentages are difficult to calculate, because a number of residents did not plan to go into the institute until after their residency and military obligations were completed. However, one-fifth of the cohort studied applied to the institute in the second year. This figure is large when one considers that institute training lasted from seven to ten years, at an estimated cost of $100,000.

The aspects of the first year which supported a psychodynamic approach, such as supervision and individual psychotherapy, con-

tinued and increased in the second year. Residents who ended their
first year skeptical that they could be effective in getting patients better
changed their tune within a few months. They came to believe that
they helped patients through analytically oriented psychotherapy. This
seeming "conversion" appeared to be merely the surfacing of what
doubting residents had absorbed in the first year. As a second-year resident with a sense of irony said:

> Many residents who were somewhat skeptical begin to feel there is re-
> ally something in psychotherapy, because they see the success of their
> first-year long-term patients. In fact, the patients they stick with are the
> ones they see as improving. They forget how many did not. And they
> selected their long-term patients because those patients had a chance of
> getting better from therapy; so they forget their failures, and they pick
> their successes. But their investment in them is so great that they get re-
> ally persuaded by the second year that they are effective as therapists.

Another way in which residents deepened their commitment to
analytic psychotherapy was through a personal analysis. A number of
residents who were doubtful (and probably despondent) began personal analysis as a way of clarifying the personal and professional confusion which the first year of residency sometimes produced. By taking
this route instead of any other, these residents were assured of redis-
covering continuity in their training. Therefore, insofar as forces of the
first year of residency drove doctors into personal analysis, even if
those residents appeared for a time to be skeptical of their profession,
professional identity was assured.

Chronologically, the second year began in the sixth month of the
first year, when one first heard references made to it. By the eighth
month, constant references, most of them yearnings, were heard about
the second year. Expectations varied, the most universal being that finally neurotic outpatients would become available. Others wanted to
escape their present life on the ward. When a resident asked what the
others on a ward would be doing next year, one said he was going to
the Psychoanalytic Institute. Another replied, "I'll do a psychiatric
study of the stock market." A third thought he'd work with children.
A fourth said, "I may become a country psychiatrist." (March 16.)

How residents chose to spend their ten hours of elective time
reveals their priorities. A third of the twenty-six residents filled less
than five hours with electives; they wanted to relax and have more time

to themselves. Of the thirty-three electives offered, sixteen residents picked a seminar entitled "Basic Concepts of Dynamic Psychiatry." Seminars in narcissistic character disorder, neuroses, and family therapy each drew eight or nine residents. Six chose prison psychiatry (four of them from one clique), a demanding elective that alone took ten hours a week. Four took community mental health services, which consumed six hours a week. Only two chose any form of serious research, and only two chose what is now called liaison psychiatry, or psychiatry in a general hospital.

The Third Year

For some residents, the third year ended their training with an elective program before they began their first job. For others, the third year marked the beginning of a new training program in a specialty, like child psychiatry, that would continue for two or more years. This study did not follow residents into the variety of elective programs that made up the third year, though a number of third-year residents were interviewed. Beyond individual choices in elective programs, more residents applied to the Psychoanalytic Institute. Not all of these, however, were converts. Over the past ten years, senior staff at the hospital had noted a shift in applicants toward those who did not think psychoanalysis was "the answer," but who thought it worth learning about. When asked why they wanted to make such a large commitment to something they were not sure of, they would say, "It's a good thing to know. You can always pick up other approaches later, but you can only find out how good the analytic approach is by trying it now." The common assumption among residents was that behavioral therapy, milieu therapy, or community psychiatry were much simpler than psychoanalysis and could be mastered in one's spare time at a later date.

An important choice for third-year residents was to become a chief of a service. The four services had a chief, three inpatient and one day hospital. Also there was a chief of a walk-in clinic, a chief of the University Psychiatric outpatient clinic, a chief of the City Hospital unit on psychosomatic disorders, and a chief of a new auxiliary ward at the State Hospital that was to receive the new overload of old and/or chronic patients from the catchment area. Over the years, these positions had been fought over and were one of the few scarce goods for which residents competed. A word, then, on competition.

The residents chosen for this program were by that fact competitive and successful. However, in the program there was little to compete for. There were no grades. No one knew how he was evaluated, and few talked about it. Even by the end of the first year, residents did not know about their evaluation. In fact, no systematic form of evaluation existed.

Being competitive by habit, residents created occasions for competition. Conferences of any kind were the most suitable occasions, and residents attempted to one-up each other or impress attending psychiatrists with their acumen. But unlike in surgery or internal medicine, neither the structure of training nor the senior staff strongly encouraged such behavior; thus it became less intense than it would have in other medical specialties. Competition also centered around avoiding certain catastrophes. Residents tried not to have a patient commit suicide, escape from the hospital or be radically disruptive, and when one of these did happen to a resident, others would treat it as a failure even if the resident could not be reasonably held responsible for the event. Residents also made competitive comments about securing scarce resources, even if it was largely a matter of luck. Thus drawing several good patients was regarded as more than good luck; it gave the resident a competitive advantage. Conspicuously missing from this list was competing to see who could get more patients better. That did not seem to be the point of residency training.

One specific attainment for which some residents competed was being appointed chief of a service. It is no surprise to learn that in most years, about two or three times as many residents applied for these positions as there were places available. In one year, however, no resident applied for the chiefships of the Walk-In Clinic, the famous Outpatient Clinic or the service at the State Hospital. Moreover, no resident could be induced to take these positions. Overall, applications for chiefships went down because the second-year cohort wanted to leave the hospital.

Why were residents, ready for their third year, leaving the hospital? Most of them said they were unhappy with the impact of the catchment area on the hospital. They felt that patients coming into the hospital from its area of responsibility were less interesting to work with than patients at other hospitals. They still felt that their training and the program did not teach them skills necessary to be effective with patients other than long-term neurotics. They also said that the third-year program lacked strength. Most residents who stayed for a third year, they claimed, did research part-time and filled the remainder with clinical work. But very little research of any scale was currently going on, they said. Moreover, they felt the research was poor, and one was not encouraged by the atmosphere to pursue research.

What were the anticipations of residents looking toward the third year? To a large extent, they began to think practically about setting up a practice, making professional contacts, and such matters. They did not anticipate many changes, because they felt the third year was so individual. However, most residents looked forward to treating "real neurotics" in the third year. While they had the same anticipation on going into their second year, they had concluded that very few patients seen in Outpatient Clinic were really neurotics. Many residents described them as the same as their first-year patients, except that they lived outside the hospital on their own. Thus, each year the residents sought increasingly healthy patients and each year felt that they could be most effective with them. A fourth-year resident said, "I'm not sure psychiatry can do that much for the mentally ill patient, but after watching a lot I'm convinced it can really help the healthy patient. With healthy neurotics, it can make them *really* healthy people."

PART *II*

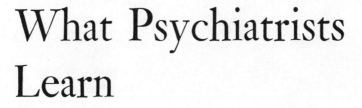

What Psychiatrists Learn

6.

Managing Patients

While the heart of psychiatric work at the University Psychiatric Center and other distinguished residencies is individual psychotherapy, managing patients accompanies therapeutic work. In ideal work with outpatients, this may come to little more than handling broken appointments and unpaid bills. In complex cases, a psychiatrist may have to work with ward personnel in a hospital, relatives, social workers and the police. Across this spectrum, decisions of management should be therapeutic; everything, the profession claims, should serve to help the patient. But when staff and residents make the distinction between "therapy" and "management" or "administration," they imply a professional fantasy wherein psychotherapy could be carried on in a social and political vacuum, with no relatives, no drugs, no hospital, no forms, only patient and therapist gaining a deeper understanding of the unconscious. Thus management by definition never gains the stature of therapy—even when it is done therapeutically.

Although managing takes place in every year of psychiatric residency, it is most intense in the first year, not only because one's first experiences are the most intense, but because the first year takes place on the wards, which by definition are a managerial structure. This is one of the basic contradictions in psychiatric work which some of the residents have already expressed in chapter 4. In the hospital, one is controlling at the same time one is doing therapy with a person. The controlling should be in the service of doing therapy; it can even be therapeutic in its own right. The profession, for example, talks of "milieu therapy" and "the therapeutic environment." Nevertheless, residents were taught that their real work lay in psychotherapy, and as we have seen, they turned increasingly toward it. Even drugs were considered part of management, though a growing number of psychiatrists, since this study was made, would argue that drugs are the essence of therapy, with psychotherapy providing support and understanding.

Despite the ideological message of the program about the importance of therapy, there was a serious effort to make management therapeutic. The center had pioneered work in milieu therapy, and various meetings on the wards were designed to foster treatment teams of nurses, aides, social workers, occupational therapists, residents, and others around the care of certain patients. Most important for training, however, the program put residents in charge of *all* care for inpatients. Thus, when a patient was admitted to the center, s/he was assigned to a resident as therapist and administrator. If the patient arrived with an older resident or outside professional as a therapist, this relationship was suspended while the patient remained in the hospital. If someone objected, they could check in at another hospital, but the rule was firm.

This arrangement caused disruption for some patients and their outside therapists, but the rule existed not for the patients but for the residents being trained, and for the hospital so that it could control all aspects of care. It paralleled similar regulations that many medical hospitals have. By putting the resident simultaneously into both roles, did the rule thereby sharpen the conflict between controlling and therapy, adding it to the other role strains that already existed, of being a physician yet not doing medicine, and of acting like a responsible professional yet having little experience?

Sociological Ambivalence and the T-A Split

One study indicates that it did. What psychiatrists learn is affected by the structure of their training, and Rose Coser investigated training at an elite, private hospital which had what the profession calls a "T-A Split," in which one resident is the therapist and another the ward administrator for a given patient.[1] Calling it an "ingenious invention," Coser shows why it is vital for effective professional work, bolstering psychiatric arguments with sociological theory.[2] It keeps the resident therapist and the administrator from having to struggle with the conflicting demands of being both a therapist and an administrator. It insulates therapy from observation and thereby allows the patient to speak openly to the therapist without putting him or herself in jeopardy by having wishes, emotions, and fantasies become the basis for ward restrictions or more drugs. Just as social groups have been found to have an expressive and an "instrumental" or behavioral leader, so the T-A Split provides one leader in expression and another in behavior.

> If the same psychiatrist were in charge of managing a patient's life on the ward *and* conducting psychotherapy with him or her, the patient would get contradictory messages from *the same person;* this would constitute *sociological ambivalence* in the core sense of this term as Merton and Elinor Barber defined it, in that antithetical behavior would be expected from the *same* role-partner.[3]

From Coser's description, it would appear that the arrangement at the University Psychiatric Center not only put patients in double jeopardy but also tied its residents into knots of ambivalance. Moreover, one can see in the T-A Split an attempt to attain that therapeutic ideal where all the worldly, administrative complexities are kept away from a pure, unperturbed relationship between patient and therapist. However, Coser is an astute observer, and as she describes how the T-A Split actually functions, another picture emerges. Though the rule is that neither side will interfere with the other, the therapist wants to know what the administrator is doing to his patient.[4] The therapist cannot even adjust the prescriptions of his patients.[5] At the same time, the administrator wants to know what is going on in therapy.[6] As Coser succinctly puts it, "the role-partner who gives support and the one who provides guidelines must be in some relation with each other if they are to treat the same patient."[7]

Moreover, the administrator is not an administrative nurse but an M.D. deeply interested in the psychodynamics of his patients. Yet s/he is not to do therapeutic work with them or talk about their behavior. This relegates administration to a mere holding operation so that therapy can go on somewhere.[8] Ironically, however, administrative decisions are considered too important to be left in the hands of a young physician resident; so the administrative supervisor runs the ward and tells the resident administrator what to do. The resident therapist, however, is fully responsible for a patient's therapy, with a therapeutic supervisor gently advising him or her what to do.[9] This arrangement implies that therapy has great status but mistakes are not consequential, while management has low status yet mistakes can be fateful.

The confusion grows when one considers the two layers of residents and supervisors. Residents find themselves part of a series of pentagons consisting of the resident therapist and her supervisor, the patient, and the resident administrator and his supervisor.[10] Relations break into a number of triangles. For example, since the resident administrator has little power, if the resident therapist wants to talk about the patient's management, s/he talks to the administrative supervisor. Using balance theory, Coser shows that this relation is inherently negative and that most other relations in the combinations of triads in the pentagon can become negative and disrupt the complex power relations that exist.

The T-A Split is ripe for manipulation by the patient, which the staff regards as "catastrophic" because it can snarl so many parts of the system that do not normally communicate very well. Moreover, a given resident is part of several pentagons, one for each patient s/he treats in therapy but who lives on a different ward from where the resident does administration, and one for each patient s/he presumably manages and who is in therapy with a different resident. The complexity of cross-cutting relations, each with their own expectations, the mixed messages about therapy and management, and the frustrations of blocked communications, make one wish for the simple but "unworkable" arrangement where one person is in charge of everything and can teach the patient the difference between feelings and acting out with full knowledge of the patient's attitudes and behavior. As the staff at UPC put it, "Administrative actions must always be integrated with psychodynamic understanding if a hospital is to nurture therapy with disturbed patients."[11]

Professor Coser spends half a book explaining mechanisms for coping with the troubles of the theoretically perfect T-A Split, most of which would be avoided by keeping therapist and administrator in close contact with each other. It appears to exist at the elite hospital she studied, not because it resolves so many potential problems in role relations, but because the hospital needs it to accommodate high-status clients without having their therapists telling the hospital how to run its wards. From Coser's observations, the arrangement pleases the senior staff of the hospital, but creates confusion, low morale, and anomie for others.[12]

But what of the "sociological ambivalence" of having residents do both therapy and manage their patients? The term, coined by Merton and Barber, assumes that conflicting expectations lead to ambivalence. It precludes the possibility of other responses by asserting that the "the ambivalence is inherent in the social positions people occupy."[13] If one begins with conflicting expectations and asks how people cope with them, then ambivalence is *one* response, and probably a temporary one.[14] From research on cognitive dissonance, and one's experiences in life, one knows that many people tend to resolve ambivalence in one way or another. What Merton and Barber's insightful essay actually is concerned with is *ambiguity;* for ambiguity lies in the situation, while ambivalence lies in the person.

Other ways in which residents handled conflicting expectations were to diminish or reject all but one of them, emphasize some over others, articulate the incompatibility and turn its resolution over to their mentors, or insulate the incompatibility by hiding it, denying it, or evading it.[15] The program's ideology was important in covering over inherent conflicts. For example, by claiming that management was therapeutic, the conflicts between control and therapy were denied at the same time that ward management was probably made more therapeutic than if no one had held this belief. By putting residents fully in charge of patient care, the program blunted criticism that the residents were only students and answered most challenges to the residents' authority. The intensity of one expectation over another and the power behind it shape the way people resolve conflicting expectations, while the structure of options determines the choice. For example, therapy was insulated from observation in this program, as it was in the program Rose Coser studied, and that constituted a major way for residents to convince others (and themselves) that they were doing professional, autonomous work.[16] Nevertheless, therapist-administrators did find patients manipulating them in therapy, as was tragically illustrated by the suicide in chapter 9. The ideal arrangement would involve a therapist and an administrator who work separately with the patient but keep each other well-informed.

Contrary to the prediction of sociological ambivalence, residents in the program handled the structural conflict of controlling their therapy patients by emphasizing one and minimizing the other in accord with their personal work style; so that managerial residents managed inpatients, and therapeutic residents unambiguously hated the managing they had to do. Likewise, residents responded to the role conflict between being untutored students and assuming professional responsibility for their patients by unambiguously shedding the former role as rapidly as possible. The most deeply troublesome conflict which created ambivalence for many residents (and, later, psychiatrists) was being a physician but not doing "real medicine." While residents resolved this in various ways—largely by emphasizing the disease-like qualities of emotional problems—their ambivalence did not dissolve easily, because being a physician had become a permanent attribute. Perhaps this is the most likely source of ambivalence, when an ascribed status conflicts with a role one is expected to perform.

Thus in learning to manage, as in learning to do therapy, residents *assimilated* parts of the job into their own work style and ways of doing things, and they *accommodated* themselves to the ideology and customs of the program. Underlying this dynamic process is conflict between residents and role partners, patients, supervisors, nurses, social workers, and other. At the personal level, there is conflict within residents between what they think they are, what they want to become, and what others expect of them. This is the central tension underlying socialization. As residents are negotiating their prerogatives in relation to others, parts of their selves accommodate to and assimilate the values and practices around them. In the following pages, this takes place in a program which gives residents as full responsibility for the care of their patients as is possible.

Accommodating to the Demands of Nurses

I was talking to [a nurse] about the new residents. They make a lot of mistakes, she said, and all her examples were about discipline. Like giving a manic patient no drugs for the first four days he is here "to see what he is like." Meanwhile he is tearing the ward apart.

(Field notes.)

Initially, nurses have power and expertise—a fact which disturbs many residents. Moreover, effective administration is a major skill when working with psychotic and suicidal patients. Yet this power and expertise are set within a psychiatric program which values diagnosis unclouded by constraining drugs more than it worries about the ward being torn apart. As full-time administrators, nurses demand tranquil patients; as therapists, residents may not want patients heavily medicated. From these conflicting interests emerges a negotiated order.[17]

Nurses' Expectations of Residents

From numerous conversations with nurses and their complaints about residents emerged a consistent idea of what they want. A good resident (or chief) is a good manager. He controls his patients so that management is easy. He should be strong, the boss, but he should be receptive to staff ideas and ask for their opinion. He should be warm and involved with the staff and not too involved with his patients, and he should have a sense of the whole ward rather than just the needs of his particular patients.

One feature of the staff culture in particular made the residents defensive and pressured them to manage their patients well. The nurses and other staff saw *the patient as an extension of the doctor,* and blamed him or her for the patient's acts. For subtle and complex reasons, this attitude was hard for residents to cope with. Residents became frustrated at the unreasonableness of this attitude. ''When the patient becomes an extension of the doctor in the staff's eyes, that is very bad,'' said a resident. ''No one blames the doctor if his patient gets pneumonia.'' Another resident added that when a patient is under a doctor's care, the doctor gets blamed for mishaps and for the patient getting worse, though he can hardly control the patient's psyche.

However, residents admitted that they often did think of their patients as extensions of themselves, or felt they were forced to by the profession. The program's emphasis on sitting with the patient and bearing his pain with him indicated a close identification. Several older residents said that they felt they could really help only patients with whom they empathized. In one discussion, residents gave examples of feeling badly when a patient did something wrong. One said he was embarrassed when his escaped patient returned, and the patient said that he reagrded himself as an extension of his doctor. This patient told his doctor, ''See what a mistake you made, letting me escape. Now I'm going to look so good that you will ease restrictions and let me out again and I will commit suicide, and it will be your fault.'' Thus all three parties, staff, doctor, and patient identified the patient with his doctor.

The nurses instruct the new residents in psychiatric care. The senior staff regards them as instructors, and the residents are told several times on their first day that they should listen to the nurses, that the nurses know more than they, and that this will be a professional problem for them. Examples of instruction can be found daily. A nurse reported that a patient was begging from everyone and filching. The resident said that at least she was a lot better than when she begged in the streets. The nurse replied with further accounts of annoying behavior, and the resident again said she was much improved. Finally the nurse said that the patient begs from patients who cannot say no and something must be done.

Nurses wanted the residents to explain why a patient has done something and/or to take action. The residents felt it. One indication of this expectation was eye contact. When a nurse reported, she immediately looked at the resident in charge of the patient in question. That she sought an explanation could be seen in her behavior when no explanation was forthcoming.

For example, one day a nurse reported that a patient was mad and was locking herself into the school closet. She looked at the resident, who did not respond. She then elaborated on her report, but the resident still did not respond. So the nurse added more material, saying the patient had had hallucinations all day and was constipated. The resident nodded. The nurse added another managerial problem, reporting that the patient woke in the middle of the night complaining of constipation. After this fourth round, the resident gave a review of the case, explaining why the patient was acting this way. After his explanation, attention turned to another case.

But the demands by the nurses for diagnosis did *not* extend to the expectation that residents teach them therapy; they acknowledged that as the residents' role. When nurses complained, as they did, that they were not being included as therapeutic agents, they only meant as *supplements* to the therapeutic alliance which the therapist and the patient had. On the other side, when nurses asked about current issues in a patient's therapy, residents were reluctant to tell because they feared that nurses would interfere with the therapy.

Complaints about being ignored as therapists led the nurses on one service to demand a conference on how more therapeutic work could be done. Below is a report of the meeting.

> The head nurse talked about nurses as therapists and their use. The residents looked bored, and although I had looked forward to this meeting, I was bored too.
>
> She said that a nurse could be useful by establishing a relationship with a patient before the resident goes on vacation, so that the patient had someone to talk to during vacation.
>
> Another suggestion was to use the nurse's relation with the patient when the doctor wanted to push the patient some way but did not want to be directly involved, so as to preserve his therapeutic alliance.
>
> Nurses could also be used when patients need a woman. Perhaps they are edgy around attendants or the resident. Or perhaps the patient's mother was important to the patient, and the therapist wants a nurse to stimulate mother-son feelings again in the patient.
>
> (Field notes.)

This negotiated order deserves attention; for it clearly shows how great the concessions were which psychiatric nurses made, concessions which also affected how residents learned to manage. Initially, residents were overwhelmed by their ignorance and awkwardness in the face of lower-status nonprofessionals who acted with assurance, if not command. But they soon "learned" from both nurses and staff psychiatrists that therapy is a more powerful tool than administration, and that professionally organized barriers prevent nurses from doing therapy but allow residents to manage. This professional ideology also means that management is not developed into a fine art. Residents learned that administrative psychiatry consists of either getting the patient ready for therapy or managing patients unable to participate in therapy. This led to profound contradictions, as expressed by a chief resident.

> *Head nurse:* Miss X. pushed a newly set window out in the ladies' room.
>
> *Chief:* You mean she didn't have to smash it? [*Jauntily punches his fist into other hand.*]
>
> *Head nurse:* Yes. The putty had not hardened.
>
> *Patient's doctor:* That sounds like a compromise. [*Laughs around the room.*]
>
> *Chief:* Did you speak to her?
>
> *Doctor:* I tried, but she didn't want to.

DOC last night: Last night I saw her. She gave the perfect Blumbergian interview, without Blumberg. [*Chuckles in room.*] How she was lonely, and lost and sad. It was the classic presuicidal speech.

Chief: That's a young, adolescent girl giving the perfect speech for the doctor, just what we want to hear. And then the day you stop listening they cut their wrists.

DOC: Well, I listened.

Chief: And got no sleep. I learned at the end of being DOC to be a meanie. Otherwise you get no sleep. [*General laughter.*]

Control and Power in Morning Report

Each day of the residents' work on the wards officially began with Morning Report. The head nurse organized reports from the three shifts of nurses and presented them to the assembled staff of residents, staff psychiatrists, social workers, occupational therapists, pastoral counselors and other interested parties. The orders of the day were negotiated, as were the relations between various parties. The report also conveyed that matters were in control; everyone knew what was happening to all the noteworthy patients and what was being done about them. For example, some residents once challenged the right of another professional to have an inpatient on the argument that the professional did not come to Report and therefore could not really know what the patient was doing.

The resident relied upon Report to know that his patients were alive and behaving as expected. For example, a resident came in to Report and asked about his patient. The nurse said the patient was not on the Report, which meant that nothing was noted about the patient by the nurses on duty. The resident was surprised, "Oh really?" Another resident said, "Perhaps she's gone." [*General laughter.*] Thus in one sense "no report is a good report"; yet the fear lingers that no report means no patient. If the patient has been upset in some way, then the resident expects continued reports, either of the same behavior or a change, and no report becomes a problem.

The items chosen for Morning Report reflected the nurses' view of the ward. The implicit issues were control and cooperation of the patient. Most items had a negative cast, although improvements were also noted.[18] The whole style of Morning Report strongly supports the inmate model which Goffman describes in *Asylums*.[19] Because of its

heavy orientation toward management, Report reflects the staff concerns about inmates in a total institution.

However, most residents did not regard Morning Report in this
oppressive, institutional cast. Rather, they thought it was important for
the management of their patients, and they regarded it as a time for
negotiating with the nurses. Because the nurses organized the Report,
residents often felt defensive. For example, it took first-year residents
on one ward six months before they felt confident enough to dare to ignore their rather imposing head nurse when she complained about how
a resident was handling a patient. Even then, the first resident did it in
Saturday Report, where only fellow residents attend. It took longer
before residents felt enough power and control to ignore items regu-
larly in the fully-attended, weekday Reports. As the sociological calendar indicates, by that time residents tended to ignore the nursing
staff as a whole.

"Report is a communal act, a ritual of a disturbed society
whereby everyone hears the problems and reassures each other that
they know what's happening," said one resident. This was true, but as
one can already see, it was also an arena of competition over control
and power.

> *Head nurse:* Mrs. Q. was up, agitated last night. She missed her
> drugs twice.
> *Resident No. 1:* I will write a restriction to keep away all visitors.
> They only excite her. [She had had visitors yesterday.]
>   . . . .
> *Chief:* If she has low blood pressure. . . .
> *Resident No. 1* [*interrupting*]: I'll give her —— [a drug.]
> *Chief:* I was going to say you might try —— [a different drug]
> We haven't used it yet, but it is good in these cases.
> *Resident No. 1* [*flatly*]: I'd have to familiarize myself with it.
> *Chief* [*nods*]: I'll give you some literature on it.
> *Resident No. 1:* Do that. [Not "Would you please."]
> *Chief* [*nods*].
> *Resident No. 1* [*nods*].

This example illustrates the role conflict residents face between
being students and being professionals in charge of patients. To show
how smart he was, the resident interrupted the chief to recommend a
drug, only to have the chief suggest another drug he did not know.
Because there are so few visible goods to compete for in a residency

full of young physicians who have spent at least the past eight years honing their competitive skills, the resident took his small miscalculation seriously and retreated behind his professional prerogative to only consider his chief's recommendation.

> *Head nurse:* Mr. T. gets angry. [*Looks mad.*]
> *Resident No. 2:* He has a pattern of getting angry at his wife and then getting drunk. Then he takes it out on someone else. So if the staff can point out to him that he is really mad at someone else—don't mention who—it would help.
> *Head nurse:* Well, he is not really *that* angry.
> *Resident No. 2:* He told me of his anger at some of the staff.
> *Head nurse:* He doesn't talk much. He keeps to himself.

Here one sees the delicate balance of power that characterized nurse-resident relations. The resident quickly responded to the nurse's report to a degree that she did not think warranted. Then the resident defended the extent of his response and its nature by suggesting that there was good reason for the staff to deflect Mr. T.'s anger. Unimpressed, the nurse added new information which indicated that Mr. T. was not seriously angry, though it contradicted her initial statement, and the exchange ended in a stand-off.

Implicit in the resident's explanation about Mr. T. is another issue of power: when can one use confidential information? The rules on confidentiality are ambiguous. On one hand, what patients say in therapy is confidential. On the other hand, the common rule prevails that "confidential" information can be shared with colleagues. Most residents did not get hung up on the horns of this moral dilemma. Whether for their own amusement over lunch or for therapeutic reasons in staff meetings, most of them talked openly about what their patients said in therapy. A minority of residents took the other position and never betrayed a patient's confidence to anyone outside of private supervision. As for the patients, it was clear from many conversations that they assumed their confidences in therapy were shared with no one.

> *Resident No. 3:* How is D.?
> *Head nurse:* She keeps her restrictions.
> *Resident No. 3:* She seems to be improving well.
> *Occupational therapist:* She certainly is in OT. . . . I put the two half-hours together and she had no trouble with it.

Resident No. 3 to HN: How do you feel about tightening her restrictions? . . . say to back of ward? [A very tight restriction.]
Head nurse: [Looks at her lap very solemnly.]
Resident No. 3: Maybe an hour a day? [*Softens the request, perhaps in response to the silence.*]
Head nurse: [Looks at her lap.]

In this exchange, the head nurse, who was more concerned with issues of power and control than other head nurses, kept strong a basically weak position in the negotiated order; for the resident could have simply ignored her and written whatever restrictions he wanted in the order book. Restrictions in this program were carefully ordered and provided a number of physical gradations: the isolation room (known as the "quiet room"), the back hall, the back ward, the second lounge, and the ward as a whole. The gradation continued with "privileges" off the ward, beginning with group trips to various activities elsewhere in the hospital, the hospital as a whole, and a variety of privileges outside the hospital. These were refined further by specifying the hours for a given privilege or restriction.

In observing hundreds of Morning Reports and other exchanges on problems of management between nurses and residents, one begins to ask what kinds of responses by residents "pass" as reasonable? Exhaustive study of field notes suggests nine responses which singly or in combination account for almost all exchanges observed.

First, the resident often gave a psychiatric explanation to the nurse, and nurses always seemed satisfied with this kind of answer. Some nurses felt they were learning about the inner life of the patient and the knowledge of the profession which dominated the culture. After all, they were *psychiatric* nurses. Because the resident was regarded as the source for psychiatric explanations, he felt pressure to give this particular kind of response. A patient was reported as getting much worse. The resident said that he did not know what caused this regression. The superchief remarked sharply, "Well, make a few guesses."

Frequently the resident would in effect continue the report which the nurse has started, thereby showing that he not only knew what she did but more. Clearly many of the other kinds of replies could be counted within this one; giving a psychiatric interpretation is continuing the report with further knowledge. However, a resident would often continue the report without adding any other information. For example, a nurse reported that a patient was "isolated and angry." The resident added that the patient had called him last night and asked if his heart was bad, because it was fluttering.

A third kind of reply consisted of putting the present situation into historical perspective. The resident usually did this to demonstrate that things were not as bad as the nurse indicated or that the patient's behavior was more stable than one would think from the report. The resident above, with the patient whose heart fluttered, gave this perspective in the second half of his reply. In another case, the nurse reported that a patient had regressed the previous day, which was her birthday and which was celebrated by her old associates at the half-way house. The resident answered that she had come into the hospital about this time last year, and that the two anniversaries together explained why she had regressed.

In the fourth kind of reply, the resident explained the behavior of the patient in terms of a stage which the patient will pass through. For example, a nurse reported that a patient made a lot of homosexual comments to other patients, and that he was depressed. The newly assigned resident replied that the patient "is testing how long I will be here and whether I will accept him. I told him that upsetting other patients is out, and the staff should tell him the same."

A fifth and frequent reply was an order of drugs or restrictions which further controlled the patient. Residents felt that this was the reply nurses always wanted, even if they didn't ask for it.

> *Head nurse:* Mr. O. is irritated.
> *Resident:* That's better than his tempers. . . . Is he OK on his medicines?
> *Head nurse:* Yes. . . . He's getting more upset. He just carries that postcard from [his vacationing doctor] and reads it over and over.
> *Chief:* That's a good lesson for the rest of you, the importance of sending your patients a part of you when you're gone.
> *Resident:* I'll raise his medicine.[20]
>
> *Head nurse to resident:* "Why did you have Sallie here last night?" [Direct questioning of a resident's action.]
> *Resident:* Well, I saw her on Tuesday [two days before] and she was on edge and kind of loose. Yesterday, she was quite paranoid and more disorganized. She told me of a hallucination she had. I didn't feel

comfortable with her going home. . . . Especially after our experience with her going to New York.

    Head nurse: [*accepting the answer implicitly*]*:* Is there something about her fear she'll become a boy? She said yesterday something about whether the barometer will go up or down. She asked me if she looked any different than the day before.

    Resident: I'm increasing her Haldol. [*Hearty laughter.*]

The resident's response to a subtle question of dynamics was so typical, such a caricature of how residents respond to problems which demand immediate attention and are bewildering, that everyone had a good laugh.

Another type of reply explained why the current policy is being maintained, regardless of whether the nurses want more or less control. A nurse, for example, reported that a patient wanted more freedom and said she thought it should be considered. The resident replied that the patient would get no more freedom, because she was avoiding many problems and was psychotic. The nurse nodded. This example also illustrates the supremacy of the psychiatric explanation.

Sometimes no one was sure what a patient's behavior meant, and the resident did not try to create an explanation. In this case, he would either be silent and look at his knees, or he asked the staff for more details.

    Head nurse: Miss R. kept her restrictions. Was hallucinating. Has delusions in the evening. Much more disorganized in the evening. [The nurse went on with numerous other complaints.]

    Resident: She was worse in the evening?

    Head nurse: Yes.

    Resident: [*Looks down at his lap.*]

An eighth kind of reply was to comfort or reassure the staff about a patient's behavior. This was rare. However, when the ward was high and the nurses were overwrought, the resident might directly reassure the staff or sympathize with a difficult situation.

Finally, the resident might divert the thrust of the nurse's report. Sometimes, one sensed that he did this as a decoy; he wanted to negotiate on his territory rather than on the nurse's. Sometimes he was only interested in one matter and replied to a report on some other aspect by asking only about his chief concern. In these replies one detected an underlying balance between the residents giving the nurses the control of patients they want yet exercising their superior position as psychiatric experts.

Evasion as a Technique of Self-Protection

Residents constantly find themselves in the structurally ambiguous position of being the expert, yet not having sufficient expertise to handle a problem, and of being professionally superior as the physician, yet lacking the experience to command the respect of subordinates. According to one study by Rose Coser, "sociological ambivalence" is more prevalent on the ward than in therapy, because the psychiatric resident also faces the conflicting expectations of patients, supervisors, and perhaps staff without the insulation from observability that psychotherapy provides.[21] One response is to be evasive. By ducking the conflict or deflecting it, one can avoid for the moment the problems of one's position.

While there is no doubt that evasion is used, each actor defines it differently. In any given episode, for example, the residents' response of continuing a report, putting it in historical perspective, comforting the staff, or saying nothing may be considered by the nurses to be an evasion. Whether they do depends on their expectations, as is the case with any other role partner of the resident. For an outsider to label a particular response as evasive necessarily ignores its contextual nature.

Coser's evidence rests largely on asking residents two hypothetical questions, rather than directly observing what residents did on the wards and in therapeutic supervision. She asked them, "If your patient in psychotherapy were to ask you whether you have supervision, what would you say?"[22] Would they address it even though supervision casts doubt on their professional authority, or would they deflect the question by exploring why the patient wanted to know? Although Coser recognizes this as a major technique of therapy, she still calls it evasive and thereby rejects the examination of motives as a legitimate technique of therapy.[23] Coser's second question was, "If a patient on your ward were to say to you, 'You're a nice person to talk to, but you have no authority here anyway; you are no help to me,' how would you handle it?"[24] Leaving aside the way this question confounds the issues of authority and being helpful, the following response was rated as highly evasive: "I think you have to explore with the patient some reason why he may feel that way."

Coser concludes: "The threat to authority is defended by turning attention away from the issue and directing it at the patient."[25] But what is the issue? The truthfulness of the patient's statement? It is true that the very act of regarding the patient's assertion as the product of feelings to be examined itself asserts the resident's authority. But whether this response is a defense that evades the issue depends on one's definition of the situation. Had the resident replied, "You may think that, but I do have authority and I am helping you as much as you allow," or had he agreed that he lacked authority and was not being helpful, he would have been no less evasive and probably less helpful.

Professor Coser found that residents gave "evasive" answers to the second question twice as often as to the first, and therefore concludes that evasiveness was much more prevalent on the ward, where residents could not insulate themselves from observation, than in psychotherapy. But the questions are not comparable in tone or content, as would be the case if a patient on the ward also asked the resident if he had supervision.[26] The direct observations at University Psychiatric Center found that residents often tried to be evasive, both on the ward and in private supervision. What Coser's study points to is the pervasive belief that everything the patient says or does emanates exclusively from his or her psyche, which allows staff not to take any reaction, question or action by a patient seriously at face value. The results of this belief can themselves drive someone with a serious problem mad.

Insulation from being observed is itself a major form of evasion that residents learn to use in management as well as in therapy.[27] While managing patients is a more public activity, residents constantly keep patients from observing their discussions with nurses or supervisors, as they keep nurses from observing or hearing their conversations with supervisors. On the other hand, they often control what supervisors of management, such as the chief, know about their management decisions. Unless the conflicting expectations are so intense that they must be fully aired, much tension is avoided this way. One interesting insulator is the order book. Like the restaurant spindles where waitresses clip their orders for the cooks, an effectively used order book protects the resident physicians from having to defend themselves face-to-face with more experienced nurses, while it allows the nurses to interpret orders in their own way.[28] But like most techniques for reducing social strain, the order book can become a weapon.

The Embattled Order Book

> ". . . the doctors use the order book to be passive-aggressive to the nurses through vague orders. This leaves the responsibility on the staff. Nurses get back by mucking up things if the orders aren't explicit. So the order book is the vehicle for aggressions on both sides."—A resident.

The nurses' expectations that the residents would know what to do and should give orders were reflected in their attention to the order book, although they ignored the orders at certain times too. Their feelings about their own greater experience and competence came out in complaints about "bad" orders. If one tried to sort out from these complaints the qualities of a good order, the expected traits of clarity and utility did not emerge. One can only conclude that there were few truly good or bad orders, but rather orders which were liked or disliked. A resident, for example, complained about the administration of a difficult female patient.

> She was scared of men from the start. . . . I talked to the nurses, and we agreed that [the patient] should have female attendants. But then they used males. Why? Because it wasn't in the order book, even though we'd all agreed. So I finally wrote it.
> That's the new thing around here in the last two weeks. Everything has to be in the book. I don't know why. For example, the other night I asked the special attendant if he had talked to the patient, and he said no. Why, I asked? Because, he said, the order book says that only female attendants can speak to her inside her room with the door closed.
> Or take another. A patient recently had to see a staff member. He asked to be escorted because he was on restrictions. The attendant refused, because it was not in the order book! Imagine! Any time anyone has an appointment he is escorted.

Nurses not only refused to do what was not written, but they did not want to be responsible for interpreting ambiguous orders. A patient, for example, refused to go to school. The nurse asked the resident what they were to do, if the staff should use force, and the resident kept repeating "She has to go." The nurses got upset, because they did not know what to do. The resident said what he meant was perfectly clear: they should *tell* the patient that she had to go. No one had done that. This conflict came up in Report, and afterwards the resident told the patient she had to go to school. The patient went.

The resident's view was that one cannot think of everything, and a good nurse knows what to do. The nurse's view was that a doctor thinks of what is essential and knows what to do.

While nurses would not do something that was *not* written and did not want to interpret orders that doctors wrote, they constantly asked for certain kinds of open-ended orders which gave them the responsibility and freedom to act as they wished. But only when they requested them and understood their vagueness. Most common of these is "PRN" after an order for medicine. Essentially nurses regarded PRN as meaning "when needed." Sometimes doctors wrote PRN orders which frustrated the nurses. If one analyzed the PRN orders to discover what distinguished a "good" from a "bad" one, one concluded that a PRN is frustrating to a nurse when she has not asked for it. Nurses went further and *created* orders, especially concerning wild patients. They did this by demanding some order of the resident or of the DOC. Working with the DOC was especially easy, nurses said, because he did not know the case and would usually agree with what the nurse requested.

Assimilating Management into Therapy

In the preceding pages, we have considered how residents accommodate to the demands of management, particularly as expressed by the nurses who run the wards. By accommodating, the resident learned the ropes and resolved one structural source of ambiguity by learning how to manage his or her patients. Nurses, who gained extra status and power from the residents' initial incompetence, were left feeling both successful at having trained the residents and discarded by them. But learning administrative psychiatry *per se* generated another role conflict with which residents struggled: the conflict between managing the patient and treating the patient in psychotherapy. In the program under study, residents usually resolved this second source of conflict by assimilating administrative issues into the values of psychotherapy.

This assimilation occurred at a number of levels. From the broadest perspective, it meant that one administered in order to prepare a person for psychotherapy or because a person was too chronic to be a candidate for therapy. (The operating definition of chronic was "unresponsive to therapy.") Although residents knew that administration could improve or worsen a patient, that in itself was seen as behavioral, not "real," change. At the more immediate level of administering, residents quickly learned to think about restrictions, privileges and drugs in psychodynamic terms. This has been well illustrated in these pages by the issue of control. The nurses and the outside observer might think the object was to control the patients, but staff psychiatrists emphasized the patients' psychodynamic need *for* control. In the minds of many residents, this became an unexamined assumption. As residents became preoccupied with countertransference, they tended to keep the same frame but turn it on themselves: we are controlling certain patients in certain ways because of our own psychodynamics needs.

Perspectives on Drugs

The attitudes by staff and residents toward drugs illustrates this theme and some of the complexities surrounding it. The nurses felt that drugs allowed for more control, "so that the ward can live." But the only official, and quite pervasive, view on drugs came from the director of training, Dr. Blumberg, who was against them. Dr. Black might have had thoughts about drug use, but he was not quoted, while Blumberg's perspective was a constant presence. And with good reason; for most residents initially found his view extremely "antimedical," "medieval," and even "cruel," yet a good number of them came to agree with Blumberg by the end of their first year.

In the first week of residency, one chief quoted Blumberg while discussing a case: "You can't get into business with a person who is drunk." The nurse replied, "Oh come on. You're overdoing it. Drugs reduce anxiety." These were the two basic orientations toward drugs. Soon after, Blumberg instructed a resident about drugs at a case conference.

> *Resident:* "It cures psychosis. It takes the psychotic features away. It takes away the delusions, and it quiets the patient down so you can be with him."
> *Blumberg,* "You've studied much more recently than I have, but my impression is that there is no drug for madness. Personally I prefer no drugs, but you have to take into consideration the nurses and how the staff feel. Most drugs are for us."

The hospital staff formed a continuum over the amount of drugs to be used. Most conservative were supervisors and senior personnel. The residents found themselves in the middle, with nurses at times urging more drugs than they thought good for the patient. Thus residents felt that "drugs are played down here. The attitude is 'Well, hold off on the Thorazine,' or 'Nothing else works, so use some Thorazine.' " Yet residents constantly fought the nurses over the use of drugs.

> A nurse was telling me about the care of a certain patient: first the residents resisted giving the patient drugs, but the nurses won that one, and they gave her lots of Thorazine.
> Then it was discovered that Thorazine didn't work at all. So a new research drug was tried. That did a little to slow her down, but the nurses wanted electroshock therapy (as an administrative measure; this was a "wild" patient). The residents wanted to continue experimenting with the research drugs, but the nurses won.

Generally, about 60 percent of the inpatients on all wards received drugs in a given month. This was a regular statistic, part of the hospital's culture, and the chiefs were competitive about which service had the *fewest* patients on medication.[29]

Reasons for Prescribing Drugs

From the myriad of reasons given by residents for prescribing drugs emerged five kinds of explanation. The first one, to control the patient, spilled over into the other reasons. For example, a drug might be given to reduce the anxiety and confusion a patient felt, so that s/he could talk about his or her emotions, but the language of control will be found *wherever* drugs are used.

It was commonly said that previous drug history was itself the basis for deciding what to prescribe. When confronted with a new patient, a resident was more likely to give the patient whatever medication he or she had had before than any other. This, at least, was a widespread belief, and residents were warned against it, to little avail.

A third reason for giving drugs was that the patient had been "in treatment" (which everyone understood to mean psychotherapy) with no results. Drugs was the next choice; shock was the last resort.

A fourth reason—a reason *not* to give drugs—was the danger of suicide. Of course a patient could be given medication in liquid form, but sometimes the question of whether a patient might save up pills caused a resident to hesitate about medication at all.

Finally, decisions for and against drugs might center around estimating the patient's anxiety. Residents often used this kind of justification, because it was their domain to determine thought disorder and psychic states. On the other hand, Blumberg and senior psychiatrists frequently recommended reducing drugs so that they did not cover strong emotions. Behind these exchanges one sensed a state of optimum anxiety. The object of both sides was to put the patient into a state where he felt his anger, anxiety, or sadness enough to talk about them in therapy but was not so overwhelmed, either by these feelings or by medication that he could not talk coherently. With this goal in mind, supervisors recommended less medication "to get at the anger," while controlling the patient administratively with tighter restrictions. It was also common to initially give no drugs (regardless of how difficult the patient was) to "see what she's really like," then prescribe enough "to show who's boss," and finally let up on the dosage until one reached that optimum level of anxiety.

Patients also believed that drugs reduced anxiety, as illustrated by the following case. A chief asked a resident if a patient's "meds were up." Yes, he said, to 2400 units of Thorazine a day. Really???!, the chief exclaimed.

> The resident told a story to explain why. The patient asked if he could see him the previous day, and when he was there he said he felt like running; he had to go somewhere.
>
> After the interview, the patient asked the resident to see him again. "I told him we could meet at our regular time tomorrow. He said he could not wait; it was important. We went into the office and he said he was afraid he might hurt someone. Then he ran for the door, opened it, holding it in a funny way, by the edge. Then he did a strange thing. He shut the door on his fingers. There he was, his fingers turning blue and I was worried.
>
> "Then he ran out the door and a nurse stopped him. She blocked and he held her for a little, and she told him he would have to go back to the quiet room. He let go and asked me if that was right. I said it was and he went back.
>
> "In the quiet room he said if she hadn't been a girl he would have killed her. I asked him what he wanted, and he said more medicine. So I gave him more medicine. . . . In five minutes he had calmed down, which shows the *psychological* effect of giving a drug." [Italics added.]

Most of the advertisements by drug companies in psychiatric journals claim that they pull a patient out of some morass. Mellaril pulls the patient out of tension and agitation. Stellazine remotivates as it reduces anxiety. Serax relieves anxiety and tension. Tofranil relieves primary depression. Librium (double-page ad) relieves severe anxiety. Haldol is antipsychotic.[30] This curative tone contrasts with the five reasons why residents gave drugs.

Underlying these reasons for administering drugs is the criterion of control. The control of inpatients and the smooth running of the ward was a prime focus both of the nurses and the residents. The residents were less inclined to consider the ward's mood as a whole, but from the first day they were told that one agitated patient impedes the therapy of many others. In reviewing the first year, an old resident said that mainly he learned more about ways to control patients, and he favored the use of drugs and administrative rules if they aided therapy. Even a disciple of Blumberg stated, "The ward is as high as we've ever seen it. There are six homosexuals walking around; X. is eyeing the door; Y. is getting patients mad. If there is a question of how much medicine to give, use more."

As one might suspect, a rich language surrounded the use of drugs, with an overtone of control regardless of context. It also conveyed a distinct image of the patient:

—You use Thorazine as a *squash*.

—1200 milligrams of Thorazine *isn't enough to hold him*.

—He was on 2400 of Thorazine plus 24 of Stellazine and it *didn't even touch him*.

—Then it was discovered that Thorazine didn't work at all. So a new research drug was tried. That did a little to *slow her down*.

—Do you think the medicine will *pile up on him* by the end of the day?

Another interesting perspective commonly found was that drugs "cover up" the issues, if not the person. "I decided a while ago to take him off drugs, to see what he is like."

Patient accounts of what drugs feel like both physically and psychologically fit the model implicit in the residents' language, although most residents denied that such a model is in their head. One patient said of drugs, "It hurts inside." Most patients considered first medication or increased dosages as a clear sign of their own deterioration. The announcement by their doctor that they were "going on [a drug]" shocked them and their self-esteem.

Similarly, patients considered getting drugs as reflecting a loss of trust. It altered the relationship between psychiatrist and patient, from a therapeutic to a more medical and therefore inferior one. One patient said that when a patient gets drugs, it is the final sign that he cannot be trusted, and he may also lose his trust in his doctor. Residents also reflected the lower status of drugged patients. "When she gets off Thorazine we can start real therapy."

Jack: Managing a Crisis

In considering different elements of resident training in management, this chapter has necessarily presented actual experiences in fragments. The incident concerning Jack brings these elements together into a complex whole. Because of the controversy it fostered, the case also highlights certain basic issues that underlie training in administrative psychiatry.

Yesterday occurred what a veteran attendant said was "the biggest panic I've seen on this ward." Jack was sitting on the floor by the ping-pong table, when the ball went under his legs. Another patient who was playing asked for it.

"Get it yourself," said Jack. The player leaned down over Jack's legs for it, and Jack "went for his throat." The other player, an attendant who is greatly respected by the patients, broke Jack's grip on the patient's throat, threatening Jack with his paddle. Jack let go, got up, went down the hallway out of the ward, down the stairs and into the inner courtyard.

The attendant followed Jack, calling for help, and stood watching him in the wall-enclosed courtyard. Six men eventually assembled and started to go for Jack to bring him back to the ward.[31] Just then, the chief arrived and stopped them until he could summon Jack's resident; then he went out to talk to Jack, as had the attendant before, but to no avail.

The attendant had concluded that Jack had "a homosexual panic" when the other patient reached for the ball. A nurse was called, on the basis that she would be less threatening. Jack kept saying that he had to kill someone, anyone, and asked to be attacked by the attendants. The nurse succeeded in getting him to sit down and said he would come in on his own.

Jack's resident finally came, and tried to talk to his patient, who was still there.[32] Jack kept repeating "Leave me alone. Leave me alone.

I'll come in on my own. Trust me.'' The resident said this really touched him, he wanted to trust Jack, and wanted Jack to think he was trusted.

The resident gave Jack twenty minutes to come in voluntarily. When the twenty minutes passed, he did not order the attendants, standing by, to get him, but went out to talk to Jack again. Jack repeated what he'd said before, and the doctor gave him another twenty minutes. The first attendant said this happened three times, and by the end Jack was practically fainting from anxiety.

This veteran attendant said the whole incident took four hours, whereas such cases usuually take twenty minutes at the most. Finally, said the attendant, nine men went across the grass at Jack, who was wielding a chair over his head. As they got near, he said, "Forget it. I'll come," put down the chair and walked in, escorted. The resident later reiterated many times how pleased he was that Jack had finally "come in on his own"(!).

As Jack entered the ward, all the hall doors between rooms were shut, and all patients had been put in two back rooms for close watch. Jack went to the Treatment Room, where he refused medication. They wrestled him to the floor, injected Thorazine, and put him in one of the Quiet Rooms (stripped bare, no handle, door is wedged shut). He kept shouting and yelling; so he was given much more Thorazine. Finally he grew sluggish.

Attendants' Meeting.

They met with the chief the next day at their weekly time, and were upset at how Jack had been handled.

"There's no need for four hours."

"Jack's resident knows nothing, he did everything wrong. He can't help it; he's new."

"Yeah, you [the chief] should have known better, though. You shouldn't have let it go."

"Learning is fine, but this is going too far. You can learn when it doesn't put the entire ward on its ear."

The attendants complained that Jack's resident was very nervous and anxious, being so torn between *trust and control*. He made Jack much worse. Patients always act out their inner conflicts toward a doctor or the service in general, they said.

The attendants in the meeting showed they knew it was coming. Two or three said they had seen signs in Jack. The tone of all their remarks was to complain that they had not been consulted and that they knew more than the doctors and could handle things better. They said they had never seen the ward so anxious.

Two other young males with homosexual feelings said they were afraid they were going to panic too. In general, the attendants said that patients felt themselves going out of control when they saw someone else out of control. They became more aware of their weaknesses.[33]

After listening a long time, the chief spoke in the attendant's meeting about learning. "You have to learn first-hand. I did it for [Jack's resident]."

The chief maintained that "these patients are begging for control" [a constant assumption here]. When they say they have to kill someone, they are saying keep me from killing someone. When they say they want to commit suicide, they are saying keep me from killing myself. The same is true for Jack. His resident had to learn this, which he did.

The attendants did not seem convinced. The attendant who first tried to control Jack said, "It's quite simple. When a patient comes here does he control the staff or does the staff control him? Jack controlled the staff for four hours straight."

These opening notes define the major perspectives, which were always in tension and with which residents must contend at all times. For staff opinion can shape the status and reputation of the resident. The staff, mainly nurses and attendants, always talked in terms of what was best for the ward, which almost always coincided with what an observer would think would be most convenient for the staff. If the patient affected the ward at all, then what was best for him happened to coincide with what the staff said was best for the ward. The resident, who thought of his patient primarily in individual rather than ward milieu terms, often conflicted with the staff on the therapy versus management axis. However, dynamics and management met in a basic belief of the hospital: if a patient asks for drugs or control, he is asking for control; and if he threatens to go out of control, he is asking for control.

Ward Meeting (two days later).

Jack's resident says that he is very pleased that Jack came up on his own. The question was control.

A patient says that Jack responded to his environment. He was confused, as we all are, by the many changes in personnel during the last two weeks. [This incident occurred during the second week of July, when new residents come in.] Who is in authority? Who is who?

Jack's resident asks the patient, "Do you mean the environment of inner feelings?"[34]

The patient replies, "No, the environment on the ward."

A patient of long duration supports the resident's interpretation and cuts down the patient by saying it was agitation inside Jack that made him do it.[35]

During the ward meeting, many patients express sympathy for Jack. The chief notes this to the group and asks if anyone is angry at Jack. One patient replies, "We can't afford to be angry at Jack. He is a patient just like us. We might do the same thing tomorrow."

After every ward meeting, all members of the staff (except for attendants and a nurse or two) took their folding chairs back into the staff conference room, closed the door, and analyzed what the patients had done and said during the ward meeting. This mass migration was taken as a natural process, and one rarely heard a resident ask what patients must think of this practice or how it affects what they say during ward meetings.

Staff Evaluation Meeting.

During the ward meeting no staff had spoken except for Jack's resident. The chief asks why? He says, "It is like thirty observers and thirty participants." [No wonder patients don't feel like talking.]

Various staff say that they were very scared.

The chief replies, "Well, say that then."

Others question whether saying it would not scare the patients, since they look to us for stability.

Jack's resident says that there were two messages about Jack in the ward meeting. 1. You have to trust a man. 2. You have to control a man out of control for the sake of the ward.

Another resident adds that one patient in therapy with him gave another message: do the doctors know and care about their patients?

During a meeting with the superchief, the residents were told that when you control your patients you help your patient, who is asking for control, and you help the other patients, who are frightened by someone being out of control. Jack's resident said he got the message and for the first time apologized for not controlling Jack.

Morning Report (four days later).

The nurse reported that a patient scratched herself lightly with a bottlecap. The resident replied, "Yesterday is the first time I haven't seen her."

The chief said, "This is the time of testing. She is testing you out, and you don't want to be seduced into seeing her more."[36]

The chief continued, "You can't ignore the incident. That would make matters worse. But you can't give in. You must see the patient, show her that you know she scratched herself because you didn't see her yesterday, and you must let her know that this kind of behavior must not happen. This is the second thing," he continued. "The first is seduction; the second is control. You have to see her to control her, to show her what expressions of anxiety and anger are permissible and useful."

This is the major rule residents learned which routinized mild crises. If there is some tension between control and therapy, there is even more between seduction and control; for to control may be to seduce and not to control may mean you are *being* seduced. Patients told me that they would get themselves into the hospital, or if already hospitalized, get themselves on tight restrictions so that they could see their doctor more often. These accounts came largely from patients who had second-year residents as therapists.

During the Saturday meeting of the residents and the chief, the discussion got on one's feelings about one's patients.

Jack's resident said he knew his person came into his work. "I grew up with a lot of control on me, and when he said, 'Don't force me; let me come in on my own,' I knew just how he felt."

A week later, a case conference was held about Jack. As a result of this conference, it was decided to discharge Jack. Thus the conference discussion is important in understanding how this decision was made and how the residents saw the case psychiatrically. First, as is the form, Jack's resident presented the case to the assembled doctors, nurses, and other paraprofessionals.[37] Then the visiting interviewer, a senior psychiatrist on the hospital staff, asked that Jack be brought in. Much of what is presented below is the relevant part of the discussion after the interview ended and the patient had left the room.

The interviewer, after some discussion, talked about Jack. [He alluded to him always as "this patient" or "the patient," never by name.

Jack's problems began in childhood, which was very disjointed, family moving around, no one caring for him, and so forth. He felt that he had not been loved. As a child, his defense was to see himself as someone special who had been abused. The only alternative would have been for him to hate himself, and so this was not a bad defense.

The trouble, the interviewer continued, is that he still has this defense, and it is a foreign body in his adult life which messes up every relationship he starts. He goes out of his way to get people to reject him. Everyone is picking on him, and he has no idea that he is doing things to provoke it. So if you give him the slightest trouble—or he'll pretend you have—he will get angry and accuse you.

Finally, the interviewer concluded, Jack will not say he is angry, but that *you* are angry at him. "You bastard!" he says, and he strikes out at this angry, picking world. But he is quite charming, until you cross him in the least.

The only way to handle him is as an outpatient. Any limits here will drive him into paranoic psychosis, and you will be in for a lot of trouble.

This conference is a good example of how more serious administrative decisions are based on the dynamics of the patient. The problem began with an extreme managerial disruption, was diagnosed by the psychiatric staff in terms of the patient's dynamics and illness, and was solved by a therapeutic recommendation which happens to be administratively compatible with the needs of the hospital.

That difficult combination, called "therapeutic management," must be carried out by the resident in his relationship with the patient. Discharging Jack turned out not to be easy, because he first agreed and then changed his mind. The resident did not interpret this therapeutically; it was as if the discharge conference had also discharged him from treating Jack as a therapeutic patient. But the administrative supervisor continued to assimilate management into therapy; he saw the resident's "by the book" response as countertransference.

The resident told his supervisor that he really got angry at Jack when Jack suggested a compromise—night care—after he and Jack had agreed on a discharge. After the conference, Jack agreed to sign a three-day paper which, if unopposed, would result in his being discharged. Now he wanted to work days and come in each night for night care.

Resident: So I said we decided it was best for you to go yesterday, and he jumped on my throat. He said, "We! What do you mean *we? You* decided. You don't give a shit what I think." So I asked him if we can work out something, and he says, "No. *we* can't. Either I control my life or I don't."

Supervisor: He is incapable of conceiving of compromise. Any decision or opinion you give is seen as a control.

I'm just furious at him.

Did you express it?

No.

You should if you can, as much as you are able.

I was not sure what I felt then.

That's it. You've got to be in tune with your feelings at the time.

Resident [*seemingly ignoring what the supervisor just said*]: But we had just decided that he would sign the three-day paper! [*Whine.*] And every time I remind him of something we discussed together, he flatly denies it. I'm just fed up with him.

So are you going to consider night care?

No. It is too late. He should have brought it up before.

Why is it too late?

Because the three-day paper has been signed. And the wheels of the institution have turned. [One can retract a three-day paper at any time during the three days.]

The next day the nurse at morning report said that Jack was withdrawing his three-day paper. His resident replied, "He is still leaving today." He went on to explain, as he had in supervision, that discharge had been agreed upon, and then Jack had suddenly dreamed up night care, but that the original plan was being carried out. The superchief commented that it would be a mistake to have Jack here at night. The report continued with other items.

In this case, one finds a number of sociological patterns that characterize administrative training. Two concern the partial conflict between teaching residents and managing the patients well. Early in the crisis, the chief decided to let the resident handle the crisis so he could "learn from the experience" even though he knew that the seasoned attendants could probably do it better. Power relations were also important here; for the attendants could have acted swiftly and effectively, as they finally did, but they had to wait for orders. Ultimately, however, they won, not only in the narrow sense of finally taking Jack the way they had wanted to, but in the broader sense of having their view of the crisis prevail and of having Jack's resident finally admit his bad judgment. What the resident (and his peers) learned from this experience was to "obey" when the nurses and attendants really urge some action *but* to understand it psychodynamically: patients want control.

Yet ironically, the psychodynamic frame shaped the entire event by adding layers to the utilitarian view that a patient had bolted and needed to be controlled as quickly as possible. For the chief wanted the resident to learn about himself as much as about managing a wild patient, and the resident so much wanted the patient to learn from the experience that he interpreted Jack's surrender as self-mastery. Both of these complications turned the crisis into a general panic and an intolerable affront to the ward staff. Someone had to go, and it could not be the chief or the resident.

The crisis also had redefined Jack. While before self-control had been part of a larger problem of getting people to reject him, which was itself only one of his problems, Jack's momentary outburst, followed by a desire to get away and cool off, had been escalated by others until he was regarded a different person administratively and therefore therapeutically. While none had been planned, a case conference was called. A consensus formed: since Jack turned everything into a battle of control, the only way to help him was to treat him as an outpatient. This conclusion essentially neglected the problems of living which had led to Jack's being hospitalized in the first place. But it did show how residents learn to accommodate to the demands of management while assimilating them into their new concepts of illness and therapy.

7.

Diagnosis

Learning how to diagnose is a skill which psychiatric residents must learn before all others. The logic of science demands it, and these young doctors have learned the importance of accurate diagnosis in their medical training. Paradoxically, however, as residents become more seasoned practitioners, diagnosis no longer retains this preeminent role; one learns to formulate a plan of treatment more by feel and common sense. But this may be no paradox at all if "feel and common sense" have by that time become imbued with the psychiatric mode of diagnosis. This suggests that the intense concern with diagnosis in the early part of residency reflects an intense need to get one's bearings, and that learning to diagnose socializes one into the prevailing ideology. Through diagnostic terms, one learns not only a theory of mental disorder but also an interlocking set of relationships. Let us begin with a case.

One summer evening, Miss Heider was admitted by the executive resident for the night, and the doctor on call (DOC) received a message that he had a new patient on his ward. I accompanied him as he went downstairs and brought Miss Heider up to the treatment room of the ward. She was big and strongly built, but not fat, and wore an old, plain dress and oxford shoes. The resident offered her a seat and asked if she wanted something to eat. She did. Later the resident said,

"While I'm probing with one hand, I like to feed them with the other."

The woman lived in a nearby working-class neighborhood and had been brought to the hospital by the police. The resident asked her several questions about her background and why she was here, and her answers went on for some time, interspersed with many side stories and anecdotes. While she gave no direct answers, the following elements emerged from her account: she lived with her parents and brother (she was over thirty), and one day came home to find a bottle of very cheap wine under a chair. She knew it was cheap wine because of a number of past experiences, experiences which she told as leisurely asides. In short, she was quite sure her brother or his friends had brought the wine into the house, and only winos drink such wine. Why, the whole family, even the whole neighborhood could deteriorate into a bunch of winos if this sort of thing kept up. She had seen winos and knew how bad they were, and she was furious, she said, that this bottle was in her house. So when her brother came home, "we had a fight over that bottle. And someone called the cops to break it up and get me."

While she gave her long account she was relaxed, drinking, chewing on a cookie. "The cops are always after me," she said. "This is not the first time they have had to break up a fight in our house."

The resident took some notes while she talked, and then at the end turned the patient over to a nurse in order to get her ready for bed. All the exchanges were very friendly, and the patient was almost happy to cooperate.

The resident and I talked about the case. I asked what was wrong with Miss Heider. He said she was paranoid, because she thought the police were after her, and schizophrenic, because she was so "autistic." I asked what he meant, and he referred to her wandering off the subject, "grandiose ideas" about the whole family, the neighborhood turning wino. In her file he wrote her diagnosis, "paranoid schizophrenic."[1]

Miss Heider did not become this doctor's patient. He "worked her up" because he was the DOC that night, but she went to the next doctor on rotation on that service. A few days later, her assigned doctor said in Report that she had graduated from Barnard, where her father had a maintenance job. The DOC resident said he was surprised, although he knew what was wrong with her. She was a paranoid schizophrenic. "I mean," he said, "she sees one bottle of cheap wine in the house and thinks the family is going to turn into a bunch of winos. That's pretty bad."

This "work-up" contains a number of themes in psychiatric diagnosis. First, unlike medicine, psychiatry characterizes the whole person by the observed disorder. Miss Heider did not *have* paranoid schizophrenia; she *was* a paranoid schizophrenic. This is the response one always gets to the question, "What's wrong with her?" One wonders how residents can so easily make this basic switch from medicine. Perhaps the fact that these new kinds of patients do not look sick helps to overcome a difficult problem in socialization. There is an eerie feeling to working with unsick sick people, and this practice of considering them as the full embodiment of the illness may bring comfort through compensating exaggeration.

By characterizing the whole person, psychiatric diagnoses also neglect the rest of the person and evidence about her. Here, for example, was Miss Heider, committed to a hospital by the police, and she was not paranoid during the interview. The resident, moreover, did not have any other evidence of paranoia or schizophrenia, and this is typical. One instance will do. In this case, I do not think Miss Heider believed the police were after her; she merely pointed out that it was not unusual for the police to break up fights in her household. But even had she been clearly paranoid over the wine, there was certainly much more to her. Although harsh, it is accurate to say that in most cases, psychiatrists learn to diagnose from anecdotal material, with little training in the rigors of psychological inference which historians or other professionals who work with case studies use. Residents do spend long hours diagnosing in case conferences, supervision, and the diagnostic seminars, but usually without this rigorous training. Part of this personal orientation is a general disdain for psychological testing. One learns to call for it, but one ignores it unless it bolsters one's own impressions. This characterized nearly all of the psychological consults which I observed.

If psychiatrists learn to diagnose through anecdotal material, they also learn to look mainly for pathology.

> The case record . . . is apparently not regularly used, however, to record occasions when the patient showed capacity to cope honorably and effectively with difficult life situations. Nor is the case record typically used to provide a rough average or sampling of his past conduct.

> . . . Early acts in which the patient appeared to have shown bad judgement or emotional disturbance will be recorded.[2]

When there are no signs of pathology, the patient is described in such a way as to leave open the question of undisclosed pathology.

> Even with considerable pressure she was unwilling to engage in any projection of paranoid mechanisms.
>
> No psychotic content could be elicited at this time.[3]

Moreover, signs of mental disorder are often given the most negative interpretation they can bear, as seen in Miss Heider's diagnosis.

Residents do not generally see themselves as agents of incarceration or as social agents who are clapping labels on people which will stigmatize them in the years to come, though that's what sociologists have been telling them for years. They seem irresponsibly naive about the impact of what they are doing, in part because they do not take these labels seriously themselves and forget that others do. Even further from their minds is the Kafkaesque view of Goffman's betrayal funnel, where psychiatrists seemingly ally themselves with the new patient as a sympathetic professional while, through administrative and verbal tricks, depriving him or her of civil rights and relationships with the outside world.[4] Yet anyone can observe residents doing this every day in an effort to make their job easier. In most commitment procedures observed, the patient did not know what he was doing or what was being signed, even though an alert observer could hear the resident "explaining" everything he was supposed to explain by law.

Finally, the case of Miss Heider illustrates the focus on the individual in psychiatric diagnosis. At the height of community psychiatry and family therapy, this residency implicitly taught that the unit of diagnosis was the individual, that the only necessary evidence was the individual's actions and accounts in the presence of the therapist, that one therefore did not normally seek information from nurses, social workers, relatives, attendants or other therapists who worked with the person,[5] and that the individual's relation with the therapist was indicative of his or her major problems.

The Diagnostic Seminar

Although residents learned to diagnose in Morning Report, supervision, and in some case conferences, the diagnostic seminar was devoted solely to learning the subtleties of this subtle art. Known as "Diagnostics," the seminar was held weekly for ninety minutes, usually led by a younger psychiatrist active in the Psychoanalytic Institute. Each seminar began at the first of the year and included only a few residents, so that the opportunity to learn was ideal. The people diagnosed were "fresh material," not patients of seminar members. The Walk-In Clinic supplied cases, and someone always seemed to be complaining that there were not enough good cases. A "good" case was known as a person who, having been interviewed in the walk-in-clinic, presented either a complex technical or practical problem. The person must also be able to wait for an opening in the seminars and thus not be in need of immediate attention.

As the seminar I observed began, a resident was sent to the outpatient clinic to get the person's file. He returned and the diagnostician (let us call him, hereafter, the psychiatrist) read it. The "work-up" in the file said that the girl was sent to Diagnostics to determine whether we should spend time with her in therapy. She had broken therapy before. No diagnosis, as such, was given, although bits about her family life were included. Just before the patient, whose appointment had been arranged by the clinic, arrived, the psychiatrist said he would not introduce her to us.[6] We sat in four large wooden chairs along the wall of a dim, bare, spacious office. The psychiatrist sat at his desk, leaving one chair alongside the desk for the girl. Our chairs faced the guest's, with the psychiatrist at right angles to both but nearer to the person he would be interviewing.

Below is a rather accurate transcription of the interview taken by one of the residents. The accuracy was possible because so few words were spoken and because long silences separated each exchange, which the reader should supply.

The well-dressed girl entered, and the psychiatrist began:

> What's your understanding [of this meeting]?
>
> *Girl:* Diagnosing.
>
> You're here to find out what's wrong.
>
> I'm not—no.
>
> [*Pause, gaze*]: Who is?[7]
>
> [Silence.]
>
> *Psychiatrist:* Do you share responsibility?

Girl: It's partly my responsibility. Partly. I'm trying to find out.

You've been attributing responsibility to your family, responsibility for not finding help.

If it will help me, I'll accept responsibility.

We have no guarantee it will help. If you want only it, then we'll be in a stalemate.

[The tension had gotten quite high, at least for me.]

Girl: You're twisting my words.

[Silence—Psychiatrist looks constantly at girl, who sometimes looks at him, at her lap, or around the room.]

Psychiatrist: What can we expect from you?

It's not a definite no (that I'll not cooperate.) I want it for relief.

Of what?

[Long pause.]

I just want to be happy.

You'll have to be more specific.

How?

Take a try at it [*sarcastically*].

[Patient looks down, shaken]: You seem to have my attitude fixed before I came here. [*Pause.*] I don't know what you mean by "more specific."

If *you* don't know, who does?

Relations with other people, with myself [*pause*] that's all I can think of.

I can't make much of that. *You* don't give, I won't give. I'm looking for responsibility from yourself.

How do you know?

From the record.

What is in the record?

I won't tell.

I think I've taken a lot of responsibility coming here.

I think you haven't.

I do.

Now where do we go?

[Pause. Girl looks at psychiatrist, looks down. Sad, but not very.]

Psychiatrist: There is no point our waiting the whole time. If this is your decision, go now.

I want to talk but. . . .

. . .we're not going to do any more for you.

I'm not happy with people. . . . Do you want instances?

What do you think I want?

I never enjoy myself with people my own age.

How come? What do you think?

I don't know.

How come?

As soon as I go out I want to come back.

You feel safe at home?

I don't know.

What's your theory?

I don't know.

What's your theory?

I'm comfortable with Mother.

With guys what are you afraid of? [*Hard tone*] I'll do the work for you.

I didn't hear you.

Now you don't hear me! [*Exasperated*] With *guys,* what are you afraid of?

I don't know. [*Pause*] I guess I'm afraid of them—involved.

Involved.[8]

Becoming dependent on them . . . for friendship.

Who's going to knuckle in first? Are you a stubborn person? [*Pause*] Can you wait a long time?

Why do you think I'm not taking responsibility?

Whether you'll take more initiative. Whether you'll clam up [*snappy, bored tone*].

I already said I'll take responsibility.

We sort of got stuck on your being unhappy. I asked for specifics. Then you clammed up.

I don't know how to be more specific.

Then we're stuck again. The point is, we won't be any more specific than you are.

[Pause.]

I don't know how to be more specific.

You've got some time left. [*Looks at watch.*] Think about it.

[Long pause. Girl looks at floor, doctor at her.]

Girl: Can you word it differently?

If I knuckle in, *then* will you give ground? Do you get into tug of wars at home?

I'd say something. . . .

. . . if I do the work for you.

No, if I knew what you were getting at. . . .

We want you to take the initiate.

I can't. . . . I don't know what to say.

You don't—hmm—do you want me to know for you!

[Three-minute pause!]

The exchange to this point took *forty minutes*. This suggests the great tension which had prevailed.

The girl finally began to talk about her feeling that bodies and their secretions are dirty.

Girl: Last week I had a date. He wanted premarital sex relations [*smile*].

Why did you smile?

Embarrassed.

Rape me. Your whole attitude today was force me. It seems you are intrigued as well as repulsed.

True. It felt good to be hugged—though I was just somebody else.

Did you want him to go further?

Yes and no. I felt dirty.

How much further. . . . I think you did.

No.

I think you wanted him to force you. Then it's *his* problem.

Maybe.

What's so horrible about experimenting?

Other girls are having a ball.

You wonder where you got the feeling of revulsion.

I never had affection at home.

Never?

When Mother stopped kissing my brother, she just stopped.

Never kissed by your father?

Never. I feel guilty.

Could you be guilty for yearning for father?

I never did.

Never?? Should we believe that?

I never wanted to be kissed. Am I lying?

It's hard to believe—You don't want to remember, because maybe it's too disgusting.

Although the foregoing is only part of the second half of the interview, about as much was said in the last twenty minutes as in the first forty. In the discussion that followed, the psychiatrist said that this was one way to interview, to force the patient to take some initiative. Resident No. 1, however, felt that the interviewer had broken many of the silences and had finally started to do the work for her. The psychiatrist vigorously denied this, despite instances that were cited by the resident. Resident No. 2 thought the interview was great, and that you could only do that kind of forceful interview after you had experience and confidence; he seemed to admire the psychiatrist's ability to stare the person down into silence.

After the seminar, the residents spoke more about the experience. It was their perception and response which were important, and the interview provided model and reality to which they reacted.

Resident No. 3 noted that during the second half of the interview, the psychiatrist not only cooperated but pushed the girl rather hard, the reverse of the first half. He wondered why the psychiatrist had not pointed that out.

Resident No. 1 was skeptical of the accuracy of the data squeezed out. E.g., he cited, she did not remember having had one pleasurable experience with her father. The interviewer had said, "You can't remember *once* when he did something nice with you?" Silence. "You never once. . . ." She then remembered a walk they had taken. The resident compared the technique to brainwashing. "We have no idea how this girl behaves. We've only seen her under very unusual circumstances. I would let her be for a while and see what kind of person she is."

The next day, a second-year resident said that the interviewer was brilliant and equally aggressive and hostile when teaching the second-year residents. A few weeks later, another psychiatrist who runs a Diagnostics was described in a similar manner.

A week after the first interview, the same girl returned for a second interview. Persons coming to Diagnostics are typically seen two or three times. The girl responded with the same manner, had the same "resistances." The "material" was about her father and then her boyfriend. At the end, the psychiatrist recommended she join a group, as a way of getting to know people with similar problems. She said she wanted to think it over. He ended, "You won't take a group. You are stubborn, aren't you? It doesn't seem to matter a hell of a lot that that is what I recommended and that I spelled out reasons for it."

Then the psychiatrist invited the residents to ask questions. They asked two about dating.

After the girl left, not to return again, the psychiatrist talked about the case in a friendly and charming way which contrasted sharply with his manner during the interview:

. . . she was most interested in having the family rejected. She showed that she was not so interested in herself; other girls like her are depressed, more open, not so stubborn and full of fight. She came here to get us to say to her and her family how bad they had been.

Resident No. 1 said immediately that she had gotten him quite angry, and detailed how. Another added that she seemed to be enjoying it.

At the end, resident No. 1 offered his diagnosis: "immature, inexperienced, and behind."

Right, said the psychiatrist. "Adolescent adjustment." There was no further discussion.

After this second seminar ended, the residents reacted further. Resident No. 2, who had been enthusiastic the previous time, said the psychiatrist satisfied his sadistic urges by being so cold and angry with the patients. He said he would have no idea what to ask; he wouldn't know where to start. Resident No. 3 commented that to push the patient is much sicker than this girl is. She should have been left on her own.

At the next Diagnostics, another person, known to the psychiatrist, was interviewed by one of the residents. The resident was gentle; yet the patient refused to discuss delicate details, such as sex, details essential for going beyond generalities. Near the end, the psychiatrist broke in with an aggressive, annoyed tone:

You haven't changed a bit in these years, have you?

Young man: Yeah. I think I've changed a lot. I'm a lot better now.

Why didn't you come in sooner?

I was doing OK. I had a friend. [The patient seemed surprised by the hostility, got defensive, hurt. Yet, as always, the psychiatrist had a central truth about his not wanting to open up for help.]

You have been lecturing us for the last half hour.

Have I? Gee. [*Shakes head in disbelief.*] I sure didn't know I was going over that way. Well, that just goes to show ya. . . .

Psychiatrist: You're angry.

No, I'm not. [*Each stares.*] Prove it.

No, I'm not in that game.

But isn't that why we have minds? You say I'm angry and I say I'm not. So I would like you to show me why you think I'm angry.

It seems to me you're in a rut. You won't *submit* and you're not smart enough to be the psychiatrist.

In the discussion that followed, the psychiatrist gave his comments in his friendly, collegial manner.

He is "paranoid with great counternoise" [the diagnosis], which means a lot of claims at being open.[9]

This type is so depressing, said the psychiatrist, because he is so hard to treat. No relation can be established. Group might be better for him, but then you get into the embarrassment thing again. The advantage of group is that he is not sure what is normal [which the man had said], and the group will give him some bearing.

On sex, said the psychiatrist, he thinks only women have needs. Men don't. He is really hurting, and he probably cries easily.

The interviewing resident commented on a certain sequence in the man's life. Little else was said. Afterwards, the interviewing resident said he did not know what to do when the psychiatrist broke in. He felt baffled.

By the end of July, one resident said that he overlooked the angry side of the diagnostician when he went to the seminar "because it interferes, and he has something valuable to say." He emphasized that the psychiatrist used his angry personality to therapeutic advantage, to get the patient to express anger. "So," he said, "you can learn to use your flaws to advantage." Resident No. 1 said he still turned the psychiatrist off altogether, but by Christmas (four months later) he said he really liked the psychiatrist, considered him very fine, very smart, fun, relaxed, very supportive and warm. He makes suggestions without being harsh when we make mistakes in interview. The others, the resident remarked, like him too.

The young man did not show up for his second interview. The seminar members talked.

Resident No. 3: "He *was* given a rough time last time. Maybe that is why he didn't show. But being kind is no good either. Paranoids respond to kindness with suspicion. The problem of transference is getting out of hand."

The psychiatrist discussed paranoia, turning the seminar into an intellectual one. He cited different literature and theories. He concluded that no one knows the underlying dynamics of paranoia.

Freud, he continued, thought paranoia was homosexuality, but at least a third are not, and many homosexuals become paranoid only when they stop their practice. Paranoid schizophrenia has the best prognosis, only second to catatonic schizophrenia—for the schizophrenic traits. But the paranoid traits are hard to reach.

It is best, he concluded, to see paranoia as a problem in object relations, where a person can let you down.[10] There is paranoia in all normals under stress. And in fact paranoiacs *have* often been lied to and let down in the past.

The only way to get into business is to stay away from the dynamics and support the paranoiac.

Afterwards the residents were enthusiastic about the meeting and noted how supportive and considerate the psychiatrist had been.

Altogether, eight psychiatrists conducted diagnostic seminars. At the end of January, residents changed seminars, thus exposing each resident to two diagnosticians in the first year. Of the eight, three psychiatrists received general admiration. Two of these used a tough, harsh style in interviewing potential patients, but residents saw this manner as an effective technique in both cases. Two others of the eight were generally condemned, and residents who had them advocated an end to Diagnostics. However, the resident association did not take this suggestion seriously. At an evaluation meeting of the association, one active member said, "There is such terrible teaching of diagnostics in the system, that we at least need the Diagnostics."

In conclusion, the major characteristics of diagnosing are seen again—the exclusive search for pathology, the loose use of anecdotal evidence, the reliance on what the person says while being interviewed, and so forth. But two additional features are evident. First, one is struck by the silence of these select young professionals in an ongoing group of only four people. Even though participation varies from group to group, the almost Victorian sense of status hierarchy, reaching from mentor to residents to patient, is surprising. It is part of a larger quality, the uncritical nature of psychiatric training. Second, residents learn, here as elsewhere, that almost any style can be regarded as professional and useful. Even anger and aggression against the patient have their uses. What matters is that one recognize what one is doing. The heart of psychiatric socialization is not, as in the Marines, to change behavior, but to recast present behavior in a certain interpretative framework or belief system. Ironically, the result observed in senior psychiatrists is the opposite, a blindness to the effects of their style. To take the case at hand, the psychiatrist was so intent on being stubborn with the first patient that he denied that he broke silences and finally did the work for her, even though resident No. 1 had written down a verbatim transcript. Throughout the year, a consistent pattern was found at case conferences, that if the visiting interviewer assaulted the patient, defenses appeared; and if he lent the patient a sympathetic ear, the patient opened up—hardly a surprising discovery. But either style was taken to be characterological of the *patient,* and no interviewer commented on the patient's style as a product of the interview itself. More broadly still, the residents and psychiatrists observed were surprisingly unaware of their own personality and its effects on others, despite the great attention to this very phenomenon.

Social Structure and Types of Diagnosis

Up to this point, we have focused on the process of diagnosis and neglected its structure. This neglect is natural and reflects the world view of the psychiatrists and residents. Diagnosis is spoken of as a single entity without a structure beyond the psychological structure of mind which lies behind the terms used. Diagnoses are regarded as "out there," terms published in a manual, and as "in here," things going inside the patient. This is illustrated by the discussion at the end of a case conference.

> As soon as she left the room, a very lively conversation about her diagnosis began.
> "She's not 'schizophrenic.' A schizophrenic is not with her contacts, while she is with every one of them. [I.e., a schizophrenic does not keep up with the conversation, is not coherent.] She's 'hysteric.' "
> Several agreed about her hysterical character and talked about whether she is like the "classic psychotic hysteric."
> "No, she's a borderline hysteric."
> "What is a borderline?"
> "It's the depression of ego defect at the time you see the patient."
> "She's narcissistic. And a borderline is narcissistic. She sees everything as all or nothing."

A resident tried to introduce "manic-depressive." Some said they can't see it. He said her wild side, her grandiose ideas, wild ride in the car are manic.

The minister said she seemed like a nine-year-old, which is when she lost her father.[11]

"Her problems are very primitive. Masculine-feminine. Dominance."

Finally the superchief spoke. She is manic-depressive and very narcissistic. No more debate.

What strikes the observer is that so many "objective states" could be found in one patient without anyone considering that how he diganosed the patient reflected his own response to her!

The irony of this mentality is that it trains psychiatrists to become partially blind to the social nature of diagnosis. As Thomas Scheff has written, "It is almost a truism, however, among social psychologists and students of language, that the meaning of behavior is not a property of the behavior itself, but of a relation between the behavior and the context in which it occurs."[12] This blindness goes back to the interviewer's obtuseness about his or her impact on the patient, a blindness which has a specific rationale that residents learn.

The patient came in [to a case conference on him], sat down, looked at the psychiatrist and said, "Do you want to put me on display?"

The psychiatrist was offended and got angry, protesting that of course he was not that sort of person. (The issue, of course, was not his personality but the structure of case conferences.)

Near the end of the interview, the psychiatrist told the patient that he had made him angry. He said, "Getting me mad is not important so long as it can be put to good use. What is it in you that makes others angry at you?"

The psychiatrist sees self as a scientific instrument. His feelings don't matter except as a presumed measure of the patient's feelings. On the other hand, the patient could not legitimately ask why the *psychiatrist* got mad nor presume that his feelings reflected the psychiatrist's emotional state.

In the discussion later, the psychiatrist explained how the patient "avoided facing his anger. The patient goes out of his way to get people to reject him. When they do, he gets angry, but says that it is you, not he, who is angry. *Then* he gets angry at you for being angry at him.'' The psychiatrist, by not examining why he himself got angry, here portrays himself as the passive victim of the patient's neurotic manipulations, an instrument by which one can measure the patient's disorders.

Besides the social character of diagnoses at this interpersonal level, use of the terms reflects the social structure of the hospital and the organization of work. First, there are normal pathologies, just as David Sudnow found normal crimes in the district attorney's office.[13] Like each criminal, each patient is unique; but there is a strong tendency to label most patients with a half-dozen pathologies, despite the great amount of time and personnel available in this hospital. It seems that this tendency does not merely stem from the pressures of an immense workload, as it appears in the D.A.'s office, but also from the more basic need of people in all walks of life to normalize their work.[14] But going beyond this first-level relation between diagnoses and social structure, one finds not one but four types of diagnoses. Each one is concerned with a different sphere of professional action. Each one has different expectancies, and thereby reflects the organization of work.

The first and most familiar group of labels are the *APA diagnoses* and their embellishments. The American Psychiatric Association issues a book with these official diagnostic terms. Each patient, for legal and statistical purposes, must be assigned to one set of terms.[15] Even though they see a wide range of patients, the residents use only a fraction of these terms. For example, a resident might call a patient ''an obsessive-compulsive personality.'' Very often a resident would speak of a ''schizophrenic'' without elaborating on which of the nine subtypes he had in mind. In most conversations observed, his listener would not demand refinement. Also, a number of official terms were rarely used, if at all. For example, no reference was heard to 297.1, ''involutional paranoid state,'' or any informal variation of it. Finally, under this first family of terms fall some very common labels which, although not included in the official nomenclature, are used in a similar manner. The most notable example is ''borderline,'' which implies the patient may go in and out of psychosis.

Many residents feel that they know psychiatric terms before they come, and they make diagnoses on their first day. The major gain from training, they say, is being able to apply them faster, to become ''more comfortable with less data,'' a dubious pattern already discussed.

While in July a person might have to report a hallucination and exhibit a delusion along with some bizarre behavior to be labelled schizophrenic, by February he need only report having had a hallucination to get the same label.

Although residents learn to deprecate APA terms and to criticize their ill effects, the official nomenclature and its informal variants are the central labels used to mark a patient. A given label stays with the patient and only changes after considerable deliberation by the labeler and those around him. The residents, however, soon learn to discount this label. Often, they say it "means nothing" and is used only to satisfy legal requirements. They frequently say that unlike a true, medical diagnosis, these terms imply neither a cause nor a course of treatment. Residents also say that these terms are crude and only label the leading style or symptom of the patient. If a person hallucinates, he is a schizophrenic. If he has a phobia, he has phobic neurosis. A good example of how little of the case the term may grasp is seen by the diagnosis of "adolescent adjustment" in the diagnostic seminar described earlier. Residents often pointed out such examples.

Despite constant claims that APA terms are useless, the hospital staff and even the residents respond more to this label of a patient than they do either to the patient as a person or to any label from the three other diagnostic clusters. Residents almost always refer to their patients by these labels, usually with little elaboration. If a resident asks another what his new patient is like, he will answer with an APA label. The staff also responds to the label. Orders from the executive offices which could influence the course of treatment are written in terms of APA classifications. Moreover, contrary to belief, prognosis and treatment are often implied by the term, according to the folklore of each APA diagnosis.[16] For example, a patient was diagnosed in conference as a "process schizophrenic." Although the term is not found in the official nomenclature, no explanation was given and no one asked questions. A resident then asked what the prognosis was, and the interviewer said, "If it is process schizophrenic, that means prognosis is pretty bleak."

To summarize, this first group of diagnostic terms answers the need of the organization and the law to ask, "What is wrong with this person?" But while these statistical, bureaucratic, and legal needs provide the most ostensible link between the social structure and this kind of diagnosis, the terms become an essential, telegraphic vocabulary for the professional staff, who are constantly asking that same question. Since these terms are the fruits of painstaking research by great clinicians over many decades, one is surprised to discover their low repute as crude, inaccurate, and relatively useless. Yet it is because these labels are discounted as unimportant (though widely used) that they are allowed to influence treatment strongly without criticism or scrutiny.

A second cluster of terms concern *managerial diagnosis,* and in the natural history of the resident working up a new patient, this is the second diagnostic cluster he or she will use. Although some of the terms overlap with APA nomenclature, managerial diagnoses differ in a number of important ways. First, they arise to answer the question, "How shall we manage this patient?" Second, this is a question that may vary from day to day or even from hour to hour. Thus, the patient is constantly being rediagnosed as an object of management. Often, however, one managerial diagnosis will apply for many days, because the patient will have a certain way of relating to his or her environment. Third, these terms are strongly behavioral. Fourth, they constitute the major diagnostic communication between residents and nurses, who generally do not know or feel comfortable with the APA terms. Thus, they are found in a specific locus within the hospital's organization of work. Finally, all those involved in management consider these terms as essential to their work and highly valid.

Examples of managerial terms are "getting high," "acting up," and "being depressed." Here are some excerpts from Morning Report, an essentially managerial meeting where the head nurse reports to the residents and chief on the patients—usually in terms of problems. Diagnostic terms are *underlined.*

1. *Head nurse:* Mrs. Q. was up, *agitated* last night. She missed her drugs twice.[17]

Resident: I will write a restriction to keep away all visitors. They only excite her.

2. *Head nurse:* Mr. T. *gets angry.* Looks mad.

3. *Head nurse:* Miss R. *kept her restrictions.* Was hallucinating. Has delusions in the evening. Much more *disorganized* in the evening.

4. *Head nurse:* Mr. O. is *irritated.*

Resident: That's better than his tempers. Is he OK on his medicines?

Head nurse: Yes. He's getting more *upset*. He just carries that postcard from Ken (his vacationing doctor) and reads it over and over. . . .

Resident: I'll raise his medicine.

5. *Head nurse:* Mrs. Rhodes is getting louder and louder and louder!

Resident: She is leaving today.

Head nurse: She strikes me as getting *higher*.

These vignettes convey much more than mere examples of managerial terms, but for the moment let us focus on them. The terms overlap a little with APA classifications, such as "depression," but are applied to current behavior in a managerial situation. Thus, a depressive patient (APA family) is to be distinguished from a patient who is depressed at the moment (managerial family). Sometimes the terms get fancier, such as "he has a fragile ego," i.e., the patient should be handled with kid gloves. Nurses more than residents used management terms such as "kookie," "screwy," and "bitchy." A resident would be more likely to call the latter a hysteric, reflecting the resident's attachment to APA terms.

"Crazy" is an important member of this cluster, used by residents and nurses alike. While used in a managerial context, "crazy" characterizes the whole patient, and psychiatric staff must learn how to detect craziness, even in the guise of normality. "Suicidal" is not an official psychiatric term, despite its centrality to treatment and prognosis, but is a prominent term in managerial diagnoses.

This set of terms has all the features of a diagnostic group. Much like the APA terms, it describes main characteristics of the patient and, more directly than the APA nomenclature, suggests care for the patient. In the minds of residents and nurses, some of these terms are almost synonymous with drug dosages and restrictions as seen in the nurse's reports above. If one asks a resident how a patient is, he could say the patient is "wild" or that he is "restricted to the back of the ward" and convey the same message.

A third family of terms is used by residents when talking about therapy with their patients. They constitute the *therapeutic diagnosis*. This group fills the same need for talking about therapy as the managerial group does for administration. But while both of these sets have the manifest function of facilitating work with the patient, inherent in their very terms is the latent function of blaming managerial and therapeutic failure on the patient. This is done quite simply by psychologizing staff-patient relations in terms which describe only the patient's degree of cooperation or engagement. Of course, the residents or other staff can point out how they contributed to the patient's therapeutic or managerial state, but this is extra work beyond the terms themselves.

A common term is "business," and much could be written about the mentality of business and work found in American psychiatric language. To be "in business" means that a patient is engaged in therapy and understands what therapy is about. Another common term is "reality testing," as in "You should be reality-testing with her." This advice means that the patient is not ready to explore psychic associations, and the resident should focus on statements about the real world. If a patient asks her therapist if he is married, he reality-tests by saying yes. Otherwise he would reply, "Why do you ask?"

Therapeutic terms include adjectives not found in the APA classifications but important for describing what kind of mind the therapist has to work with. Patients were said to be "rigid," "austistic," and "perfectionist" in contexts analyzing what approach would be most therapeutic. These terms appear less variable than managerial terms but more so than APA labels. Style is more stable than behavior, and since the therapist basically sits and talks with the patient, her style of responding is more stable than her behavior in a twenty-four-hour period under the nurse's care. For example, a schizophrenic woman will probably be so labeled during her entire stay at the hospital even though she emits schizophrenic behavior a very small fraction of the time. At the beginning, she might display "flat affect" in therapy, which, in the mind of the resident, impedes progress. However, in time she might be able to express more affect, thus losing that therapeutic label. At a managerial level, one basic characteristic of therapeutic diagnoses is that they imply her labels could change at a variety of speeds.

The fourth family of classification is *dynamic diagnosis*. In the minds of residents, this is the skill they come to learn, and this is the diagnosis which really matters. Besides APA diagnosis, this is the only kind of diagnosis which staff and residents openly recognize. It is, in this case, rooted in psychoanalysis, and it contrasts sharply with more behavioral diagnoses. After a "nonsuicidal" patient made her first attempt, for example, the therapist said there was no dynamic change in the patient but it might take two years to find out why she did it. Dynamics is defined by residents as the structure of the unconscience, the defenses and fears which determine how a person relates to the world. They are found in the historical antecedents to current malaise.

> Ned Reich and I talked about making a dynamic assessment of a patient. He defined this as determining the patient's strengths and weaknesses, when they work, how they break down, and what happens.
>
> I asked him how this was different from a layman doing the same thing. He answered that we practice more and know the right questions to ask. I said I was surprised he did not mention that dynamics were based on an elaborate theory of mind. He replied that we really don't know.
>
> I asked if he did not want to be an analyst (as he had expressed before). He said, you make a commitment of faith, like a monk, and he did that long before he came here.
>
> Had his experiences here helped him to see whether there is reason for his faith or not? He answered that he could not explain how, but yes. He was surer there was something to analytic theory. But on the whole, he thought, the difference from a layman is that we make a lifetime practice of understanding each person's way of building his world.

At University Psychiatric Center, dynamics reduce to only a few basic issues, work and love, anger and loss. But discussions of a case are more elaborate and idiosyncratic. The entire structure of an interview is determined by its central interest in dynamics. The presentation contains bits of history which might supply "clues" to the patient's dynamics. The interview and discussion often concentrate on how the patient handles stresses as a reflection of his or her unconscious defenses and deprivations. Often the dynamics are quite elaborate, consisting of a little story which highlights the patient's personality structure. A weak example, because it is so descriptive and lacks an interpretative framework, is the psychiatrist in the diagnostic seminar telling about the girl's interest in having her family rejected or about the young man denying his sexual needs. A strong example, which encapsulates the patient's central problem in a theoretical statement, is given by the clinical director, Elvin Blumberg:

> I'm very glad we had this case, because it is good to talk about chronicity. Chronicity is the result of not resolving the first regression. Each sub-

sequent one has the same elements. The ego wants to try to integrate the conflicting elements again and again.

The death of her husband is not a loss, but has the tone of a sexual frustration. He left her sexually high and dry again. He abandoned her too.

The dynamic diagnosis, residents learn to believe, is the key to patient care. It is the most personal and most sensitive of the diagnostic classifications. It is also the only diagnosis which attempts to penetrate symptomatic evidence.

> *Resident No. 1:* In dynamics, you are interested in the *hammer* that smashed the crystal.
>
> *Resident No. 2:* No. You are interested in the *structure* of this crystal, why it broke the way it did. That's why Blumberg goes back to the first crisis, because subsequent ones have the same pattern.
>
> *Resident No. 3:* But when you make a diagnosis you end up with much less than with what you started. In contrast, look at the theory of crystals in physics. Here, we merely describe the *end state,* with not much implication about how it got that way.
>
> *Resident No. 4:* There's not been much progress. We just label the dominant symptom or sign.

Ironically, dynamic diagnosis is the only one which has no labels, no set terms, despite the theoretical machinery which underlies it. Therefore, as part of patient care, it remains weak. Finding labels necessary for communication, the residents and staff fall back on APA terms. But this necessary compromise has more permanent effects; for through daily use, APA terms become their language for patients, whom they then see as disease entities.

Despite the importance of dynamic diagnosis—or perhaps because of it—residents showed no critical awareness of its inadequacies. They got caught up in the endless game of speculative interpretation, using a tautological system of propositions about how the psyche works, trying hard to be as subtle at the game as their mentors. While they were learning it, two psychiatrists from U.C.L.A. were reporting their research at the national meetings of the A.P.A. on what they called "a psychiatric ritual."[18] They found that psychiatric residents and staff were no more likely to make a correct diagnosis from dynamic formulations than would be expected from chance, and they concluded, "The thinking process associated with the creation of dynamics formulations appears to represent a misuse of deductive reasoning typical of the psychiatrist's semantic efforts to play the scientific game."[19] This can be particularly confusing for residents, they argued, because "the psychiatric resident may present a given patient to several supervisors, each of whom has widely divergent views with respect to dynamics and may give markedly contrasting advice."[20] Examples of this difficulty are the two assessments of Mrs. Tucker in the chapter on case conferences.

Dynamic diagnosis completes the set of four diagnostic clusters. In working with patients, there is the need to catalog or quickly label them, to talk about their management with the ward staff, to talk about their therapy with the professional staff, and to explain the basic nature of their disorder. Each level of diagnosis carries its own set of expectations and organization of work. For example, management terms are learned from the nurses, and residents learn slightly different sets on each ward. Nurses, on the other hand, never seem to learn APA terms well, and they rarely presume to talk about the dynamics of the patient. This organizational separation of language has little to do with the intelligence or experience of nurses. Social workers, most of whom do therapy themselves, use APA terms and therapeutic terms but rarely dynamic vocabulary. Each set is used in different settings for different purposes: the APA set for basic labeling and policy, the managerial set for administration of patients, the therapeutic terms for supervision and individual psychotherapy, the dynamics for causal roots analyzed by psychiatrists.

The priority which residents give to the different diagnostic sets reveals their value system. Highest esteem is given to talk of dynamics, reflecting the great value residents place on the psychoanalytic model. This value is sometimes unconscious, as when residents who say they are not yet sure whether they will use the analytic model are at the same time using this talk, whose language allows them to think only in psychoanalytic terms. Next, residents value managerial and therapeutic sets, because each marks symptomatic behavior in an important sphere of activity. Residents claim least interest in labels and thus in APA terms, although they may be most trapped by them.

A great deal of "feel" is evident in how diagnoses are made, and residents learn how to "feel" while still appearing professionally precise. One example is calling a talkative, insistent woman an "hysteric." This was often synonymous with "an hysteric bitch," which conveyed the feeling more clearly. Taking another example, I spent a long time trying to find out when a patient with an "acute" diagnosis is labeled "chronic" and sent off to the state hospital. The answer quite simply is, when the therapist gives up trying. "Character disorder" is frequently used as the synonym for chronic among neurotic patients. If you feel the neurosis is embedded, you call it a character disorder. Finally, a striking example of feel is telling a sociopath from a schizophrenic, a difference so great that most people would not imagine it to be a problem. A female resident said that she could tell a sociopath from a schizophrenic by how she *felt* when he threatened her. If she felt he really meant it, he was a sociopath. If not, he was a schizophrenic.

Two particular problems of feeling out the diagnosis are deciding when a person is crazy and when a person is lying. Like everyone else, psychiatrists use the word "crazy," by which they mean psychotic. At the end of a case conference, the staff discussed this issue.

> Immediately after the patient left, the occupational therapist, who worked closely with the patient, said: "I can't see her as crazy. I guess it's my own feelings that keep me from seeing her that way."
>
> *Resident No. 1:* Yeah. How could she go through so much and look so good? It's hard to believe her fantasies. [She imagined that she and a movie star were in love and having a baby.]
>
> *Resident No. 2:* It's amazing that she has any affect left. She doesn't look crazy. [Note the main diagnostic category is "crazy."]
>
> *Resident No. 1:* If there's a constitutional disposition to schizophrenia, then she must have a constitutional disposition against it.
>
> *Chief:* She has an ego problem. She has trouble with her autonomy. She said she didn't mind if people took her things. [In the interview, she spoke of a certain patient who took her things. She said she didn't mind, because that patient only took from people she liked, and because she knows that the patient needed people. She said that it was nice to possess something that is now a part of someone you like.]
>
> *Interviewer:* She is *very sick*. It is just *because* the reasonable statements about the fantasies come so naturally that she is. [The main lesson.] . . . I recommend that treatment be as reality-oriented as possible.

After this conference, several residents talked excitedly about the case. They said that they had learned something, how deceptively normal a crazy patient can appear. In the case below, a resident "discovers" that his patient is psychotic.

At the conference she really came across as *crazy*. Up to then I was not so sure. I mean, she made a lot of sense sometimes; she was hangin' in there.

And I kept changing my diagnosis. When she first came in, I thought she might be schizy, but then I put down *borderline,* then *hysteric.* I wanted to put down the best thing with the best prognosis. I really did not want to believe she was crazy.

Even if no question arises as to whether the patient is sick or normal, there is constantly the question of whether the patient is telling the truth or "malingering." This problem is never resolved except by the viscera.

[Excerpts from the interview. The interviewer seemed to be intentionally harsh, to test the patient's authenticity.]

You think your marriage is all washed up?

Yes.

What have you learned with your therapist?

The way I go about getting things is no good.

How did you get things? [Note past tense.]

Devious. I was dishonest. [*Pause.*] I cheated my husband.

What about the hospital? Do you use the same devices?

I can't think of any examples.

What about the time when you . . . ?

Oh, yes. I forgot. Thank you, you're right.

EVALUATION

Interviewer: "When you decide whether they're ready to go, you're really playing God. There's no insurance."

"She says all the right things. She's learned all the right words to make us feel comfortable."

"I've decided to believe what the patient says, even if you have the sneaky feeling she's lying."

Feeling plays such a large role in diagnosis and treatment of mental illness that professional practice reflects the practitioner.[21] In psychiatry this interrelationship is strongly recognized, as evidenced by great focus on countertransference in the therapist. For example, the residents greeted the news that a man with twelve years of analysis had been admitted with hoots of laughter. Someone suggested he be interviewed by his analyst (more laughter). The residents rejected the suggestion, because the interview might become a mental status of the analyst rather than of the patient! After so many years, they said, a patient *is* his analysis, which in turn reflects his analyst; so that a diagnosis of the patient would be a diagnosis of the analyst. Yet the residents were never heard talking about their own personal and social biases. They declared patients to be ''crocks'' or ''fascinating,'' with no self-reflection. While they were being trained, researchers at University Psychiatric Center investigated biasing factors in the way second-year residents diagnosed and disposed of people who came to the outpatient clinic.[22] Like many researchers before them, they found that upper-class applicants, regardless of diagnosis, were offered treatment at the center, while lower-class applicants were referred elsewhere. Patients whom residents liked were offered psychotherapy more often and hospitalized less than patients they did not like. Summarizing these and other findings, the authors of one paper concluded:

> The results of this investigation clearly demonstrate that social position and interviewer attitudes are linked to the diagnostic process and to the allocation of available services.[23]

But they also found that residents were not aware of these biases, even though they are an inherent part of diagnosis. Despite the emphasis on self-examination in psychiatry, diagnosis remains an unselfconscious assessment by one group of people who ''know'' they are experts on another group of people who they ''know'' are ignorant.

8.

Case Conferences

One of the great arenas for learning about diagnosis, therapy, and administration is the case conference. Like a tribal ceremony, this dramatic ritual brings together nurses, student nurses, social workers, ministers, attendants, psychiatric residents, guests, psychologists, chiefs, superchiefs, and other staff to watch a senior member of the profession evaluate a patient. Here residents compete to make insightful remarks before their elders, find professional models of diagnosis and therapy, display their disregard for other members of the therapeutic staff, and resolve difficult issues in the care of patients. Case conferences at UPC took place in large rooms with chairs in rows on three sides, while the fourth wall served as a backdrop for the interview. Besides their formal purpose, conferences were a meeting place for busy staff who otherwise did not easily find one another; so clusters of people talked with each other until the chief arrived with the interviewer and announced that the conference would begin.

The patient's resident opened with a presentation of the case which included key events, crises or problems that led to holding the conference, the patient's psychic history, and the major aspects of psychiatric treatment, if any. There was widespread consensus that a good presentation took ten minutes or less. Often, however, this ideal was exceeded.

The chief complaint about case conferences was the length of presentations, and residents focused their criticisms on the social worker, nurse, and psychologist, whose reports followed theirs. (Psychiatrists "present"; others "report.") In cases where it applied, a social worker reported on the patient's family and on therapy she had done with the family. This could and often did overlap with the resident's presentation, and residents often complained about the social workers being redundant and lengthy. But often the same residents had made no effort to coordinate with the social worker on the case—a pattern which tells much about learned status, the primitive state in this program of "the therapeutic team," and the state of family therapy. One relegated the family to the social workers (whom, in this hospital, I found extraordinarily talented) and got on with "the real business of treating the patient."

The report of the psychologist raised another status issue, the discrepancy between longer, more rigorous training in psychological diagnosis than psychiatrists received, and the penalty of second-class citizenship for not having a medical degree. Unfortunately, many psychologists saw the case conference as an occasion when they could display their expertise. They gave long, jargon-filled reports on their tests which made the residents groan. If some laymen regard psychiatry as a parody of common sense, then psychiatric residents consider some psychologists as parodies of psychiatrists. Quite often, no psychological report was given, either because it had not been done or because it had not been requested by the resident, an omission which the psychologists resented.

Other reports might come from nurses and/or attendants who described the patient's behavior on the ward, his or her relationship with other patients, and problems of management. Once these were over, the interviewer (usually a guest) sometimes discussed the case briefly before signalling for the patient to be brought in.

A new resident presented for the first time Mrs. Tucker, a sad lady in her fifties, to Dr. Blumberg, the director of clinical training. In his presentation, the resident explained that her husband had recently died. He said she was "self-centered" and "unable to grieve." "She is aware that she can't grieve and complains that she might not be normal. But I think it is a device to gain my sympathy and get me to help her."[1] No diagnosis was given, except reference to her "recurrent depressions," which had been noted in the outpatient clinic.

Patient entered, shook hands with eyes down. Looked around at us. "What do you gentlemen want of me today?" Sighing, tired voice. "I seem to be deteriorating here [*rubs forehead heavily with hand*], I don't know. I forget things."

. . . .

Tucker: You can't see into a person's head here, can you.

Blumberg: Not really. And we can't really look into their hearts either.

Silence. She looks steadily at him for the first time.

Tucker: You mean the real heart?

Blumberg [*smiles*]*:* I think you know what I mean.

From this point on for thirty minutes, Blumberg got her to talk of her first lover, who had dumped her. He kept asking her, "What did you do with that feeling of excitement?" She finally revealed (it felt like a confession) that she had later slept with another man.

Suddenly she riveted her eyes on the audience of thirty and snapped, "How can I undress before all of you?!" She had not been looking at us before.

Blumberg: So the two of us [note "two"] can see what has to be seen.

Tucker [*immediately resigned and again only aware of Blumberg*]:[2] I hoped you could patch me up in a week or two and send me out as good as new.

Blumberg [*nods*]: That didn't work the first time, did it?

Tucker: No. Nor the next or the one after that. [*She suddenly turned to a resident*]: You don't have to smile about it! It may be funny to you but it's not to me. [Resident's face flushed.]

Blumberg asked her another question, as if the outburst had not occurred, and it succeeded in pulling her back to him and their conversation. He repeated his earlier question.

Tucker [*turning sharply to a nurse*]: Are you enjoying this? I'm sorry. I don't mean to be antagonistic.

Blumberg: But you'd rather be antagonistic than answer my question.

Tucker began to talk about her first experience at "self-relief." She also said she did it after her lover abandoned her.

Blumberg: Is the tendency for self-relief what causes your snapping?

Tucker: I don't know.

Blumberg: Is intimacy better than relief?

Tucker: Yes, with my husband, at least.

Blumberg: How about the first time you relieved yourself?

> *Tucker:* In the earlier years of our marriage, my husband was better.
>
> *Blumberg:* Does your doctor know how troubled you are about sex?[3]
>
> *Tucker [looks at her doctor]:* I think so. *[Doctor nods.]*
>
> *Blumberg:* Can I talk to your doctor about these things?
>
> *Tucker:* Do you need my permission?
>
> *Blumberg:* I'm asking you.
>
> *Tucker:* OK. *[To her doctor]:* Can you do anything for me? *[Doctor nods.]*

She doesn't want to leave. Blumberg thanks her for coming but she lingers on. She asks, "Do I have to go now?" She says something about the outside being nothing, void. She leaves slowly. The door closes behind her.

EVALUATION

The patient's resident asks why Blumberg had focused on the early years. It is clear that he has been focusing on the recent grieving over the lost husband, and later he says that he thought he was being classically analytic in focusing on "object loss."[4]

Blumberg says he was not convinced that she enjoyed her husband more than self-relief. He says she is trying to recapture the first experience of pleasure.

"That's why people get themselves into that psychotic state we call love, where no one pays any attention to what the other is doing."

The residents loved this folk wisdom of Blumberg's. Some thought it was corny, but over time Blumberg wore well with the residents as a wise analyst who was not caught in the jargon of his profession. His "looking into hearts and heads" exchange also appealed to them, and many tried it as an early technique.

All of the residents considered this interview to be a first-class example of psychoanalytic insight. Blumberg had uncovered new, early material on which he built the entire pathology of the case. The resident therapist, an analytic type, decided to change the focus of therapy to early sexual experiences. Nothing was said about the public humiliation which the patient had suffered.

The Social Functions of Case Conferences

Case conferences serve a number of purposes, some more recognized than others. In the early phases of psychiatric socialization, they provide a frequent source of microtechniques for groping residents to try out on their own patients.[5] Later, they provide whole models of psychotherapy, though not as satisfactory as supervisors, with whom a resident can work over a longer period. At all times, case conferences illuminate the techniques of interviewing. Visiting interviewers are also a source of personal psychoanalysts and therapists for the residents, particularly as countertransference issues and the professional culture move them toward psychoanalysis. Here, as a number of them mentioned, they can watch leading analysts in action and imagine themselves as the patient.

Ostensibly, case conferences help the presenting resident solve problems of diagnosis, therapy, and management. Residents also say it is useful to sit back and watch someone else work with one's patient. But for residents in the audience, the case conference is a forum of wits, a chance to outguess the interviewer and to show up one's peers in the presence of senior staff. For the audience staff as a whole, the conferences serve to reaffirm everyone's role and status in the patterns of seating, the structure of the presentation, and the discussion of the case. The next few pages detail some of these eight functions.

Learning to Interview

Case conferences are not the only place where residents learn to interview, but they provide a steady stream of new ideas and examples. Unlike at a medical conference, the interview is the core of the case conference; it is primary data for the analysis. Eventually, residents tire of conferences as they gain confidence in their interviewing ability. Their attention turns from the particulars of interviewing to the techniques of the therapeutic hour or week,[6] and for this the vignettes of case conferences are much less helpful than supervision.

The interview begins with seating, which in the case conference consists of two chairs in the middle the "stage," about five feet apart. One learns as a therapist that one should sit still. Shifting positions conveys a sense of uneasiness and even weakness; the man of strength does not move. One sits back, not forward with elbows on knees like an athletic coach. One learns to look steadily at the patient, with full concentration. These attributes alone would make it easy to distinguish the therapist from the patient in a silent movie, even if both were dressed and groomed alike.

One technique of sitting so intrigued the residents that it deserves mention. It was Blumberg's position. Essentially, he reclined in the chair, with his body sloping away from the patient, so that he would turn his head and talk to the patient over the chair's arm nearest the patient. This brought Blumberg's head a foot closer to the patient than the rest of his body. If Blumberg had swung around, bringing his whole body a foot closer as well, the patient might have squirmed. The position created an atmosphere of intimacy without imposition.

Another technique of interviewing is to keep the patient focused on the interview, and in the public forum of a case conference this general problem becomes greatly accentuated. The patient and interviewer are to pretend that the others do not exist or that the interview is taking place in a storage room full of mannequins. If a patient talks to anyone else in the room, that person will remain silent and try very hard to show no facial or emotional response. If the patient insists, the member of the audience (often the patient's own therapist to whom he or she turns when unsure about something in the interview) will say something to direct the attention of the patient back to the interviewer. However, the protracted silence which follows the patient's turning to speak to some familiar member of the audience whom s/he sees daily is enough to make him or her turn back to the one person in the room who will speak. Residents do not like this artifice but say it is the only practical way to get on with the interview. In any case, a large number of patients do seem to forget that anyone else is in the room.

Many residents believe that how one opens an interview is critical to what follows. Usually the interviewer opens the conversation. One interviewer impressed me and one resident as especially natural:

> *Interviewer:* Why don't you sit down?
>
> [Patient does, in the first chair.]
>
> *Interviewer:* Do me a favor, uh, and sit over here. I need the ashtray.
>
> *Patient* [*smiling*]: I need it too.
>
> [Interviewer lights her cigarette.]
>
> I've been hearing some things about you, and I guess you've had some trouble. [Straightforward and honest yet suggestive.]
>
> Yes.

Tell me about it.

From the beginning?

Well, start wherever you want. [An outpouring followed.]

Another interviewer who knew the case began, "How are you getting along?" (Oh, fine. . . .) "What's been happening to you since I last saw you?" He was very direct and moved in very fast.

In a final example, the patient came in the room rapidly and quickly sat down. (Male patient, female interviewer.) The interviewer began, "What's your trouble?" Her tone was soft and one sensed that she had completely engaged the patient and that they were oblivious to the rest of the room. The patient replied, "I've commited suicide several times. I haven't changed since I came here."[7]

Many of the openings, however, struck me as quite silly, if not insulting and offensive, though the residents did not comment on it. On the other hand, several patients did.

For example:

OPENING NO. 1

Interviewer: Won't you sit down? [Patient sits.] I think you know everyone here. [Patient looks around, which he had not before.] What do you think this conference is about?

OPENING NO. 2

Interviewer: We've been talking about you.

Patient: I figured that.

What do you want us to figure?

I don't know.

Are you at peace with yourself?

Yes . . . but I get nervous with lots of people around. [*Looks at audience.*]

So, [*leans back*] you aren't at peace with yourself. [Patient does not reply.]

OPENING NO. 3

Patient comes in, shakes hands, sits and looks away.

Are you nervous?

Yeah.

So am I before crowds. Why don't you look around you and see how many familiar faces there are. [Patient does so briefly.] As best as you can estimate, what is the purpose of this interview?

To figure out plans for the future.

Do you have plans?

Yeah, Go into the community and work.

What would you do?

I'd be a file clerk.

Have you worked before?

Yeah, in factories after high school. . . . Why are you asking me all these questions?

I want to know how you did before you came here.

It brings crazy feelings.

Crazy? . . . Can you tell us about them?

No. [Patient continues neither to face the interviewer nor to look at him.]

A good interview gets through the defenses of the patient, exposes basic aspects of his problems, and reconstitutes him so he can leave the room, all in about twenty minutes. Residents most admired those who they felt "get at basic material" without ruffling the patient in the slightest.[8] Less subtle but also admired is the interviewer who strips the patient before the audience, as Blumberg did in Mrs. Tucker's first interview, and patches the patient's emotions up enough for her to exit. To the residents as to other psychiatrists, "basic material" consists of events and feelings about sex, intimacy, and loss. The analytic ideal of "getting at" lets the patient take herself there through multiple associations, but residents showed more interest in quicker techniques, like those of Blumberg.

As deviant cases will, one interview highlighted some of the normal features of conference interviews. In this case, the psychiatrist looked away from the patient about 60 percent of the time. In most interviews, the doctor looks at the patient without ever losing eye contact, almost scrutinizing the patient. Also, this doctor told the patient about his problems very early and very extensively. After three minutes he had told the patient that he was "a very sick man" and the reasons why. He even alluded to "your weird smile." Residents said they admired this doctor for his sincere honesty and concern for the patient. Finally, this interviewer talked about two-thirds of the time, while most interviewers talk as little as possible.

In his effort to get at basic material, the interviewer has great advantages over the patient. He or she knows about the patient's weak points and major defenses before the patient enters. Also he or she asks the questions, and most patients allow the interviewers to probe as far as they wish. The pressure can be great. For example, one patient was quietly protective of the probes the interviewer made into his sadness, his depression, his troubles. After several attempts, the interviewer, who knew this beforehand, flatly said, "Your penis isn't working right, is it." He continued to press upon the patient all the negative things in his life, such as his failure with women, which he also knew from the resident's presentation, until he succeeded in "bringing out" the patient's sadness. Residents constantly discussed and thought about ways to break down defenses. Some residents thought this interviewer had been too crude and inconsiderate; others replied that the technique had worked.[9]

Finally, the interview must end. From observation and residents' discussions, the main purpose is to get the patient emotionally reconstituted and focused on how he or she can improve. Often, for example, the interviewer will begin the close by asking the patient if he or she has any questions. The interviewer has no intention of going into them, but this prods the patient (who has been *responding* for some time) to take the *initiative*. The close also redirects the patient from the interviewer to the therapist, as when Blumberg asked Mrs. Tucker, "Does your doctor know how troubled you are about sex?" And although Mrs. Tucker saw through the artifice, he also asked, "Can I talk to your doctor about these things?" In private therapy, the analogous task is to turn the patient from the particulars of the session's discussion to the task of living until the next appointment.

Solving Problems—Types of Conferences

More than any other factor, the presenting problem of a case conference determines its shape. Based on this variable, there are six types of conferences. *Analytic* conferences focus on the person's psychic history and psychodynamics. This, of course, is a kind of diagnosis, but these conferences differ from *diagnostic* ones, where the chief concern is to formulate a specific diagnosis. (Is he a schizophrenic or a sociopath? Is she crazy or just courting our sympathy?) In analytic conferences, diagnosis at this level is already known; yet the resident or his chief feel there is need to understand more about how the psyche works. The style of such conferences is more leisurely and exploratory.

Occasionally, *neurological* conferences are held, because it has been decided that the patient's problems stem largely from some disorder in the nervous system. These are the only conferences with a strong medical flavor. The residents delight in them; at the few ones observed, there was an excited atmosphere of being back home again. Questions came forth with unusual eagerness. Few transformations are so dramatic as residents' attitudes toward a patient "lagging" in psychotherapy when it is discovered he has a neurological deficiency. Suddenly issues of "working with the patient" disappear. The cause of disorder is physiological and thus fated. The patient-doctor contract changes; immediately "problems of therapy" become irrelevant. Residents talk only of administrative arrangements; for there are no longer questions of psychodynamics. In these cases, medicine is embraced like a lost friend.

Therapeutic conferences, by contrast, are concerned solely with the problems of doing therapy with the patient. The focus is usually, but not always, either on the present or on certain blocking points in the therapy.

Administrative conferences concern problems of management, such as disruptive and unresponsive patients. Of course, these could be and should be considered as therapeutic problems, but such conferences have a distinct, administrative tone which indicates that what to *do* with the patient is not the same as how to *treat* him or her.

Finally, *discharge* conferences are distinct from other kinds of administrative conferences because they carry in them the tone that the patient is being dumped, rejected or the tone that the patient has recovered enough to leave. However, most cases selected for discharge conferences do not represent successes but the knotty problems of failures.

The Ethics and Language of Judgment

Residents quickly learn how to use psychiatric language to disguise their feelings toward a patient. We have already seen examples of how residents and psychiatrists talk to gloss over ambiguities and to simplify—perhaps oversimplify—a person's problems. A good example is the first conference of Mr. Downs.

> Mr. Downs, the resident began, was a quiet, sober, silent patient, unresponsive to personal therapy. He could not handle loss or potential loss and had been in and out of the hospital for several years. He lived alone and was in his fifties.
>
> Before coming to the conference, the resident reported, Mr. Downs was very worried about being presented. "They'll trap me," he said. The resident looked at his colleagues: "The sounds paranoid, doesn't it?"
>
> . . . .
>
> The resident ended his presentation by saying, "He has been believed to have involuntary psychosis with paranoid features. His defenses are largely obsessive-compulsive."[10]

After the interview, the senior psychiatrist asked the resident for his recommendation, and the resident said he had "been going back and forth on EST." On one hand, he said, it is "barbaric," and Mr. Downs would lose his memory, which was important for his regular job. On the positive side, he continued, Mr. Downs is not "really" getting better using other "modalities."[11] The resident said he had just seen EST and did not think it was so barbaric. Moreover, the EST physician had told him you can do shock without memory loss. At this point the audience laughed. The chief intervened. "He is chronic. EST, like everything else, does less well with chronics." Since the effective definition of "chronic" means "unresponsive to therapy," the chief was right, but like most psychiatrists, he made the diagnosis "chronic" as if were scientific and had some existence independent of the therapist's frustration at getting the patient to respond. The resident replied that the EST physician had gotten "some spectacular results with chronics on EST. EST is not optimal, but it's the last thing we have to offer before giving up."[12]

Five months later, there was another conference on Mr. Downs. This time the presentation was stronger. It began, "This is the eighth

admission of this fifty-nine-year old, white man. . . ." The same resident intensified the impression of hospitalization by saying that recently the patient had been in hospitals two-thirds of the time and that
the intervals between remissions were diminishing. The presentation
was shorter and led to two questions.

> One, is this hospital with its capacities and talents best for him? Are
> we contributing to his deterioration? [Resident shows file which is two
> inches thick.]
> Two, is he good from the view of teaching residents? We have him
> as administrators, and we seem to be witnesses to what's going on
> without being able to influence treatment.

Following this statement, the resident went into the family history,
therapy, present state, and current treatment. The patient, he said,
"blocks EST completely." [13] Everything has been tried. "Nothing
works." The patient was now on Mellaril. The interviewer interrupted
to say that prolonged use of Mellaril affects the eyes. The resident
looked surprised and said he did not know that. (An implicit criticism
of the chief?) On the first treatment of EST after the July conference,
the patient "responded dramatically . . . and his stay was very short."
But Mr. Downs had to be readmitted, and this time he became very
demented after the fifth EST. Mr. Downs, concluded the exasperated
resident, is a person with "involutional psychotic reaction with loose
and paranoid ideas who is becoming a chronic patient." [14]

The tortured discussion which followed reflects the profession's
ambivalence over dirty work. These good men must care for persons
society cannot tolerate, but at times like these the task exceeds even
their tolerance. Their obligations to the patient, to society and to themselves had become irreconcilable.

> *Staff Psychiatrist No. 1* (Interviewer): Before discussing the ques-
> tions, how does he affect the people around him? How does he make you
> feel?
> *Resident therapist:* He seems so helpless. . . . I feel I have no con-
> trol over his stay here. [15]
> *Old Therapist* [unusual to have a patient's old therapist at a confer-
> ence, but in this case he is at the hospital]: When I had him he seemed
> helpless at first and I wanted to do something for him. But more and
> more I got angry. [For the therapist to get angry is a criticism of the *pa-
> tient*.] In general, the service feels frustrated. We've tried everything
> with no results.

Interviewer: Downs is being *asked* to perform and he knows it. The residents show it and he knows it and freezes up. I suppose it is true that a teaching hospital has these demands [on the patient], but I want to show how these attitudes are harmful.

Resident therapist: I've taken the other side, that he should go slowly.

Interviewer: I also think he may come here so he can avoid the lonely lunch and have a nice resident to talk to. He got out of the state hospital fast when he was there for ten days.[16]

There are two ways of thinking about transfer. One, as therapeutic. Or as just throwing in the sponge.

Resident No. 1: It's not therapeutic. Once he knows this place is not available, he will give in to the state hospital instead of getting out.

Resident No. 2: Are we talking about long- or short-term therapy? Transfer might be short-term therapy if it shocked him out of his dependency on hospitals. Long-term would be getting him a home with foster parents.

Superchief: For over two years he has had his way. Nothing has an effect. He would never leave if no one mentioned it to him.[17]

. . . .

Resident No. 2: Are we thinking about us or him?

Interviewer: You should have him required to do occupational therapy. Scrub the floors for an hour. [!]

Chief: I cannot separate our anger from his.

Interviewer: I wasn't going to say this, but this is a way of the ward expressing its anger at him in a way that might help Mr. Downs.

[Near me, resident No. 2 is whispering to a nurse about lobotomy.]

Interviewer: One thing is lobotomy.

Resident No. 2 [laughs]: That is just what I was saying. He is classic. We said we tried everything, but we didn't state the obvious conclusion!

The interviewer then told stories of *successful* lobotomies. The second staff psychiatrist mentioned that VPC had two in ten years.

Resident No. 2: First I think we should raise the themothyazines some.

. . . .

Chief: Why not try more shock treatments? It did some good before.

Interviewer: You might send him home too. Push him out and see if he can make it.

Resident therapist: That contradicts what you said before.

Chief: When you push Downs, he just collapses.

Resident No. 2: It's funny. After the gruesome idea of lobotomy, we turned to all these optimistic alternatives.

Resident No. 3: All this has been on whether the decision is therapeutic. Should we throw in the sponge?

Interviewer: Definitely not.

End.

Seemingly the conference had no conclusion. Several weeks later the therapist talked about the conference. "I was ready to transfer him at the conference, but when a big gun like that tells you to try harder, you think twice." But while the resident therapist was trying again, the chief and superchief decided to transfer Mr. Downs, and the resident agreed.

Learning to Be Comfortable

As these examples show, residents learned there were many ways to handle a patient. While at first they tried to figure out which techniques were the most effective in what circumstances, this scientific frame of mind necessarily faded as they realized the data were too vague for such precise solutions to their anxieties as young therapists. The answer was to use the approach or techniques that were most comfortable for you, the therapist. Consider the second conference with Mrs. Tucker, in which the resident presented all the history of her sex life which Dr. Blumberg had brought out. The resident had been inspired to continue therapy with her, but she was always deprecating herself and he couldn't get her motivated. The interviewer, a senior psychiatrist invited to review the case, made the following analysis.

Your approach is all wrong. Agree with everything she says about being rotten, lazy, helpless. Do it to the end. When she says she is deteriorating, say, "Yes, you probably are. I'm not sure how much improvement we can expect for you."

[The suggestion excited the room. Excellent gamesmanship.]

"The patient is ambivalent about her worthlessness," Blumberg explained. "Otherwise she would commit suicide instead of talking about it. What she does is to transfer her intrapsychic ambivalence to her interpersonal relation with her therapist. She says how bad things are, and those around her play out the positive role. But if you support her statements of woe, she will start to say, 'Well, I'm not all *that* helpless.' Then you tell her you're not sure she is right, and she'll answer, 'If I try I can get better.' "

Resident No. 2: Won't this reinforce her depression and lead to [*draws finger across throat, saying krrrr*]?

Interviewer: No. Also, this way you are not arguing with her about the state of the world. Your relation is better.

Resident therapist: I'm getting to learn this technique through sheer exasperation.

This therapeutic interview contrasted sharply with the first, analytic one in the therapy recommended. The resident therapist liked both equally and felt he learned something vital from each. Both interviewers made dramatic interpretations which kept all of the residents on the edge of their chairs. This interviewer's lesson in brinksmanship gave the residents the thrill of cliff walking and the fear of disaster.

Over time, the essential message of therapeutic conferences and experiences in one's own work is that almost any approach can be defended as professionally respectable. In this case the resident had experienced two reversals of treatment with no indication of what would work. His original focus on current loss may have been as sensible as the other two; all three approaches were based on sensible arguments. Also, this second conference with Mrs. Tucker was one of several points at which residents learned that their anger, resentment, and disgust with a patient could be expressed and be considered as "therapeutic." What mattered most was that one was in touch with one's feelings. The goal of work on countertransference is not so much to eliminate the therapist's neuroses from therapy with patients as to make them conscious.

Matching Wits and Gaining Status

By force of habit acquired in high school, college, and medical school, residents are very competitive. Yet competitive structures and clear rewards are conspicuously missing from psychiatric training. In this program, residents knew that in some way supervisors were rating them; but how, on what, to whom, and with how much effect on the future was hard to know. Even being selected as a chief in the third year did not necessarily imply distinction. Many residents did not apply, and part of the culture said that ward chiefs were residents who never grew up and wanted to return to their first year. In this vacuum, the case conference stood out as a forum for competitive display. It was superior to other staff meetings because of its size and because a star psychiatrist was visiting. For the presenting resident, this meant composing a perfect synopsis of the patient's problems, the relevant history, and the main questions for the interviewer. No fat, but no meat trimmed. For the audience, the conference provided material on which to try one's wits. Thus the conference is full of whispered asides to one's neighbor. But if one wants to gain status, one has to come out in the open. One resident especially adept at such gamesmanship explained over lunch how it works.

> There are the case conference games, which are very different from therapy games, and which are linked closely with your status in the hierarchy. The object is to impress your colleagues, and the rules for doing this vary from place to place.
> For example, at University Psychiatric the in thing to do is to show that your patient is *healthier* than the next doctor thinks he is. We rarely emphasize the healthy aspects of the patient, and it is always cool to prove the validity of what is not normally considered.
> At the Veteran's hospital where I used to work, the in thing was to make your patient out as *sicker* than he seemed to the next guy. For example, you took what the patient said as "an oral manifestation of genital feelings" or of anal needs, regardless what he said!
> There are different degrees of sophistication to this process. Another resident at the table agreed. The simplest is to state that while everyone else thinks your patient is X (e.g., sick) he is really Y (e.g., healthier). Even better is to describe all the steps and history needed to demonstrate this statement. Most subtle of all is to show that Y really *includes* X, which of course makes rebuttal impossible from the other side. If you are talking with a superior, this is a way of showing the superior that he was really saying more than he thought he was!
> Let's say someone in the conference says we have to be tough with this patient. Doctor B one-ups by saying, why are you talking about being tough? Are you angry at the patient? (There's nothing so cool as pointing out another resident's unconscious countertransference.)
> Then you speak up as person C and say, "Why is everyone talking about anger? What this patient needs is tight restrictions. Reality testing is the real issue." Reality testing is in here. You challenge the whole premise of the conversation.
> To top that, you say that by setting limits for the patient we are really giving something to the patient, and by the current lack of restric-

tions we are showing our anger at the patient. That way you include all their discussion into your argument. Of course you can do this in reverse just as easily!

The irony of this primer on professional one-upmanship is that both residents at the table were very involved in their patients' care and made sincere pleas for specific treatments, only to be one-upped by a more detached colleague.

What is a Good Conference?

From numerous conversations emerged the residents' image of a good conference. It is, above all, dramatic. Either by revealing some new facet, such as Mrs. Tucker's early sex life, or by putting matters in a fresh light, such as recommending that one agree with Mrs. Tucker's despair, the conference opens up new perspectives. A good conference is never long; presentations are crisp and brief. Attendance must be good, and the patient must show up. The interviewer must be good, well-matched with the patient. Much time was spent trying to match well. For example, Blumberg believed that most psychiatric problems came down to loss; so the whole hospital brought him patients with problems of loss, which affirmed his wisdom. The interviewer must never be condescending, never use the "when you've had more experience, you'll understand" line.

Patients' Response to Conferences

That some patients were suddenly not outside the conference door when their therapist went to fetch them—despite precautions against this happening—and that some patients responded, as did Mrs. Tucker, to the audience, deserves attention. As with "normal" people, patients vary in their taste for conferences. Some love the display; others loathe it. However, quite often a patient would be reported as "decompensated" or agitated soon after a conference.[18]

Both patients and residents were uneasy about a coming conference. Depending on the resident and on scheduling, a patient could know as much as two weeks in advance when he or she would be presented. Often, however, residents did not find out until near the date because of last-minute arrangements, or might not want to tell their patient. Residents felt a betrayal at exposing to the public a private, confidential (seemingly), therapeutic relationship, and at forcing the patient to speak before a crowd. Sometimes residents admitted that they had not prepared their patients for the event—another example of what psychiatrists call countertransference.

Thus both psychiatrists and patients school themselves to evade or deny the more painful features of public conferences. One patient said that her doctor had mentioned the conference two weeks in advance. She didn't think about it at all until the night before, when she got nervous. That morning she couldn't eat and felt very nervous—could not stop walking around. It was the thought of all those people that upset her. She said it was not fair to have a patient go in front of all those people. But when she walked into the conference, she tried to block out the presence of the others, and it worked pretty well.

Other patients faced the reality of conferences and dealt with them maturely.

> I was talking to John, a patient, about his conference. I asked him what he thought.
> "It's a rather coarse situation, don't you think?" he said in his refined accent. "I mean, do they really expect anyone to give them much information about themselves under those circumstances? I'm not going to tell some man I've never met before about myself, with no chance to know him, and I came in there with no intention of doing so."
> I said I agreed.
> He asked how they reacted, and I said they knew what he knew, that he did not want to say much. I did not tell him that this was used to portray him as "extremely defensive."

At the beginning of residency, the therapeutic-type residents (see p. 52) felt like John, and even volunteered such opinions once or twice. Otherwise the subject never came up. Later in the year therapeutic types, when asked, felt badly about it and said they tried to forget it. The other two types said that patients here pay a price as objects for training in return for good, cheap care. "It's a price they pay for coming here."

Some patients are more explicit about not cooperating. To do so takes more courage than most people, especially troubled people, can muster. A few patients simply do not show up. If they do not want to go through the risks involved in running away, they slip into a crevasse of the basement until lunchtime. Below is a case conference of a patient who openly refused to cooperate.

> *Interviewer:* Is this your first time here? [He knew it was not.][19]
> *Patient:* No.
> *Interviewer:* What ideas do you have of what we want?
> *Patient:* You want to ask me questions about what's wrong with me and why I am here.

The main theme was that she said she would not talk. He asked if she kept things to herself? No, she said, she shared them with her therapist, but she did not want to confide in a stranger. "You aren't relevant to my therapy, and I don't know you."

The interviewer persisted doggedly. He would repeat what she said, putting it in a question. She would just keep saying, "That's right." For example:

I'm not relevant to your therapy?

That's right.

[*Pause*]: Do you really think I am not relevant to your therapy?

That's right.

Next, the interviewer changed to "You fend me off."

I'm sorry. [Said sweetly.]

You push me away every time I try to help you. [Note, he assumes that he was close to the patient to begin with, and has the *right* to be.]

I don't mean anything personal.

Did you plan to do this to me even before you met me?

Yes.

Well, you defeat me. I am at your mercy. Why won't you talk?

It's none of your business.

EVALUATION

As she left, a resident let out a big sigh. "Gee whiz. When she first started I thought she really had a point. It's really amazing that patients can come in here and talk as they do to strangers.

"But then when you pleaded and offered her your help, and she pushed it off, it seemed to me that any normal person would have responded. She was very cold."

Her therapist: "Well, I didn't think she would talk *that* much. We had a big hassle on whether she would come at all."

The discussion was entirely on the material in the presentation, deciding whether she was "oedipal" or "oral" or both.

No diagnosis was given, but all agreed that her basic problem was *trust,* which went back to her not feeling loved.[20]

This unusual patient, by being neither contemptuous nor deferential, brought out the moral character of the case conference. After the interviewer had tried every technical tactic, trying to corner her with her own material, he turned to the moral foundation of psychiatric practice.[21] Patients, who are ignorant and weak, should seek the wisdom and strength of psychiatrists.

The structure of the conference itself accentuates the power of the interviewer, as two patients observed as they talked about their conferences.

What made conferences so powerful and scary are certain techniques, they said. Your therapist can continue to make you self-aware of your feelings but after the beginning he can't ask blunt questions, because he knows the stuff already.

But a new man, they continued, can and does. For example, one of the patients had cut his wrists, and the opener at his conference was, "How are your wounds?"

"Wham! That really knocked me flat."

They both said they disliked the audience, but a good interviewer will concentrate so much on you "that there are only the two of you and you forget the rest."

One of them illustrated how powerful this was. He was deep in an interview with [an admired interviewer] who got him to talk about very sad things. Suddenly the interviewer sat back, turned to the room and said, "When you get the patient to this point, you should not let him wallow in his sorrow, but pursue further into the roots of his sadness." Then he quickly leaned forward again and in the soft, intimate tone which he used with patients, continued to interview as if nothing had happened.

The patient said that he was mad inside, but he did not admit it to himself, and the interviewer was able to engage him immediately where he had left off and make him forget again that the audience was there. [I am reminded of brainwashing in *Manchurian Candidate.*]

After the conference, the patient said, he went to the back window and looked out until tears streamed, he was so mad at the interviewer. But he never told his therapist.

Although residents sometimes felt embarrassed about the public display of patients' private lives before strangers, at root they believed that no supplicant is a stranger among priests. To politely reject the opportunity is to be a cold, abnormal person. The profession responds through diagnosis, by considering the rejection itself as further evidence of how pathological the patient is and therefore of how much he or she needs their help.[22]

9.

Treating Suicide

Few acts disturb the peace of men's minds as does suicide. To many it seems less understandable than murder—or perhaps too understandable for comfort. More than any other major profession, psychiatry grapples with suicide. Ironically, it often succumbs to suicide as well. Suicidal people and those who try to help them assume that psychiatrists are experts in suicide care, possessing special diagnostic and therapeutic tools.[1] Yet the observations of this study and reports on suicide care indicate that such an assumption is often not warranted.

Residents learned in a haphazard way how to treat suicidal patients. They would get them by chance, and they would be supervised by junior staff assigned to the service where they were working or by one of their regular supervisors who was free to discuss the case. Each of these supervisors, however, had learned the same way, haphazardly from others who had worked out their own folk theories of how to handle suicidal patients. These ranged from very conservative practices of restriction to liberal beliefs that suicidal people must be given all the chances possible to take responsibility for their own lives to dramatic tactics where the psychiatrist would confront the patients with their own ambivalence and thereby help them to pull themselves together. Residents could—and did—get different advice on a case from each supervisor they consulted. In short, the blind led the blind, and there was no true expertise about treating suicidal persons. Although there is a common body of knowledge and techniques that specialists in suicide care have shared for a long time, it was not taught.[2]

This lapse in training would not have been so appalling if psychiatrists did not see themselves and were not considered as having the professional and medical expertise to treat suicidal persons. Given that the residents, like those before them, graduated from training as sure of their own folk theories as those who had graduated before them, there is no reason to believe that this generation feels any less qualified or is any more in need of systematic training than the generation who taught them. Alan Stone, professor of psychiatry at Harvard, has written that ". . . many psychiatrists possess no systematic or comprehensive approach for dealing with suicidal patients."[3] A research team at U.C.L.A., where more work has been done on suicide care than anywhere else in the nation, concluded, "In short, then, one might expect that the major personnel of psychiatric hospitals are not optimally suited by predisposition, training or experience to deal with the issue of suicide in a rational and objective fashion."[4]

Suicide Care and Psychiatrists

As noted in chapter 2, psychiatrists score high on death anxiety and therefore may not be suited by predisposition to handle suicidal cases well. Many studies note how terrified psychiatrists are by suicide, and during residency one learns in a deep irrational way to dread the prospect of having a suicide on one's hands the way one learns to cringe at electroshock therapy. Summarizing interviews with over two hundred psychiatrists whose patients had committed suicide, Litman wrote, "The reaction of therapists as therapists emphasized fears of being sued, of being vilified in the press, of being investigated, and of losing professional standing."[5] Other investigators have described the initial response as similar to a traumatic neurosis.[6]

Treating suicidal people, then, requires a certain kind of personality and expertise. Since suicide centers were first begun at the turn of the century (by ministers and social workers, because physicians refused to treat them), a consensus has arisen about how best to help suicidal people.[7] This includes being warm but fearless, so that the threat of suicide does not distort one's work. Suicide workers emphasized active support and intervention, unlimited availability, a willingness to take risks with death, a team approach to therapy, and network therapy that mobilizes significant others in the person's life. Countertransference is particularly dangerous; practitioners advise others to handle only one or two cases at a time and talk over the cases with a colleague or supervisor.[8] Harvey Shein, a national authority on training for suicide care, concluded in 1974: "However, it is my impression based on discussion with many residency program directors, that such comprehensive education is now being provided in only very few residency training programs."[9] The situation has not improved since then.

Given indications of poor training, one should not be surprised that a prevalent theme in the studies of suicide care is that the patient has been mistreated. One begins with evidence that therapists make a number of errors in their work. They often fail to ascertain the extent of suicidal danger[10] or they commonly write off nonlethal attempts as "manipulative gestures," a term that connotes an unserious, irritated approach by the therapist. Considering how many attempters commit suicide later, this is an irresponsible distinction.[11] In addition, doctors prescribe a variety of drugs to suicidal patients. Davis found, in a study of over two hundred people who committed suicide with barbiturates prescribed by physicians, that over two-thirds had a history of previous suicide attempts.[12] Another study showed that one-third of the persons killing themselves in the San Francisco area used prescription drugs.[13] Mintz concludes, "One might indeed ponder what kind of a nonverbal communication the suicidal person must feel he is receiving when he is handed a prescription for a potentially lethal quantity of drugs."[14]

More detailed studies support Mintz's suspicion. A study of thirty patients who committed suicide as inpatients or soon after discharge showed that 30 percent had attempted suicide before. It found three patterns of therapy which contributed to the suicidal act.[15] First, some therapists did not recognize an event or crisis of great importance to the patient.[16] Second, a number of therapists were pessimistic and discouraging to the patient about the progress being made in therapy. Third, therapists refused to tolerate the "infantile" demands and dependency of the patients. This last pattern was found by seven others and appears to be the most common.[17] In a review of thirty-two suicides over ten years at a clinic, Victor Bloom found "that each suicide was preceded by rejecting behavior by the therapist."[18]

The clinical material on psychiatrists rejecting suicidal patients describes a powerful sequel.[19] Coming to someone as a last resort, the suicidal person finds an initial concern that gives hope. The person begins to lean on the therapist as the therapist begins to analyze defense mechanisms which the person uses to barely keep going. This leaves the person even more vulnerable and dependent on the helper's support. The therapist feels this pressure, calls it infantile regression, and pulls back. Problems of countertransference loom large. Therapy is reduced without explanation; the helper "forgets" to give a phone number; he or she goes away without notice; the therapist's manner in treatment becomes more curt. Feeling abandoned by the one individual who seemed strong and supporting, the patient commits suicide.

Training that perpetuates the myth that all staff are equally competent to teach residents how to care for suicidal persons contributes to such therapeutic tragedies. Moreover, psychoanalytically based therapy, with its emphasis on deep probing and nonintervention, is just what most suicidal persons cannot tolerate and contrasts sharply with recommended procedures.[20] But to admit this and the need for a special program would require the staff to admit their ignorance and the limitations of their techniques.

Beliefs about Suicide

The unspoken pact of fear and ignorance that keeps residents and staff from dealing openly with the special problems of suicide results in beliefs and rituals that reflect on all psychiatric work.[21] When residents worked with suicidal patients, they believed that suicide gestures or statements were "a cry for help," an expression of the healthy part of the patient that wants to overcome despair. After suicide, residents and staff talked about how the desire to suicide comes from an irrational, inaccessible part of the psyche. In treating suicidal patients, concerted—even extreme—efforts were made to stop it, such as confining the patient to a small, bare room and having a staff member sit at the door twenty-four hours a day watching the patient. After suicide, residents and staff talked about how "you can't stop someone from committing suicide if they want to die." During treatment, residents were taught to show the patient how s/he is responsible for his or her life and were counseled to mollify their overwhelming sense of responsibility.

Seasoned therapists unambiguously articulated this point of view to residents. Yet both staff and resident therapists used restrictions, involuntary commitment and drugs to prevent suicide. After a patient killed him- or herself, the double message was still there, but in new language. Staff and residents believed that the patient was responsible for his or her life, but they deeply felt that it represented therapeutic failure. In these shifts of belief before and after suicide one sees how suicide is the chisel which splits apart the tenuously joined halves of psychiatric identity, between the responsible physician who cannot help and the helping therapist who does not wish to be responsible.

The interaction between symbols and social situation represented by altering beliefs and the social functions they serve are partially illustrated by the case of a young man whom we shall call Daniel Forman.

> The chief walked straight to his chair next to the nurse at the front of the horseshoe of patients and stated like a news item at six o'clock: "The reason for this special meeting is that there is some sad news: Mr. Forman is dead."
>
> Immediately, from a patient: Who is he?
>
> *Chief:* He committed suicide probably over the weekend in the [place] where he worked.
>
> Gasps throughout the audience.
>
> Who is he?
>
> *Chief:* He was admitted on the [date].
>
> Oh, was he the one with curly hair?
>
> How old was he?
>
> What did he look like? [All these questions were by female patients.]
>
> *Chief:* Apparently, he [chief describes how Forman killed himself.]
>
> *Patient:* It makes you so scared. You need help and you can't even get help here.
>
> *Chief:* It certainly shows the limitations we have on helping.
>
> *Patient* [*whisper*]: Amen.

The first meeting was quickly filled with a search for clues, even though everyone knew Daniel Forman had said he planned to kill himself. For example, one patient said, "I'm partly responsible for his death. He left a note to the electrician that the *light didn't work,* but it did and I threw the paper away." Patients as well as staff entered the search, at the same time wondering aloud if *their* clues would be noticed.[22]

This is the first of four stages that have been identified in the response to suicide. Numbness and disbelief characterize the initial reaction, quickly followed by anger, fear and a sense of betrayal by the therapist(s). These often noted feelings are grounded in the social definition of the therapeutic relationship. Therapy is presumed to be a joint effort based on mutual trust. This does not always happen; even new residents quickly sense great distrust by their patients. But if therapy has been going for a while, the therapist often feels a relationship has been established and plans the course of treatment. In this context, suicide elicits intense feelings of betrayal, especially if the therapist feels progress was being made.

Another strong feeling is anger, not only from being betrayed, but also from conflict that seems built into many therapeutic relationships. As Goffman has observed, the nature of professional work is such that the expert must get the client to accept his point of view. The psychiatrist constructs an understanding of the patient's problems which often differs from the patient's viewpoint. Much therapeutic work centers on the therapist getting the patient to see things his way. The use of confidential records, disclosure practices, and the belief that nothing is due to accident are elements of the psychiatrist's efforts.[23]

Anger comes not only from the patient betraying the bonds inherent in the therapeutic relationship but also from the relationship's imbalance that allows the patient to express hatred and rage but muzzles the therapist. "Indeed," writes one authority, "the problem of tolerating the hatred from the patient and accepting the hatred in oneself may be a core problem in the treatment of the suicidal patient."[24] A number of clinicians note that the feelings of anger and loss resonate in the therapist, who resents the patient's license to vent them when he cannot.[25]

Fear centers on being villified. The therapeutic relationship implies that the doctor is in charge, has expertise, and is responsible. Suicide thus implies gross negligence. Yet rarely is a therapist in full control of a suicidal person; expertise is often lacking; and aside from cases where the therapist contributes to suicide, it is unreasonable to hold him responsible for someone else's act. These false expectations, however, are built into the doctor-patient relationship.

The third phase of response to a suicide is a tendency to deny more painful aspects of the failure it represents, as reflected in the shifting beliefs mentioned before. In this case, a series of ambiguous messages were interpreted in a way to deny certain aspects of the case.

Mr. Forman (as the psychiatrist called him) had told everyone that he was going to kill himself in the middle of the month. In an interview, Dr. Kent, his therapist, explained why he let Forman off the ward.

> He and the chief decided it best for Forman to work at what he liked and to be with friends [who shared a pad with him in Cambridge]. They all knew the dangers, he said, "but we felt that there was a good relation between him and myself, as good as you get in three weeks." [Work privileges were given to him in the first week here.] Moreover, the work could be used as a therapeutic issue. The first week went fine. He returned punctually; therapy was good. When a suicide [on another service] was announced, Forman smiled. Kent confessed they had not talked about it in session. But "I think something was going on, in therapy. I still think so."

An important belief emerges here: that when a patient communicates with his therapist, the patient is involved and a "therapeutic relation" has been established.

Experienced therapists say that this is a myth.[26] Another myth, which may have been followed here, is that if a therapist talks about suicide, like the suicide on the other service, he will further implant the idea of suicide in the patient's head and implicitly sanction it. What happened in this case is that the therapist interpreted all early ambiguous signs as indications of a strong therapeutic alliance. Like other beliefs that prevail before a person commits suicide, it deepened the commitment of the therapist to help the patient and emphasized the therapist's power to help.

As the case was discussed and the search for early clues continued, two beliefs emerged. First, Mr. Forman was determined to die. The chief even brought in Mr. Forman's previous therapist, who told the entire ward that Mr. Forman had planned suicide for a long time. This was one of the principal reasons why he had been admitted. "It was only a matter of time," and "You cannot stop someone who wants to commit suicide.'' Mr. Forman had been a quiet person who did not draw too much attention, which was noted as an indication of how he had gotten the staff to ignore him. Second, the staff believed that Dr. Kent had really "reached" Mr. Forman in therapy. Mr. Forman had left a suicide note which included the names of several physicians and other staff but not Dr. Kent. This was universally interpreted as evidence that Kent meant so much to him that he could not write his name along with the rest. The opposite inference could be made, but the overall conclusion was that the therapist had not made a mistake. He had failed (to keep the patient alive), but had not erred. This crucial distinction in professional work separates professional standards (doing good technical work) from lay standards (solving the client's problem). The beliefs which arose after the suicide protect the profession, because they "show" that *despite* the therapist's power to help, the patient's impulses got the better of him. They also "show" the power of diagnosis, that suicide was *retrospectively predictable*. The fact that the psychiatric staff let Forman out to work during the day on the grounds that he would not attempt suicide until the middle of the month rather than ten days ahead of schedule faded into the background. They had planned to return him to full hospitalization a week before his proclaimed suicide date, but he beat them by a few days. Only one person, a patient who had been a mental health worker, refused to forget.

> *Chief:* We felt he was balanced enough to go out.
> *Patient:* How can you tell a balance in a month on something that has been going on for years? That seems like a contradiction to me. How could you let him out?
> *Dr. Kent:* He seemed to be able to talk.
> *Patient:* I can't see why he was left out on weekends. I mean he wasn't watched then.
> *Dr. Kent:* He had a lot of work to do, and he seemed to like his work.
> *Patient:* Well, did you search for him immediately? Did you look at his place of work?
> *Dr. Kent:* He was supposed to come home at 10:00 P.M. and we started a while after that.
> *Patient:* But you don't wait!
> *Chief:* If a man is late, you give him some leeway.
> *Patient:* Not with a suicide. You never waste a minute with a suicide. You make no assumptions.

The Suicide Review: A Ritual of Reaffirmation

The fourth stage of response is the suicide review. Unlike mortality and morbidity conferences in medicine, the suicide review takes place many weeks after the suicide, long enough for most people involved to talk out their feelings until they tire of the subject. But like such conferences in medicine, the suicide review is a tribal ritual intended to bury the case and reaffirm the professional standards that may have been shaken. Suicide is always a failure; the question is whether anyone made a mistake. Daniel Forman was reviewed in December.

The presentation was very long, detailed and dull. It seemed designed to show that, from the patient's history, suicide was inevitable.

Two patterns emerged in the history. First, that he went quickly into a rage. . . . Second, the pattern of people rejecting him, especially psychiatrists. Not straight rejection, but passing him on.

Then he came here, and in less than a week went from ward restrictions to group privileges to hospital privileges to night care so he could work.

Mr. Forman was described as "brilliant" and other such adjectives, so much so that finally the reviewing psychiatrist interrupted. "We've got to save the dumb ones too." [Everyone laughed sheepishly under their breath.]

In the discussion, the senior reviewing psychiatrist analyzed the case. First, we were the next ones to brush him off. The reviewer made it sound pretty bad; then he added that he was not condemning the staff. "Heaven knows, I've made so many mistakes. . . ."

But the lesson of the day he gave was that what makes a man a professional is that he does not react to a situation as a layman does. If you faint at blood, you get out of surgery. Here, you have always to say, "Am I reacting the way everyone else did? Do I fit the pattern?" To do this, he said, you have to withdraw from being a human and see your humanness through professional eyes. For the reviewing psychiatrist, this is the most important lesson. . . .

Second, no one took the previous suicide attempts seriously. Most psychiatrists who had treated Forman previously thought they were merely manipulations.

"Why did they see the attempts this way?" asked the consulting psychiatrist. "Because the patient used a common technique of deprecating his actions. 'I'm nothing, don't take this stuff seriously.' And you don't; then he kills himself."

Again, the lesson is that a patient is a prism through which you see his life, and as a professional, you learn to correct for distortion.

In the discussion, another member of the Review Board said that had Mr. Forman been kept in the hospital, he would have regressed, so it was not clear that the wrong thing had been done. Then several people in the room and finally the main speaker agreed that Forman would have committed suicide anyway. . . .

Later, the chief said that last year's Suicide Review Board found two common patterns. . . . The second was the person who convinces the doctor that his work or something is the only important part of his life. So the doctor lets him go out to do it, and he kills himself. . . .

To understand the suicide review in its stated capacity leaves one disappointed and confused. On one hand, the reviewer had implied that the staff were rank amateurs who had killed a man by not being professional in their relations with him. Moreover, the mistake was one found to be a pattern in suicide reviews of previous years and the most common pattern recorded in the general literature. The degree of malpractice implied is considerable. Yet everyone left feeling relaxed and fulfilled. All the doctors said that this had been a very fine conference. Afterwards, they mainly chatted about the *reviewer* and his performance.

It is difficult to sustain belief in the manifest function of suicide review—to determine what was done wrong and to learn from it. Not only does the audience respond to other features of the review, but the lessons drawn are not communicated in any serious manner. Psychiatrists generally do not know what patterns previous reviews have found, and what is learned is only communicated to those present on one ward.

Like other acts of reintegration, the suicide review is a ritual designed to reaffirm the profession's worth after doubt was cast upon it.[27] Beside suicide, many problems in psychiatric work raise doubts about competence. Accounting professionally for decisions on these problems is a latent function of regular case reviews. Like many of the informal acts which begin when a problem such as suicide occurs, the review must strike a precarious balance between the individual and the profession. It may protect the practitioner in matters of blame, but only at the risk of jeopardizing the general standards and cohesion of the profession. If, on the other hand, it judges the individual member to be wanting, the profession may reintegrate itself, but at the cost of embarrassment and admission of lax self-regulation. Thus it serves the organized function, mentioned at the beginning of the paper, to spread and allocate losses. Perr put it well when he said he felt he needed a jury of peers to say he was not guilty.[28]

The suicide review attains a proper balance by diminishing the significance of the suicide and then by effectively removing it as an issue. Its main features support this inference and follow many rituals of judgment and contrition. The presentation is very long. In it, much evidence points to the inevitability of suicide, much more so than presentations made by the same therapist about the same patient at conferences while he was living. The senior reviewing psychiatrist "explains" the suicide and talks about what can be done to become better professionals.

Often, the analysis of the case and the criticism are based on thin evidence, but the collage of bits into some whole is what impresses the audience. As in other aspects of psychiatry, storytelling is important. At the end of the review, the main feeling is one of being impressed by the reviewer, a reaffirmation of how fine psychiatry is; for in its darkest hour, a clear lesson can be drawn by a model of the profession (the reviewer), implying that, had the best men in psychiatry been handling the case, it would not have happened.

Recently, Charles Bosk has found many of the same features of the suicide review in mortality and morbidity conferences at a leading residency in surgery, characterizing them as "the transformation of negative evidence into a positive display of an attending's skill."[29] In surgery, however, many of the decisions in a case are not made by the resident but by the attending physician. Nevertheless, in both cases the surgeon or the senior reviewing psychiatrist steps in to interpret the evidence in such a way as to bring about this transformation. In both cases, the resident is protected; his errors are passed over or forgiven. In both cases, actions which are not supported by research or accepted practices must be explained, and in both cases this is usually done by citing the special circumstances of the case and the clinical judgment of the reviewer. If a mistake has been made, it is excused by the act of admitting it, a practice which encourages residents to be open about their own mistakes. Moreover, the suicide review, like case conferences and supervision, teaches physicians how to transform what even a colleague might regard as a mistake into a matter of interpretation.

10.

Supervising Psychotherapy

Central to any training program is the supervision of rookies as they attempt the roles they will later assume. Supervisors fulfill a number of social functions in training. They provide role models of how to act, what to feel, and how to judge difficult situations. They oversee work and control the impact of mistakes. This requires a delicate balance between letting the residents have responsibility enough to learn from mistakes they make and taking over so that serious errors do not occur. In psychiatry, supervisors almost never take over and residents are given great responsibility from the start, implying that there are not many serious mistakes to be made. When a mistake is made, the resident is forgiven and remembers not to do it again, while the supervisor forgives but remembers that the resident made a mistake. This puts the resident in the supervisor's debt and tightens his bonds with the group.[1]

Supervision is a way of transmitting tribal wisdom, known in medicine as clinical experience. By implication, supervisors indicate that clinical experience has greater worth than scientific expertise, because they draw on their experience to frame and modify the implications of research or theory to the case being treated. Although a profession is based on a body of scientific and esoteric knowledge, its actual work strongly tempers that knowledge with each individual's first-hand experiences with clients.

218

Emotionally, psychiatric residents want all the supervision they can get, and they tend to identify with one or perhaps two supervisors they particularly admire. This craving for more intense supervision stems from the heavy emphasis on psychotherapy, which itself is emotionally intense and bewilderingly complex to those being trained. The residency program at the University Psychiatric Center particularly emphasized psychotherapy. Dr. Blumberg, its clinical director, defined it as ''the process of feeling oneself into the patient's dilemma to discover the painful experience, ideas and affects avoided by the fragmented ego.'' Only through such empathy, Blumberg argued, could one make a good diagnosis and go on to show one's caring for the patient.

While all supervision has elements of dependence and therapy, the demand to empathize with crazy, defensive, and sometimes hostile patients heightens the therapeutic aspects of supervision.

> Psychotherapy is probably the most complex of all human relationships; during its course the therapist participates in a variety of roles both spontaneous and studied. Additionally, the therapist is burdened with responsibilities, and is subjected to an assault by the patient's neurotic strivings from which there is no retreat, and towards which he is expected to react in a manner that will be of therapeutic value for the patient. No matter how extensive his training, the beginning therapist will find it difficult, without support and expert guidance, to stand up under the unreasonable demands and violent projections of the patient.[2]

One continues to hear this viewpoint throughout residency and well into psychoanalytic training, six or seven years after residency training has begun. It is paralleled by fears that supervision will turn into therapy, that sound advice about countertransference (the therapist's projection of his own neurotic problems onto the patient) will turn into an examination of the trainee's unconscious.

This parallel has several implications. First, it suggests an extreme example of the ideal that professionals dissociate their personal feelings from their relations with clients; for here is a profession which attempts to do this while using personal feelings as a major tool of analysis and treatment! Small wonder that resistance to learning and interference with therapy are commonly cited problems.[3] This makes supervision far more intense and intimate in psychotherapy than in surgery, law, or engineering. Second, the parallel between overcoming countertransference in therapy and avoiding therapeutic transference in supervision indicates how similar are the relations the patient has with the therapist to the relations the therapist has with the supervisor. In both the goal is to replace ". . . dissociations with associations, disconnections with connections, unconsciousness with awareness and insight."[4] Third, the parallel helps overcome what Chessick calls the "crucial triad of difficulties": professional identity, the anxiety over psychological-mindedness, and the conviction that psychotherapy is meaningful.[5] Supervision provides professional identity and makes psychotherapy meaningful not so much through results as through personal involvement with it.

The Organization and Variety of Supervision

Each training program organizes its supervision differently, and in this short space one can hardly attempt to cover all the complexities of supervision. To begin with arrangements, University Psychiatric Center had an unusual amount of supervision, about six to seven hours a week for each resident. Supervision had two basic forms, the continuous following of one case and the general review of many cases as they come and go. Some supervision explicitly took the first form; some the latter. Specifically, administrative supervisors reviewed a range of constantly changing cases, but in keeping with the integration of management with therapy, they also advised residents about the psychotherapy of the same patients. These psychiatrists, such as the chiefs, the superchiefs, and full-time senior staff, worked in the program. The arrangement contrasts with what Rose Coser describes at a nearby residency, where therapeutic and administrative supervision were kept apart and where administrative supervisors essentially told residents what to do.[6] At the University Psychiatric Center, supervisors did not directly intervene in residents' care of patients unless they thought the situation was dire. More commonly, these supervisors served as the court of appeal in disputes between nurses and residents, when the issues of administrative control versus therapeutic insight arose between them. But on the whole, the administrative supervisors would respond by clarifying the alternatives and issues rather than by taking matters into their own hands.

Supervision itself usually took place privately in a hospital office, but there was some group supervision, especially with Drs. Blumberg and Black. Residents claimed that supervision differed from that in medical school, where the supervisor wanted the facts in detail and responded by citing the relevant literature as part of an intellectual analysis of the problem. Sometimes this happened, especially with supervisors who were candidates at the Psychoanalytic Institute. They were consistently described as ferociously, almost obsessively, intellectual and process-oriented. Two analytically-oriented residents explained.

> The best kind is process, where you tell what happens in the process, blow by blow, and the supervisor listens and then comments after the full flavor is given. But few supervisors do that, both agreed. Some supervisors, they said, cut in after the first sentence. They do great with it, but can't go too far . . . perhaps because they can do better with a minimum of evidence, because their theories are so much better than their understanding.

Process supervision, however, had its price. Reviewing his first year, one bright resident said that

> he had missed any serious discussion of what really goes on in therapy over time. They learned a lot about the blow-by-blow technique, but not the overview.
> "Good supervision" usually entails detailed analysis of interaction. We learn how to play the piano, but we have no idea of what we're playing, or what notes make up a sonata, or whether what we are doing is beautiful.

Notably absent from supervision in this program was first-hand knowledge of the patient. In most cases, the supervisor had never met the patient, though a few residents urged a supervisor to interview a particularly puzzling patient. There were no tapes, no videotapes, no one-way mirrors or other forms of direct observation. This did not seem to bother most residents or supervisors. One resident, however, who was very interested in polishing his technique, started taping his therapy hours but then realized there was no one to listen to them. Finally he put his machine in the car and listened to his tapes as he drove home each day.

Note taking was more common. It appears that a fair number of supervisors asked for them, and very few discouraged them. This in itself was regarded as semimedical.

I take notes on every session with each patient, but the process is spotty. First, it depends on whether the session is interesting or different than previous ones. I may write simply: "[name of patient]: More on his sense of uselessness."

Second, it depends on my mood. With one patient there are swings. For a few weeks, I will write very little. Then I'll write in great detail.

Thirdly, it depends on the supervisor. If I have a supervisor who goes over the notes and who is instructive that way, I will write notes for him. For Dr. ———, however, I write notes but poor ones, even though he emphasizes notes and detailed interaction. He is poor.

I keep very fine notes on Patient A. I'm committed to him. I'm also very committed to Patient B., but with her it is a matter of support and love, not therapy. A. can benefit from therapy. Also, A. changes [not necessarily the same as improving] so you can see the changes over time, while B. is always the same.

Structurally, the absence of the patient or of detailed information about what happens during therapy meant that supervision focused heavily on the resident. Socialization rather than patient care was the main concern. However, this program was not an extreme example of this structure; for some programs actively discourage any note taking. They consider it a form of intellectualization that keeps one from closing one's eyes and *feeling* what went on during therapy.

What makes a good supervisor? In part, the answer in psychotherapeutic work is a good person. "It is precisely what he is in the depths of himself—his real availability, his receptivity and his authentic acceptance of what the other is—which gives value, pungency and effectiveness to what he says. . . ."[7] M. Grotjahn asks, "How to teach patience and devotion, tact and timing, decency and tolerance, empathy and intuition, modesty and respect in the face of supporting loyalty and keeping distance, carefulness and courage, honesty and frankness?"[8] The answer is that the resident identifies with the supervisor, who presumably has all these qualities.

Among the supervisors at UPC, residents identified certain types. There was the Grand Master, the sage who said little but was important to everyone. There was the pure analytic type who responded to a case with a very intellectual analysis of the dynamics of the patient or of therapy. Residents described young analysts and institute candidates this way. Whether residents liked this or not depended on how psychoanalytic they themselves were. One protested: "With some supervisors, they won't let you get three sentences out when they interrupt and start telling you how this goes back to the oedipal problem, and go on about all the problems of the patient in infancy. God! I can't stand that stuff. It leaves me cold.''

But another resident said: ''——— is a very good supervisor. He is very dynamic; he sees dynamics in everything.''

The third type of supervisor described by this second-year resident is the countertransference one. He is always focusing on you and how you feel. In reviews at the end of the year, two residents remarked about such supervisors.

> *Resident No. 1:* Many supervisors use Freud's analogy. Two porcupines try to get close to one another, but each time they do, they prick one another and push each other off, hurt. It's like two people with their defenses.
>
> *Resident No. 2:* [My patient] taught me the great truth of this.
>
> *Resident No. 1:* I used to hate Adam for his pet lines: ''What do you think? What are your feelings? It's your responsibility.'' But now they are the words I use the most on all my patients.

From observing supervision first-hand, I noted three types of interaction—a different way of distinguishing among the varieties of supervisors. One kind, the *director,* took over after five minutes of reportage by the resident and instructed him. This supervisor decided what would be discussed in the supervision; he defined the problems and offered solutions. The content could be either analytic or managerial, but was rarely countertransference.

> The resident briefly described a schizophrenic boy who was soon leaving the hospital.
>
> The supervisor said, ''You are not to see him very much after July first. You are to visit with him for half an hour a month, no more. Show interest in his progress, but do not indicate great interest. I say this for the sake of your well-being and your family. He could really drain you.''
>
> The resident resisted. He said he was quite involved with the patient and planned to see him more often.
>
> The supervisor replied by quoting two senior staff members on limited attachment. He added, ''There is no transference with these types.''
>
> The resident said that the patient saw his father in the way he treated the resident, indicating transference.

The supervisor appeared ruffled and said in a resigned sigh, "OK. Do what you want. But a word to the wise."

A second kind of supervisor listened carefully and made occasional but well-placed remarks. Residents were comfortable with this type of supervisor and felt he was sympathetic. The *listener* style lent itself to discussing countertransference, because the resident exposed himself so much in talking. This style most closely resembled a therapeutic relationship, though the supervisor could use humor and other devices to keep this relationship more professional.

> A resident presented a case familiar to Dr. Blumberg. He had recommended bringing up transference issues, and the patient had begun to talk about her feelings for her old therapist. The resident had asked her if she had similar feelings for him, and she said no.
> "You planted seeds," said Blumberg, "and they will grow." The resident stopped presenting, wordlessly staring up at Blumberg.
> Blumberg continued, "Pretty soon she'll be talking about you."

A third type of supervisor served as a *consultant*. Here, the resident determined the agenda by asking direct, concrete questions which the supervisor answered in a business-like way. This particularly characterized supervision about administrative matters.

Learning to Interpret

Central to all therapy and a major goal of supervision is learning how to interpret. This seemed particularly difficult to the residents, in part, I suspect, because they were so close to the cases. As an observer of supervision, I often found myself silently interpreting the case being presented the same way the supervisor did a few minutes later. Yet if the supervisor first asked the resident to make an interpretation, he would often stutter, fumble, or make an ill-considered analysis. This contrasted with the residents' usually articulate, intelligent manner outside of supervision.

Another aspect of interpretation is learning when to do it, as illustrated by the following supervision with a widely admired psychiatrist.

> The resident launched into the case, his only adolescent one since September, and refreshed the supervisor's memory with some telling anecdotes. He continued by reading from a steno notebook in which he had hand-written notes about therapy—about a page and a half for each session with the patient. He saw the patient twice a week.

After reading notes on five sessions, the resident described his returning from vacation to find the patient mad. He asked the patient why he was angry, and the patient did not know.

"Are you angry because I have been away?" The patient said no.

For the first time the supervisor broke in. "That was not the right thing to do. You went too fast with that interpretation. You were expecting a boy who lacks narcissistic control to interpret his own behavior immediately or to see it if it is pointed to him." [Contrast this response with Blumberg's response above when faced with a similar case.]

The supervisor suggested that the resident should have encouraged the patient to free-associate about his recent life. He had just moved, and he felt like a stranger in the new neighborhood. Ask him if he felt alone. He would probably say he had been confused and that there was no one to help him with his problems in the neighborhood.

After going through this material, the supervisor continued, one could then suggest that his anger had something to do with the vacation. By then it would be clearer, and one could point to his sense of loneliness, his sense of abandonment. This would be an important lesson in learning about how he responded to deprivation and might improve his "object-relations."

Once a patient is neurotic, you can get more cognitive in your work. The resident's error, he said, had been to focus on the *content* of his anger rather than the *process*.

At several points, the supervisor emphasized that one must not get entangled with the "surface material." One must see what is happening in the relationship as the surface material is being produced.

. . . .

The resident described an upsetting incident in the therapy. He told the patient that if he was to do therapy, he had to stop taking drugs. The resident also prescribed some Thorazine. The patient was to come in the next day.

The supervisor said, "If you don't give him what he wants, he will get more and more agitated, until you do. I told you the story about the patient who strangled me? [*Pause.*] He was choking me and I punched him. He immediately calmed down. That's what he wanted, *control*, and once he got it he was satisfied." [I.e., give the patient what he wants, and what he wants is for you to control him.]

The supervisor said that the resident had given the patient three gifts. 1. It's either me or the drugs. 2. My medicine is better than yours (the prescription). 3. I'll take care of you (come in tomorrow).

The resident continued, reading about the next session: "When the patient arrived, he looked great." [The supervisor smiled, satisfied with his prediction.]

226 □ Becoming Psychiatrists

But, the supervisor said, "You gave too small a prescription. Patients want to be limited, to be structured and cared for. Control is a gift, Don't give twenty units. Knock him out with a thousand. It won't hurt him. The point is to *show him who's in control*. Then you can let up the dosage."

This passage illustrates an important lesson constantly taught in residency: how to interpret to the patient so that the therapist can always be right and persuasive. The supervisor emphasized that "a very important skill is to read between the lines, understand what is unsaid, and listen with the third ear." In talking about psychotic patients, he pointed out that everything they say is an association even though they don't know it. No one questioned that the patient was angry because his therapist had gone on vacation. When the patient said this was not the case, he was denying feelings he could not face. What the resident failed to do was to lay the groundwork for the interpretation. Had he gotten the patient to talk about a recent trial in his life (moving to a strange neighborhood), the therapist could have suggested that the anger had something to do with his vacation. If the patient insisted his loneliness and frustration were caused by the new neighborhood, the therapist could have asked: "You mean you were in that strange neighborhood and you didn't even once wish that you could talk with someone about your feelings?" If the patient had not produced such material at all, but had said that the recent past had been fine, the therapist could have remarked: "If things are going so well, then how is it that you're angry?" The lesson to be learned again and again was how to get the patient to produce some material which could be used to support one's prior interpretation.

A second lesson which all three of the experts from supervision conveyed was not to get "involved," "entangled," "manipulated," "seduced." This reflects the basic tension between the expectations that a professional will maintain enough dispassion to keep his good judgment in spite of the inherent intimacy of a treatment that uses the therapist's emotions as a major tool.

Handling Supervisors

Many residents complained that there was little "systematic supervision" and that supervision was "largely a waste of time" because so many of the supervisors were not interesting. At first, out of insecurity, residents cling to supervision for moral support, one of the main uses it has for them. But this soon wears off. Many residents also resent so much supervision, while at the same time extolling this program precisely because it offers so much supervision. As one resident said,

> They're not very good this year. I mean, supervisors are poor, and they don't have pizazz. They're not bright, most of them, and they have no strong point of view, no clear response. When they say something, you already know it.

Considerable energy goes into handling this problem. An unusual but total solution is not to contact a supervisor, or to call up and say you have nothing to present this week. Some older residents never meet with an assigned supervisor *at all,* even with ones they have never met, because of their poor reputation in the residents' subculture. Sometimes, the supervisor is too embarrassed to blow the whistle. Another technique is to tell the supervisor that you only have a half hour in your schedule, or that you can only meet every other week. Residents may also use these tactics out of anxiety, and even if they do not, that would be the psychodynamic interpretation of their action.

Among residents who meet with their supervisors (the vast majority of cases), other techniques prevail. Residents create problems where none really exist. This preserves the pupil-tutor relation; it is a social kindness by the resident to the dull or vacuous supervisor. The more confident residents chat. An item or two may be discussed, but otherwise the conversation may range from keeping cats to discussing R. D. Laing. This changes the relationship and residents report that it makes an otherwise tedious appointment pleasurable.

When supervision works, it seems to work within certain confines. For example, residents complained that supervisors would hear only certain kinds of cases. They would discourage residents from presenting sociopaths, psychopaths, geriatrics, and other cases which were often the most troublesome to the resident. This was particularly true in the first year, when the program's responsibility for a catchment area produced inpatients as far from the supervisors' experience—past and present—as could be. Residents often reported that most supervisors had nothing to say theoretically or practically about inarticulate, uneducated, usually black patients. For this reason, and because supervisors are people to impress, supervision was largely seen as an occasion for presenting one's "good" patients.

A good patient is described as one whose "dynamics" are complex and subtle, and who is responsive to psychotherapy. According to the residency subculture, a good patient is also one in whom the therapist is involved, and thus the case is rich with countertransference issues. In the first year, good patients are more rare than in the later years; so that residents end up presenting their "only good case" to their "best supervisor" over a long time. In a few cases, a resident would have a very good patient whom he would keep to himself and present to no one—a rich case of countertransference if ever there was one.

These observations make it clear that *process* supervision is what residents learn to value. Their idea of a good patient and a good supervisor centers around long-term treatment and examination of the therapeutic relationship. Residents only wish there were more good process supervisors and patients to present to them. Central to this kind of supervision is the *supervisory alliance*. All the major texts on teaching psychiatry emphasize the importance of establishing this alliance, so that the resident has sufficient respect and trust to respond when the supervisor points out blind spots and resistance. What the texts do not consider is the structural pattern of the supervisory alliance. If a resident has four or seven supervisors, can he or she ally with all of them? Given the wide range of styles and advice among supervisors, how would the resident handle so many cross-cutting alliances? The professional role set would be riddled with conflicting expectations. To these speculations, I can contribute only one informal observation from the study: most residents have one or sometimes two supervisors with whom they strongly identify. Regardless of who the supervisors are in one instance or another, each resident by some magical process "discovers" that one supervisor (and occasionally two) is just what he or she has been looking for. Further investigation might well find that this is a way in which residents solve the structural problems of multiple alliances, and a way in which they acquire a clear professional vision to cut through the fog that surrounds them.

Katherine: A Case Study

Some of the complications which arise in supervision and from in-hospital psychotherapy are illustrated by the case of Katherine. As a case, it is in no way typical, and like the rest of this account of supervision, it cannot hope to cover the full range of issues which psychiatrists have raised throughout the years.

The resident assigned to Katherine was an analytical type. He had suffered through medical school and internship just to enter psychiatry; naturally he was very pleased that University Psychiatric Center had accepted him. Among first-year residents, he was one of the few who rated therapy as the prime modality of treatment, though management and control entered the relation weekly.

Katherine had been in the hospital for some time and had worked with one of the previous year's new residents.[9] She briefly met the incoming resident on the first day and, coming back from his office, said to a friend, "I hate him." A week later she said she liked her doctor OK, but was not sure whether she could talk to him about personal things. She said they had been talking about the loss of her old resident (which the residents of transfers are told to do at the start). "But I don't have much to say, because we never got along."

A week later at a staff meeting, her resident said Katherine was tied to the therapist *before* last year's resident, and that the latter never shook off this attachment. He wondered if *he* could, and said he would "put it on the line tomorrow."

During the residents' meeting with the chief in the third week, Katherine's doctor wondered what would be left if you took away the fantasies of a patient.[10]

> One resident answered with the classic line—with sick people you have to root their life in concrete realities, and they will appreciate this.
>
> Another mused that there is pain in fantasies too. Imagine the pain for Katherine each day when her earlier therapist did not come. You can teach her that she can have a beautiful memory which is real and not lost, while at the same time living in the present and forming new relationships.
>
> The first resident felt we were talking about ourselves and our own feelings about the patients.
>
> The chief pointed out that for a whole year Katherine had found it worth the pain to keep her earlier therapist in her mind and not relate to anyone else.[11]
>
> Katherine's doctor made the leap to talking just about residents' anxieties, where the conversation remained for the rest of the hour. He mentioned he knew his person came into his work.
>
> The chief said, "You find, in the middle of your second year, that

the patients you still have or who are still in the hospital are those who have the same problems you do.''

Another person said he wanted to keep his patients dependent so he could be independent.

"Yes,'' said the chief, ''you keep the ones you need and get satisfaction by curing the others!''

In the next week, the resident did not mention Katherine to his chief in supervision. At the staff planning conference, a nurse said that Katherine had told her that her doctor did not understand her. "He does not pick up distress signals,'' she had said, ''and that scares me.'' At the fourth staff planning conference, the resident reported that his patient suspected him of telling her parents about her and feared he was ''sabotaging.'' The chief suggested he ask her why she was here. The resident said there was no point in asking that and described what therapy with Katherine was like. If you asked her that, she would typically come back with: ''Why are you asking?'' ''Why should I tell you?'' ''What will you do with the information?''

The following day I asked the resident about the nurse's report that Katherine feared he was missing distress signals. He said that he took any information from the staff about her as a potential message to him indirectly. He sensed Katherine might be right, which was why she told the nurse. He also told me that he was pleased with his work with her.[12] She came every time and stayed for the full half hour, which meant she tolerated him. Since the start, there has been progress. "As she comes to trust me more—and she likes me a lot, I think—she also withdraws. She doesn't want anyone to know that she is coming closer.''

The next few weeks centered around what might be called *The Little Prince* episode. Most of the supervisory hour in the fourth week was taken up with another patient. However, at the end the resident mentioned that Katherine had brought him a little book, *The Little Prince,* which he had not read before. She also mentioned *The Red Balloon.* The chief asked, ''What did you do?'' The resident said he was not sure what to do at the time; he stalled during the whole meeting so he could have time to think about whether he should read the book or not, or take it or not, and what each alternative would mean to her. At the end he said he would read it in the next week.

The supervisor suggested that the resident ask her what it meant to her, what is significant, what giving the book signifies. He himself interpreted it as a way of Katherine getting more of her doctor while she was not there in his office.[13] He ended by saying he was pleased with what the resident was doing with Katherine. The supervisor impressed me as quiet, supportive, gentle.

At the fifth staff planning conference, the resident reported that Katherine was concerned about his taking her earlier therapist away from her. This is the therapeutic issue, he said, but he added that things were picking up with her, because now she came to therapy three times a week.

In the sixth week, the nurse at Morning Report said that Katherine had been upset during nurse's group and had cried over the loss of another patient, a great amount of expression for her.[14]

During supervision with the chief the following week, Katherine's resident thought he was "getting engaged" with her more. The day before, she had told him she felt "a big hole inside." The resident added, "and that was big stuff for me." He said that he treats everything as open. On the first day, for example, she said, "When do you want me in?" "This implied that I wanted her, but I told her when I would be around and said it was up to her to come. When she left early from a therapy session, I asked her why she was leaving, but didn't tell her to stay." He continued, "She says she can't trust me, and I ask her about that."

Katherine had also been seriously misbehaving, and the two doctors decided that the chief would be the "authoritarian and ogre" while the resident as her therapist could be sympathetic. "Fine," said the resident. "I'll ask her what the chief said to her."[15]

"Oh," the resident continued, "and you know what her favorite book is?"

> The one she gave you?
> *The Little Prince.*
> Who's it by?
> Saint-Exupéry. And it's all about friendship. This guy from another planet is looking for a friend, and he comes here and meets a fox. And the fox teaches him how to have a relationship. And the fox says, "Everyone is always shooting at me and chasing me. But we can be friends. Your hair is the color of the fields, and when we are friends I will remember your hair when I look at the fields." In other words, if we have a successful transference, everything will be fine.

The supervisor repeated twice that he thought the resident was doing well with Katherine, and the resident was pleased to hear him say that, because he felt so too.

In addition to the initial therapeutic relation, serious problems of administration had arisen. Katherine refused to cooperate with the nurses and occasionally caused trouble on the ward. During the Feelings Meeting in the eighth week, her resident said that she had been misbehaving since her resident of last year had left. In general, a patient would be discharged or transferred for her actions, but she told him that she did not fear being expelled, because she had gotten away with it before. The resident said to the group that he had talked this issue over with his chief and an administrator, and they agreed to wait to see how she acted—"whether she is asking for more punishment or whether she is willing to negotiate." The resident felt that her wanting to run away and the deep material he felt they were exploring in therapy were connected.

The next Saturday's Feelings Meeting focused almost exclusively on Katherine and her deviant behavior. This time, another resident asked how she was doing. Her doctor said, "Katherine is very fragile," and continued:

> She has a two years' history of running away. Now she stays in therapy three times a week for half an hour. And she talks about her deviance, which she never did with last year's resident. These are real gains, and I think I've gotten further than her previous therapists.
>
> But I don't feel I can tell her to stop [her misbehavior], because she'll just run out and do it anyway.
>
> The big therapeutic issue is *honesty*. I want her to tell me when she does it and how she feels. But then she says, "Why should I tell you? You'll only kick me out." My only advantage is that she does not like doing it and it gets her down.
>
> *Resident No. 2:* What you described is a long history of *manipulation,* and that is what she is doing now. You should tell her you want to help her by getting her to stop something she doesn't like to do. Then you restrict her so she can't do it any more. She will be angry, but you have to take that.
>
> A number of the residents saw Katherine as having made an accomplice of her doctor. If she told him—as he wanted her to—about her activities, he had to tell the chief. But then he was a squealer. One suggestion was that she deviate only after she has asked permission, "acting in" (toward the therapist) rather than "acting out" (away from the therapist).

Her resident said, finally, that this issue was *all he had to work with*. She didn't tell him much of anything else. This was *the* issue. The chief told him all right; just hammer away at it all the time. Katherine's resident said that suggestion was very interesting to him.

Complicating this problem of misbehavior was the previous resident's failure to punish Katherine for her deviance. The other residents said one must start with a clean slate, set one's own rules. They first gave examples of how they had put their foot down and controlled the patient, then examples of the opposite, when patients had broken the rules *more* or had *left* therapy.

By the end of the meeting, the resident felt frustrated and bombarded from all sides by contradictory advice. "To hell with you guys; I'll do what I want to."

The supervisors' assessment of Katherine's therapy was somewhat different from that of the residents. For example, in the ninth week, Katherine's resident was in a three-way supervision with another supervisor, but Katherine's case took the entire hour. The resident began to read from notes made after therapy with Katherine. The supervisor also took notes and listened without interruption, except for questions of clarification. For several weeks, he said, the primary interest, aside from her deviance, had been her saying she has "funny feelings." When asked what they were like, she said they were feelings of distance, being scared, and fear of going crazy; her deviant acts relieved them. Her therapist added that he thought the acts replaced an earlier stage of acting out, when she did not have these feelings. As for *The Little Prince,* she was not able to say what was significant about it for her. He said her style in therapy was to speak a maximum of three or four sentences and then say, "I don't know." Or "I can't think of anything."

The supervisor's first comment was to recapitulate what the resident had said about *The Little Prince,* that Katherine had brought up the book three times, that she wanted a response, that he gave a "safe" one, and that then she clammed up and wanted to leave the session. She had said in effect, "I'm wasting *your* time." The supervisor concluded that Katherine was disappointed in him as a therapist.

The supervisor added that she thought Katherine was uncomfortable with her freedom from restrictions. Quickly, another resident asked how this inference was made. The supervisor hesitated, started speaking several times before admitting she could not answer his question. She added, seemingly as a partial explanation, that Katherine controls the relation a lot.[16]

The resident raised the honesty issue. Katherine had admitted that she had lied to her previous resident. He told her that he knew she would lie to him too if he asked her about the deviant acts, so he wanted her to tell him about her actions without his having to ask! The supervisor questioned this approach, but said she was not sure what message the resident was giving her by this request.

In the tenth week of therapy, Katherine's resident again had the three-way supervision, and again this case dominated.

The resident read from his notes on therapy again, and several times he pointed out that Katherine did not initiate conversations or even respond very much. As an example, he said that a staff member had told Katherine's parents about her misbehavior, and the parents had yelled at her. Katherine was now mad at the betrayal of confidence, and blamed her doctor. The resident apologized and got no response. Then he asked her if she wanted to go to school and got no reply. When he pointed out that she had to go to school under the law, she said that she would go. "So you see," he concluded, "how passive she is, how she gets people to decide things for her. She won't initiate." The supervisor commented that it was a mistake to tell her she had to go to school, and criticized him heavily for being so angry at his patient and for always initiating. The resident listened but did not accept or understand the thrust of these remarks. He said, "Yes, I was angry, but I separated out my anger at her insistence at failure when she is investing herself in many ways, from my hope and expectation of her progress."[17]

The supervisor responded: "The patient's question is 'do you care?' You are being too reserved, brainwashed by the advice, 'don't get seduced.' For example, your reluctance to respond at all to *The Little Prince*."

After supervision, I talked briefly with the supervisor and asked her how Katherine's relation with her resident had worsened since the beginning because of the ghost of the earlier therapist and the resident's attempts to be neutral. She thought Katherine was "in business," as evidenced by her efforts to bring the therapist into her life. I asked, like what? She replied, like her bringing up *The Little Prince* three times; but she could not think of anything else. She went on to talk about "being in business" as a prelude to "forming an alliance" where the patient and therapist agree on what they are working for in therapy.

Meanwhile a third group, the patients, formed their assessment of Katherine's therapy, and I found it rather easy to talk with them. Katherine would talk for hours with her friends, and they openly joked about how she would string her resident along by tossing him a provocative remark now and then, like having "funny feelings."

Katherine's best friend said that Kathy could not talk to her therapist. "Of course," she said, "he is better than [last year's therapist]— anyone would be."[18] Because Katherine's previous therapist was almost universally esteemed by his peers and superiors, I inquired further about him among his old patients, and found several others who had not reacted well to him.

With equal acuity, the patients kept score on the new residents. They noted that Katherine's resident had had three patients sign release papers, which they took to be "pretty bad." One patient said that his main mistake was not being more decisive. She said that when she told Katherine about how decisive her own resident was, Katherine said she wished she had him instead.

Soon thereafter, Katherine was told by her resident that she would not stay here and would probably be transferred to a state hospital or to a school.

> The resident reported that when he told her she only had two months left, she wanted to leave sooner. She said she would show him she was ready by not seeing him any longer.
>
> He claimed he had not seen her in therapy since, even though he invited her every time. She started to mix much more with other patients and lower staff, and played games now.
>
> But he said the message she gave was the opposite. "The only thing that counts is how she is with me and whether she comes to my office and sits or not."
>
> Several days later the resident mentioned that the girl had two sides, the masochistic side we never hear from, and the fantasy side, which builds castles in the air—wanting to live from day to day, wanting an apartment of her own, being a hippie.[19]
>
> "How is she?" I asked.
>
> He felt the masochistic side was being satisfied now by her not coming to therapy. She looked happy, but was suffering. She failed here, got nowhere.
>
> I thought she looked pleased with her departure.

He said that she was. But she was feeling the failure and loss, and liked it.

In the discharge summary written by the resident some time later, the doctor wrote that Katherine had regressed in the hospital, due to her forming no significant relationship with the therapist. It was among that 10 percent of discharge summaries which listed "therapy" as the prime factor in treatment.[20]

Reflections on Katherine

Although interpretation happens everywhere, supervision is the major arena for learning how to interpret patients, and psychiatric interpretation is what distinguishes residents from nurses and many of the "lesser" staff. Harold Garfinkel would call these interpretations "accounts"; Berger and Luckmann would speak of the "social construction of reality"; and anthropologists would call them "myths." This does not necessarily mean the accounts are untrue—if truth could be determined—for the essence of a myth is that it explains why things are the way they appear and how they got that way.

The first myth, or account, of Katherine's case concerns a nurse's report that Katherine thought her resident did not pick up distress signals. The resident saw Katherine as correct by the very fact that she told this to the nurse, an example of common reasoning in psychiatric work. The stronger interpretation followed, in which the resident placed Katherine's fright and signal of her fright into a general interpretative framework: as she got closer she also withdrew. Her pulling away was a sign of increasing closeness, her withdrawal a sign of trust.

One notes that the kind of language used by residents (but not so much by nurses) casts issues of management in terms of therapy. The myth of fragility, which began with the idea that Katherine would run the closer she got, was the resident's central reason for not raising therapeutic issues nor controlling her deviant acts. To this was added the interpretation that Katherine was dependent on her deviance. The question, then, was whether this dependence was in any way good, and the resident presented a story to show that it reflected progress. At no time was it suggested that she might simply enjoy these acts. Instead, they were fitted into a total explanation of her psychodynamics.

Despite this integration of administrative and therapeutic issues into one interpretative frame, the case of Katherine shows that eliminating the T-A split in no way eliminates conflicts of interest which can arise when one does psychotherapy with patients one wishes to control. In the eyes of residents at University Psychiatric, the integrated approach made treatment more honest and often more effective, because the patient's actions and the resident's orders became part of the therapeutic encounter. They became so, of course, by being incorporated into a comprehensive, psychodynamic account of the patient's life.

In learning how to construct accounts and how to introduce them in therapy so that patients could not reject them, residents were ''being socialized.'' Yet putting this in the passive voice, as most socialization theory does, neglects how active and critical residents are. Socialization actually presents a paradox of active individual struggle and surprisingly uniform results. This is possible because, while each person tries to come to terms with the new reality before her or him, the agents of socialization provide a coherent, limited set of symbols and accounts to draw upon. Each person absorbs these common elements, yet crafts them in a way that suits his or her style. Supervisors are important for instructing residents in how to use the new interpretative frame and to showing why alternative frames do not work. They also provide a range of personal models from which residents can choose what suits their style. From an inside perspective, this gives the impression of eclectic diversity, just as an outside perspective may perceive uniformity. By the nature of the process, both are right.

PART *III*

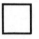

Theory
and Interpretation

Although this study raises many questions—about the
quality of the residents, the quality of therapy, the conflict between the professional obligation to always do
what is best for the patient and the priority given to
training psychiatrists, about the disdain for patients who
were poor, elderly or black—Part III will concentrate
on what happened to residents during their transformation from regular physicians to psychiatrists.

11.

The Moral Career of the Psychiatric Resident

Learning to become a psychiatrist is not easy. In a brilliant reflection of his residency experience at Yale, Samuel Klagsbrun wrote, "The physician who enters into a psychiatric residency has little information available to him concerning the personal price he will pay for his training."[1] Writing from their residency experiences at Menninger and Wisconsin, Halleck and Woods began, "The psychiatric residency is a time of extraordinary emotional stress in the life of the prospective psychiatrist, a stress which may have a profound effect upon his personal well-being and his subsequent professional adequacy."[2] The search for efficacy and the doubts about whether one is doing any good; the groping for techniques in a kind of therapy so different from those in medical school and internship; the role confusion with patients who get worse if one tries to intervene in their behalf and whose symptoms sometimes remind the resident of himself; the relinquishing of responsibilities to the patient when total responsibility had seemed an unambiguous beacon in medicine; the ambivalent relations with non-physician staff who are subordinate but more competent—these are five major issues with which our study found residents must struggle in their quest for a psychiatric identity, and which make up the sociological calendar in chapter 5.[3]

The stress and anxiety of psychiatric residency has not gone unnoticed in the professional literature, though most of the best articles have been written by psychiatrists just out of residency, and one of the problems is that teaching staff do not know what residents are going through.[4] Of late, the profession has been concerned with psychopathology among residents. As noted in chapter 2, a national survey in 1971–72 reported that 8 percent of their psychiatric residents "exhibited emotional illness and/or failing performance."[5] Another recent investigation found that 22 percent of a group of psychiatric trainees scored in the range of nonpsychotic emotional illness as compared to 3 percent for other medical postgraduates.[6] One resident interviewed his fellow residents and found that 74 percent said their program was stressful, 68 percent had experienced depression, and 26 percent of them had entertained suicidal thoughts.[7] An official Task Force on Emotionally Disturbed Psychiatric Residents was formed, and in 1973 it conducted a national survey covering 91 percent of all residents of that year.[8] The results were sobering. Nearly 7 percent did not complete the year, a rate which adds up to a considerable number over the three years of residency. Another 6 percent finished the year "despite marginal performance and/or emotional illness."[9] A quarter of those who dropped out were identified as having "emotional illness," though the public might like to know that 60 percent of these disturbed residents continued to train elsewhere or to practice medicine. The suicide rate for this group was the "highest rate yet reported for any residency specialty."[10] Of the ones who scraped by, 63 percent continued to perform "marginally" or "badly", but apparently were not dropped.

What goes unnoticed in this large study by the Task Force on Emotionally Disturbed Residents is a blurring of the training experience with personal pathology. The goal of the survey was to measure "emotional illness and poor performance,"[11] as if they were synonomous. For example, 6 percent finished the year "despite marginal performance and/or emotional problems," again blurring the two. Two-thirds of the residents who dropped out are reported as having left "in good standing"; and so the authors do not pursue them. But why did they leave? And what besides personal pathology contributes to marginal performance? In their pioneering article, Halleck and Woods prophetically warn: "While it can be rationalized that the disturbed resident would have become ill anyway, or that the experience can be a useful one, it is quite possible that the decompensation might not have occurred in the absence of the stress of residency.''[12]

The problem, of course, is that psychiatrists naturally tend to think about the stresses of training psychologically when these may be the intended or unintended consequences of how the training program is structured. In a classic study of the mental hospital, Stanton and Schwartz showed how the formal and informal structure of the hospital affected patients' symptoms and therapy, unbeknownst to the staff.[13] The effort here is the same, to analyze the structural forces which residents must confront, each in his or her own way. That there is variety the figures leave in no doubt. In the studies just cited, a quarter of the residents in one study did *not* report residency as being stressful, and three-quarters did *not* entertain suicidal thoughts. If 13 percent of the nation's residents drop out or perform marginally each year, 87 percent apparently perform well. From all reports, however, the socialization experience of becoming a psychiatrist is a powerful one, and in the end each person incorporates large parts of it in his or her struggle with it. The residents who suffer most visibly serve to highlight the latent consequences of how professional training is organized. While that organization has been shaped by history, accident, politics, and design, it seems in the end bent on altering the moral career of those who pass through it. This chapter and the next make a similar effort to uncover the informal and formal patterns that underlie the residents' initiation into psychiatry. They rest heavily on the residents' experience described in chapter 4, but it is also important to show how this analysis extends beyond the idiosyncrasies of one program. Since the description of University Psychiatric Center is already in hand, this chapter will emphasize all the other first-hand accounts of residency training in the literature, to convey a sense of what they are like, and to demonstrate how this model of the moral career applies to them all.

Ironically, the concept of moral career was first developed in a study of mental patients. Drawing an analytic parallel between patients and psychiatric residents may stretch the credulity of some; one reader averred that the deprivation suffered by young doctors could not possibly match that of the patients at St. Elizabeth's Hospital, where Goffman did his study. Yet the process of stripping and reconstituting are similar and may even be felt as intensely by some residents.

The Nature of the Moral Career

Psychiatric residents, like law students, military officers, and other professional candidates, feel anxiety and stress not because they are merely learning a series of techniques and a specialized body of knowledge, but because their sense of self is being shaken. Much of one's personal identity concerns one's career, a word which means "progress or general course of action of a person through . . . some profession or undertaking, some moral or intellectual action. . . ."[14] Thus trainees have both a professional career and a moral career, though we think less often about the latter. Yet the idea that each person has a certain moral stature, that one uses certain values for judging oneself and others, that one's moral career can degenerate or progress is not new to Tolstoy or Jane Austin or to most great writers.[15] Moreover, the concept of career binds together two perspectives: the individual's and that of the surrounding social or professional community. While a career is personal and one "has" a career, it takes place in and is shaped by the structure of that community and the values of significant others, who often form the essential network for one's professional career.[16] Thus moral career links one's values and self-image to the interests of the social or professional community in a dialectical relationship.

The study of careers naturally centers on turning points; for there the relations of past, present, and future come into sharper focus. When Anna Karenina, for example, succumbs to passion, her exemplary moral career spins and lurches downward, each chance for rescue rejected until she ends a life made wretched by the conflict between her new values and the moral community in which she lives.[17] Turning points, even good ones, are necessarily disruptive, and one feels disruption most acutely when it happens in a highly structured environment such as a training program, where those in control shape one's resources and set the boundaries in which individuals make their choices. The amount of disruption depends on the individual and on career contingencies, such as what schools a person attends, the influences of one's family on career goals and values, and whether one finds a mentor. For some aspiring psychiatrists, medical school is a turning point away from the values which psychiatry stands for in their minds and toward science and technical medicine. Since we have examined the impact of medical school on psychiatric careers, we shall not review it here.[18] But even for psychiatric residents who have no difficulty in reconciling medical school with psychiatry, the values implicit in medical routines they have been practicing until now at least appear so different from those imbedded in psychiatric work that it is unusual for the residency experience not to alter their moral careers. The specific form of these changes depends, again, on such contingencies as what kind of residency one enters and what important relationships develop. But if the particulars are limited by place and time, it does not matter; for they illustrate a larger, more enduring pattern.

The Stages of Moral Transition

In his famous essay, "The Moral Career of the Mental Patient," Erving Goffman wrote a compelling description of what happens when an emotionally troubled individual enters a mental hospital. Goffman's analysis, however, was flawed and incomplete. He was describing not so much the moral career of the mental patient as a turning point in that career, and the stages he used ("prepatient phase," "inpatient phase") reflected institutional status rather than stages of moral transition. Moreover, they only apply to patients, when the task should be to identify the underlying, universal phases of moral transition that mental patients, psychiatric residents, police officers, and other subjects of organizational socialization experience.

1. Feeling Different and Being Discredited

Coming into any new program, a novice will feel different from those already there, and the old hands will try to discredit those of the novice's ways that are not customary, even if this is done without plan or malice. While this happens to students in nursing and residents in surgery,[19] it is particularly stark in psychiatry. "The relative independence of authority achieved by the physician prior to beginning the psychiatric residency is immediately challenged upon beginning the first year. Whatever his age, whatever his previous accomplishments, the beginning resident is viewed—by himself and others—simultaneously as an expert and a novice."[20] Small wonder that "he is often preoccupied with the loss of identity as a physician attendant on the deemphasis and slipping away of the medical knowledge he has spent five years of his life accumulating.''[21] Nearly every study of residency has found this pattern. ''Our interviews of first-year residents abound with statements such as, 'I felt like a boy doctor without a toy stethoscope,' and 'I felt as though I was beginning my internship without ever having gone through medical school.' ''[22]

While these initial experiences have been often described, the structure that causes them has not. First, it is important to realize that two conditions promote anxiety: involvement or responsibility *plus* uncertainty.[23] The more involved or responsible a person feels in a situation and the more uncertain a person is, the more anxious he or she will feel. Both conditions are necessary; for experiencing just one presents no serious problem. Thus, if a program wishes to break down old values and ways of seeing the world, it will maximize involvement or responsibility as well as heighten a feeling of uncertainty.

In addition, two conditions contribute to uncertainty: lack of definition and irrelevance of past experience. The less clearly defined the task to be mastered, the more uncertain a person will be. And the less people can draw upon past experiences to cope with a new task, the more uncertain they will be. They will try to redefine the situation in light of past experiences in order to make more sense out of it, and they will try to adapt past skills so they can master the new situations.[24]

To the extent that this fails, they are left in the frightening position of having few resources with which to cope with a novel and confusing problem. From these conditions, two results follow. The people become more dependent on those who appear in command of the situation, and they tend toward closure to allay their anxieties by incorporating the nearest model that promises to restore clarity and control.[25]

Psychiatric residency fulfills all of these conditions, which provide an excellent framework for integrating almost all the studies that have been made of residency programs. Despite limited competence, ''the resident is given high professional status in the hospital, both officially and unofficially. He is regarded as a responsible psychiatrist by the public, by his patients, by the nonmedical staff, and, in a sense, by his psychiatric superiors. How shall he deal with his anxiety regarding his professional competence?''[26]

The young doctors find their professional values challenged and their identities threatened. Their pride in precise diagnosis, in swift effective action, and in responsibility for the patient's well-being, all meet frustration with these new patients. Staff tell residents to abandon "rescue fantasies," call active intervention "intrusion," warn that the patient may be manipulating the resident, and allude to similarities between the patients and the residents. "A recognition of similarity leads to a variety of responses, the most common of which is a blurring of identification with a concomitant decrease in objectivity, leading the resident to doubt his ability to handle stress."[27] Residents try to cope by drawing on their medical training. "It is well documented that new psychiatric residents tend to become obsessively preoccupied with conventional medical detail as a reaction to the impact of the first encounter with psychiatric patients."[28]

The vagueness of psychiatric principles further increases the uncertainty and hence anxiety of the resident. "Lacking the security of independent measures of pathology, he feels isolated from his previous medical experience. . . . Psychiatric concepts are difficult to teach and even more difficult to learn, since to be of value they must be both intellectually understood and effectively integrated. More amorphous and implicit than the clearly articulated and highly organized principles of organic medicine, they are more threatening to the student both in their content and in the more subjective manner of their presentation."[29]

Part of the discomfort of psychiatric principles is their application to the residents as well as the patients. In fact, it is not always clear how the two groups differ. Residents must learn to understand primitive fantasies and intense emotions in both their patients and themselves.[30] Halleck and Woods conclude: "Perhaps no psychiatrist goes through training without at one time or another worrying about the loss of his sanity. Being unequipped to understand the more subtle nuances of a psychotic diagnosis, he frequently misinterprets personality traits or symptoms in himself as having the same meaning they do in his patients."[31] Merklin and Little conclude that if "a resident does not experience anxiety and subsequent 'transitory neurotic symptoms,' it might indicate that his defenses had developed to such a degree as to prevent him from significant emotional interchange, thereby decreasing his therapeutic effectiveness and professional scope."[32]

Observations like these by many authors imply that the moral career of the psychiatric resident may not be too different from the moral career of the mental patient. As described by Goffman, the patient feels he is losing control, losing his mind. He attempts "to conceal

from others what he takes to be the new fundamental facts about himself, and . . . to discover whether others, too, have discovered
them."[33] Each resident, like other people during their moral career,
constructs "an image of his life course—past, present, future—which
selects, abstracts, and distorts in such a way as to provide him with a
view of himself that he can usefully expound in current situations."[34]
Given the deviance of the psychiatric career and its self-consciousness,
psychiatric candidates work hard at their stories for their parents, for
old classmates, and for themselves. But the structure of mental health
programs makes this difficult, "for few settings could be so destructive
of self-stories, except, of course, those stories already constructed
along psychiatric lines."[35] Although writing about the press of psychiatric structure on mental patients, Goffman might be writing about residents when he observes that "the self arises not merely out of its possessor's interactions with significant others, but also out of the
arrangements that are evolved in an organization for its members . . .
in which significance for self is made explicitly to the patient, pier-
cingly, persistently, and thoroughly."[36]

Besides creating these conditions for maximizing anxiety and
making recruits susceptible to new moral values, psychiatric residency
employs degradation ceremonies. In his classic study of degradation
ceremonies, Harold Garfinkel described their five characteristics:[37] 1.
the discredited event or actor is made to stand out; 2. it is not the specific event but the whole class of events or actors that is discredited; 3.
the moral framework requires, not allows, that the new definition of
the situation be accepted. Trying out, "reality testing," and the like
may occur but are considered morally inferior; 4. the denouncer must
be a public figure. He or she must be accepted as such and be seen as a
transcendent figure who does not speak from personal values; 5. he or
she must deliver the denunciation in the name of the tribe's values.

Psychiatric residency abounds in such degradation ceremonies,
from psychiatric nurses who openly scold a resident for misjudging a
patient or not knowing a technical matter[38] to supervisors who gently
show residents how their own neurotic preoccupations are interfering
with therapy.

2. Moral Confusion

For all but the strongest residents, the net effect of being different
and discredited is moral confusion. Anxiety runs high. Residents can

no longer tell right from wrong, as they generally could in medicine a few months earlier. Certain moral lessons come across quickly: managing patients is not very important; certain kinds of patients are not worthwhile; a high priority is to work with patients who can teach you something. Yet none of these feel very comfortable, because they conflict with old values. As Fred Davis points out, this moral discomfort originates in the sense of alienation from oneself that occurs when doing unnatural things.[39] Trying to psyche out instructors (especially when it fails) also contributed to alienation.

Residents struggle for a long time with attacks on the old moral order, which is made up of values from medicine and naive images of psychiatry. Are senior staff really serious when they say that one should not try to cure the patient? Is it right that the patient should do most of the work in therapy? What constitutes moral conduct is unclear. Is one's first duty to get patients out, or to sit through their pain and not administer drugs? Many residents are not sure from day to day why they are doing what they do. Is Carl manipulating his patient; is she manipulating him? Is Marc right that the hospital impedes therapy, and if so what are we doing here?

The mutual concealment noted before makes matters worse. Each resident (like each patient) tends to think he alone is so bewildered. He may notice some confusion in others, but he is too self-preoccupied to make the connection. "Threatened by his strange environment, his feelings of discontinuity with his past, and his lack of preparation for great responsibility, the new resident is in a hazardous position. His fears for his own sanity are more intense, as are those of people who experience cultural shock when suddenly required to adapt to a foreign civilization."[40]

3. Numbness and Exhaustion[41]

In class after class, the great researcher at Menninger, Robert Holt, observed a slump.[42] A number of other studies have since noted that lack of success with patients may lead to "therapeutic nihilism." "Residents who react in this manner often become cynical, unbelieving, and chronically dissatisfied."[43] Klagsbrun writes: "I spent three years attempting to bury a part of myself that expresses concern, warmth, and involvement with patients. I learned how to hide my feelings and prevent 'transference cures' and 'flights into health.' "[44] Speaking more generally, Klagsbrun writes that the resident "is expected to tolerate the guilt he feels for assuming a distant attitude toward his patients without having a guarantee that such an attitude helps. . . . He has learned that his feelings and reactions are not reliable guides to therapy because they are related to his own past and present life as much as to the patient's impact on him at that moment.''[45]

Nothing seems to work. Everyone is tired, and again there is a striking parallel with Goffman's description of how the patient feels at this point. He or she also lives with a bewildering array of orders and urgings from nurses, attendants, and psychiatrists. But more important is the scrutiny and exposure that finally makes one stop trying to work out an account of oneself as a moral being.

> Having one's past mistakes and present progress under constant moral review seems to make for a special adaptation consisting of a less than moral attitude to ego ideals. One's shortcomings and successes become too central and fluctuating an issue in life to allow the usual commitment of concern for other persons' views of them. It is not very practicable to try to sustain claims about oneself. The inmate tends to learn that degradations and reconstructions of the self need not be given too much weight, at the same time learning that staff and inmates are ready to view an inflation or deflation of a self with some indifference. He learns that a defensible picture of self can be seen as something outside oneself that can be constructed, lost, and rebuilt, all with great speed and some equanimity. He learns about the viability of taking up a standpoint—and hence a self—that is outside the one which the hospital can give and take away from him.
>
> The setting, then, seems to engender a kind of cosmopolitan sophistication, a kind of civic apathy. In this unserious yet oddly exaggerated moral context, building up a self or having it destroyed becomes something of a shameless game, and learning to view this process as a game seems to make for some demoralization, the game being such a fundamental one.[46]

Marc says he does not care anymore. Carl says we're no more than a traffic station. Ken knows his work is sloppy, like everyone else's. He feels he is being sucked dry, like a gigolo with too much business. Everybody says they're sad. Dave points out that there is no evidence that what we do to patients works. A great moral victory becomes getting a discharged patient coming back for therapy. "The question," says Ken, "is whether there is life before death."

4. Moral Transition

The period of moral exhaustion is a moment of truth. Somehow one must go on or quit. It is during this phase that all those neurotic symptoms and psychosomatic disturbances noted by psychiatric educators either subside or get worse. "A common reaction to strong stresses upon the resident is the development of a therapeutic nihilism which may never remit. . . . Just as serious a problem as the nihilistic resident is what might be called the bandwagon resident, who latches on to whatever philosophy is prevailing at the time and endows it with the status of fact."[47] Cynicism, conversion, and (most frequently) working out one's own beliefs within the framework of the program are all forms of transition that set the professional's moral career on a new course. At another residency during the same period, an extraordinary resident documented a transition similar to those we have observed.

> In our struggles, we rallied around a succession of theories of therapy and mental illness. . . . As each theoretical position was explored and found wanting in turn, we gradually worked our way towards a purely empirical position.
>
> We swallowed hard, put aside our prejudices, and pushed the red button on the electrotherapy machine, cringing while we watched its effect, but unable to deny its benefits. Being empiricists, we became free to manipulate the patients, their families, and even their business associates. . . .
>
> We amassed experience as empiricists and we relied on what "worked." . . . The failure of our patients often became interpreted in our minds as personal failure. . . .
>
> There are relatively few constructive defenses available to a resident in crisis. The most common solution to identity crisis during residency is to jump on a bandwagon—to borrow an identity and make it one's own.[48]

The apathy and demoralization experienced by the residents results from their trying to maintain a sense of self in the face of an alternate moral framework. But once they become receptive to that new framework, moral renewal can begin. Again, the parallel between patient and resident is striking.

> If both the custodial and psychiatric factions are to get him to cooperate in the various psychiatric treatments, then it will prove useful to dis-

abuse him of his views of their purposes, and cause him to appreciate that they know what they are doing, and are doing what is best for him. In brief, the difficulties caused by a patient are closely tied to his version of what has been happening to him, and if cooperation is to be secured, it helps if this version is discredited. The patient must "insightfully" come to take, or affect to take, the hospital's view of himself.[49]

Residents arrive at this point in their moral career at different times. One would think that those who had always wanted to be psychiatrists would start at this point when residency began, but the realities of inpatient psychiatry, combined with their medical training, delay this phase even for them. It starts when residents more or less give up on getting patients better and turn to their own countertransference as the focus of therapy. Their morale picks up.

The sheer press of work is crucial in getting residents to arrive at this point. Day in and day out they have to act like psychiatrists, enacting constructed performances that approximate as closely as they can what the program's directors seem to want. This constant role playing is what carries residents along, even though for a while it makes little sense at all. For the more one does it, the less inauthentic it seems, particularly when patients and supervisors take your performances seriously.

It's like, remember when you were a first year resident and you were scared to death of your patients and you found out that they thought you knew what you were doing? Eventually you felt like you knew what you were doing too.[50]

This daily role playing both helps to push out the residual of old perspectives and brings into conscience the new moral order, *which is embodied in the very roles one is performing.* Some catch on much more quickly than others, and here the peer culture becomes very important. For the concealment which characterized the early phases gives way to helping as peers have something to share rather than to hide.

The process of resocialization is clear. Under the conditions of anxiety, there are strong tendencies toward closure, toward the nearest model that will restore clarity and command.[51] To the extent that the search for closure and certainty in past (i.e., medical) approaches fails, one turns to those who one thinks are masters of the present task.[52] As Gary Tischler found in his study of psychiatric training, the resident makes the transition by depending heavily on key supervisors. He accepts advice as dogma and "blindly clothes himself in what he believes to be the attributes of a psychiatrist, without regard to fit or appropriateness."[53] One tends to identify with one or more of these models. One may fear or admire the model. Fantasy and exaggeration of powers play an important role in this process, not only out of high anxiety and immediate needs for coping, but also out of the tendency to reinforce oneself by imagining one has the powers attributed to the model. The ideological closure of the program and the prevalence of supervision contribute to this transition. The constant presence of patients is also important, because in a similar fashion they attribute powers of healing to the struggling resident.

As bonds of identification strengthen and individuals gain confidence, trainees begin to wean themselves gradually from those on whom they have depended. They come to perceive these models' flaws and limitations. Increasingly they attribute to themselves a sense of mastery, and this is enhanced by their working alone, away from critical eyes. Moreover, the effort put into acquiring the values and skills they now have is likely to protect them from weaning, even if they are unrewarded. "Effort justification" seems to be an important mechanism in professional socialization.[54]

The increasing responsibility which the program gives to residents in the second half of their training facilitates this stage of socialization. The residents also have more choice. The third year is entirely elective, though the choices are made soon after the first year. This timing gives residents a large sense of autonomy but in a way that ties those choices to the most vulnerable period of socialization. The structural feature of individual autonomy also facilitates a growing sense of mastery. Trainees increasingly attribute successes to themselves and failures to the patients or to difficulties of the case. This is a common pattern in the professions. The autonomy promoted by rules against interfering with colleagues' work and a selective use of powerlessness may be structurally necessary for some professions to survive in their present form.

Some trainees break away and find alternate moral frameworks. From their sense of futility, of estrangement, of disillusionment, they conclude that the tenets of the program do not just seem wrong but *are* wrong. While most residents, for example, talk about the lack of evidence that psychotherapy does much good, very few make that the foundation for a new approach. This requires great strength; for it is one thing to recognize a well-known flaw in the discipline and another to thereby reject the roles and techniques and language that surround one on all sides. More residents try this than succeed in establishing an alternate reality, because when they reject these central attributes of the profession they find themselves empty-handed. Supervisors and peers ask them, "What would you do instead? What's your theory?" Because they must go on (or quit), they are essentially being asked to develop a whole theory and body of effective techniques in a few months. Overwhelmed, they retreat and accommodate or convert.

But a few find outside help and establish a different moral order. One strong, bright resident from Japan went through the confusion and despair of early training until he realized one day what bothered him so much about psychoanalytic theory. It was based on the premise that people are neurotic and that society stands against the individual, so that the task of therapy is often to assist a "realistic adjustment" to the limitations of one's life. Drawing sustenance from his Buddhist faith, he concluded that this philosophy was morally sick. The goal of life is to grow, to attain one's potential, not to be fettered by invisible bonds and to adjust, he argued. He found a minor school of psychiatry which supported his moral views and which had worked out techniques to accompany it.

Another resident felt confused and disillusioned until he took seriously the evidence that psychotherapy was a vague, subjective and useless tool. He had read about behavioral therapy and started learning all he could. He concluded that it was the scientific, modern approach to mental problems. It had the attributes of his original self-image as a doctor—precise and helpful. He found one or two people to support him in his work, ignored most of his peers and supervisors, and he has since distinguished himself in the field.

In most cases, however, moral transition is likely to follow institutional lines because they are so pervasive in everything one says and does. In this phase of groping, testing and episodic failures that characterize any first attempts to assimilate a new set of values, professional ideology is obviously critical; for it contains the new moral precepts in a coherent world view.[55] It provides an interpretive scheme for appraising performances and communicating their "meaning" to peers and instructors. The distinguished psychiatrist Jerome Frank explains this function more specifically:

A therapist can succeed only if he has some conviction that what he is doing makes sense and that he is competent to do it. He gains this feeling first of all from his therapeutic successes, which, often erroneously, he regards as evidence for the validity of his theory. That is, a patient's improvement may actually have resulted from aspects of the therapeutic situation that escape the therapist's formulations and even his notice, such as the rebirth of hope. The success rate of most psychotherapists, however, is scarcely large enough to sustain their self-confidence. . . . adherence to a doctrine may be a major source of emotional support, and the most supportive, hence the most seductive, theories explain away the therapist's failures while letting him take credit for his success. . . . As one young psychoanalyst was heard to remark: "The wonderful thing about psychoanalysis is that even if the patient doesn't get better, you know you are doing the right thing." This is a caricature, of course, but it contains a germ of truth, and could be said with justice about many other systems of therapy.[56]

Is this kind of moral renewal at all related to Goffman's description of the mental patient? He writes: "In casting off the raiments of the old self—or in having this cover torn away—the person need not seek a new role. . . . Instead he can learn, at least for a time, to practice before all groups the amoral arts of shamelessness."[57] To a degree not fully recognized, professionals also take on a kind of moral order that from the layman's point of view is amoral and shameless. One learns it is professionally "cool" to speak openly to fellow residents about one's neuroses and fantasies. A cocky female resident in her third year was joking with male residents about the food at supper and said the peas remind her of "balls." The men laughed nervously as she outclassed them in shameless candor. A senior psychiatrist who did valued work with local patients assured his listener that helping others was not his true motivation. Freud showed, he said, that wanting to help is merely a way of sublimating desires to control others and aggrandize oneself. What others admired he "knew" to be a sham.

In professional work, turning to technique ends many moral dilemmas. There is great comfort in knowing that by doing technically good work one is ipso facto doing good. Means become ends. A moral order built on a single strand is thin indeed. Much that has been written against lawyers, social scientists, doctors, and others comes down to their brushing aside considerations of expense, pain, and the ends to which their services are put in the name of "good professional work."

Jerome Frank indicates this is the case in psychiatry, and I think it is generally the case among professions. As a moral order it not only elevates one's strength (technical skills) above all else, but it also has the advantage of freeing the professional from the difficulties of the more complex moral order from which he came. Some might call this kind of perspective "moral abandonment" rather than moral renewal. Responsible professionals guard against the dangers of this one-stranded morality, and their efforts are to be applauded. But *the structure of professional work constantly reinforces the narrow morality of technique.*[58]

5. Self-affirmation

This phase denotes the end of a dependence on models and a building up of the new world view. It signals what is traditionally called internalization, making this world view firmly one's own.[59] In a parallel study of student nurses, Fred Davis accurately characterizes the features of this phase as an assured stance toward professional work even when beset with new difficulties, an ease at articulating the kind of practice one believes in and how it differs from others, and a tendency to reinterpret past traumas and self-doubts by minimizing or even ignoring them. ". . . they suppress the frequently jarring and ego-alienating alterations in attitude and perception which, as I have tried to point out, are actually entailed in the becoming process."[60] Because of this suppression and their structural position as the agents of socialization, psychiatric educators are much less sensitive to the moral career we are describing than are residents going through it.

The moral transition in psychiatry is unusually thorough; for even in the course of training, one's personal style and problems are subject to scrutiny every week by several supervisors in the name of countertransference. If one undergoes psychoanalysis, which such supervision naturally induces one to do, one's entire life history is recast into a new world view. Because it is so thorough and takes a long time, self-affirmation may come in waves over time. That is, a third-year resident may be amused at how naive he was when he entered residency, but three years later his self-affirmation will be deeper, and he will look back in a similar way at his self-confidence as a third-year resident. Within the residency program, the importance of the latter part of the second year and the entire third year lies not in major new changes but in weaning oneself from role models and gaining a sense of mastery.[61] Each individual does this in his or her own way, but is strongly influenced by the structure of training. In a major survey, for example, of all the psychiatrists, psychologists and psychiatric social workers in New York, Chicago and Los Angeles, over 70 percent identified a Freudian or neo-Freudian ideology as their guiding orientation. At the same time the data showed that "the practitioner extensively modifies and adapts these formally learned tenets to suit his own situation."[62]

Conclusion

An occupational hazard of psychiatry is to interpret psychiatrically individual actions which are really part of social patterns. By integrating observations from major studies of psychiatric training into a general model of professional socialization, and by pointing out the ironic parallels between residents and patients exposed to similar forces of socialization despite the stark differences between them, one comes to realize that the acute emotional turmoil of psychiatric residents cannot be understood simply in terms of their psychopathology. The personal cost of psychiatric training and its moral consequences must be studied in terms of the training process itself as well as in terms of residents' personal strengths and weaknesses.

A major consequence of the socialization experience we have described is that young psychiatrists move away from being advocates of the patient and toward being technicians. The intensity of the first three stages of moral transformation results in their becoming very self-preoccupied, even if they were altruistic before. The conversion-like experience leads to premature closure on issues full of ambiguity. The well-being of the patient becomes of secondary concern, as the history of psychiatry so amply illustrates.

This study also belies the superficial nature of "adult socialization." We tend to think of socialization, particularly in the adult years, in terms of continuity, of variations on fundamental themes arrived at early in personal development. The more this is true, the more trivial by definition adult or professional socialization must be. Yet to experience it is to know that something important has happened. The recent work of Daniel Levinson has given substance to our private sense that there are major life transitions among adults.[63] His work shows that young professionals in their late twenties or early thirties are struggling to realize their dream as they look for a "true mentor" to foster their development. Yet they are also weaning themselves from parental bonds and coping with their disappointments as well as those of their parents. The transition from medicine to psychiatry often entails losing part of the parents' or the individual's dream of becoming a "doctor."[64] Most residents by this time are also learning about their capacities and limitations in intimate relations. Residency training does not help, putting great stress on a person's mate. Writing of the resident's wife, Halleck and Woods correctly observe:

> Her husband is gone long hours, is frequently upset and tends to develop ideas which she can rarely understand. In discussions with her husband and in kaffeeklatches with her neighbors, she hears psychiatric terms, interpretations and concepts applied to herself and her family which may not be flattering. In this setting many residents and their wives find themselves exposed to entirely new problems in relating to one another that they may not have been prepared for at the time of their marriage contract.[65]

Here, in the middle of what Levinson calls "Settling Down"—a period of finding himself, founding his own family, stabilizing his career and establishing a mature relation with his parents—the resident experiences therapeutic impotence, is put at the bottom of a new heap, has his values challenged, and consequently subjects his carefully nurtured self-image to reexamination. All this happens in a field of institutional forces and requires an explanation that considers both the psychological and social dimensions of the experience.

12.

The Structure
of Psychiatric Residency

Like all other trainees, the residents at University Psychiatric Center were affected by the structural features of the residency program. Yet most residents did not perceive them clearly, often attributing pressure from them as personal trouble. Nor is the structure of other residency programs usually perceived by investigators, even though they shape the residents' moral career, diagnostic bias, therapeutic ability and professional values. Drawing together a large number of studies with this one,[1] this chapter integrates the research on residency training and identifies the structural features in the residencies that have been studied.

Starting with the Sickest Patients

One of the most obvious structural features of the training program is that residents began on the wards, treating inpatients.[2] In the second year, they kept some inpatients from the first year, but all their new patients were outpatients. If one required hospitalization, a first-year resident would take over the case.

This feature seems designed to crush certain medical habits. These patients *looked* healthy; yet they were the least likely to improve under anyone. For several months the new residents wheedled, per-

259

suaded, cajoled and commanded their patients to get better—with discouraging results. When the patients were lower class and/or inarticulate, treatment became even more difficult. Speaking of another residency, two psychiatrists wrote, "The inevitable disillusionment may lead to therapeutic nihilism and severe doubt as to the wisdom of his choice of specialty. Unfortunately, it is a common practice in psychiatric training centers that the sickest patients are treated by the most inexperienced staff, the first-year residents."[3] There is a high price both to residents and to psychiatry for this structure, but it does increase anxiety and probably makes socialization more effective.

Several reasons were given for this structure. The training staff claimed that disorders and defenses were most easily seen in very sick patients; thus new residents could learn more easily the basic dynamics of the psyche. Also, psychotic patients, they said, do not cover up their great pain and rage. If the resident must learn to sit and bear the patient's pain, inpatients were the best teaching material. A chief said, "If you can sit with these patients, you can sit with anyone." With inpatients, staff argued, the new resident must face and cope with the most primitive defenses of the psyche.

These psychiatric reasons for starting residents with inpatients may be important, but they do not fathom the depths to which this structure affects trainees. First, it socialized them to a psychotic view of mental "illness." The residents' root experience was with psychotic, "primitive" patients, and they were constantly told that these very same forces existed in healthier patients, only more completely controlled and disguised. This structural feature provided a strong basis for a psychoanalytic, "medical" view of personality. Of course, this view would strongly color the doctor's future treatment of outpatients as neurotics rather than as people with problems of living. It comes as no surprise that older residents said their outpatients were almost as sick as the inpatients they had. This structural arrangement also preserved as much continuity as possible between medicine and psychiatry; for psychotic patients were more easily seen as having a "disease" than outpatients, who might be more easily seen as simply "troubled." First-year residents *assumed* all cases were sick, resulting in the rule, "When in doubt, diagnose ill."[4] In sum, the implicit assumption that the basic dynamics of the psyche were the same in psychotics as in all patients became a self-fulfilling reality through socialization.

The implications of this training are grave and may account for the tendency in psychiatrists to see severe pathology where none exists.[5] Lawrence Kubie has called the consequences of starting residents with inpatients disastrous, "a form of medical malpractice."[6] "Instead of engendering that difficult but essential balance between objectivity and empathy, we encourage the resident to dismiss the unfamiliar with easy clichés about 'psychotic' or 'schizoid' personalities. The traditional sequence of training perpetuates the invalid assumption that there is only one way to become depressed, elated, anxious, compulsive, paranoid, hypochondriacal, deluded, hallucinated, or to develop conversion symptoms."[7]

Besides providing a basis for a psychoanalytic orientation to be elaborated in later years, inpatients also crush myths more effectively than any other possible arrangement. In terms of socialization, they are the best material for bringing about relative deprivation, that state wherein old actions which were successful in a previous context are seen to be ineffective if not injurious in a new one. Residents come to psychiatry with a desire to treat people personally; many state how much they enjoyed talking with patients as medical students. For these humanists, inpatients are the hardest to get to know personally. In the first two months, many residents tried to get close to their patients and found it impossible. The patients were hospitalized because they could not effectively relate to others, and many were emotionally unable to be intimate. Moreover, the residents had a distancing amount of power and status.

Many residents also came with the desire to cure patients, to lift them from their mental torment. These desires were labeled "rescue fantasies," and the inpatients effectively proved the point. They were least likely to get better. If they did improve, it was often for no apparent reason. If patients did not change, residents tired of them. As we have seen, residents began to sense that they had nothing to do with improvement, or if they did, they could not pinpoint their influence.[8] By the fourth month one heard evidence of very strong responses to relative deprivation, as in Ken Reese's dream about his patients splashing formaldehyde on him. Another report on residency training concludes: "The inpatients he sees during this year may be some of the most disturbing people he will encounter in his psychiatric career. There are few comparable situations in medicine in which a physician is given so much responsibility in an area where he starts out with so little knowledge. Though he has usually achieved some sense of identity as an adequate physician during his internship, this is quickly threatened.''[9]

Working with inpatients while learning psychotherapy virtually determines the residents' attitudes toward inpatients. The structure and the process are irreconcilable, and since the future lies with the process, the structure gets uniformly criticized. Specifically, the residents learned that they could not do psychotherapy in the structure of an inpatient hospital, either because patients were too sick or because they were not given enough time. The average inpatient at this acute hospital stayed for four months. As one resident said, "It took Frieda Fromm-Reichmann four years to cure a schizophrenic; do they expect me to do it in four months?" A psychiatrist could treat schizophrenics in a chronic hospital for four years, but residents regarded such places as the end of the world. Thus one was not surprised that by spring of the first year, the residents had lost interest in hospitalized patients. Jeff Roche said, "This was the first time that I got a patient whom I really didn't want at all. As an intern, you reach that point some time toward the end of the year. . . ." Later, four residents compared notes and decided they had had one acute schizophrenic between them. Many residents concluded that love and care are all that the inpatients need, and the nursing or social work staff can do that competently. At the same time, the residents uniformly looked forward to getting healthier patients in the second year. Thus, starting with inpatients taught residents that the active, interventionist style which made them effective in medicine was ineffective here and even made some patients worse.

Moreover, the program was designed to contrast these inpatients with healthier outpatients, for each resident got one "university patient." These patients were selected before the new cohort arrives by older residents working in the Southard Clinic, where outpatients are seen. Every profession has its ideal client, and the older residents set aside for the new residents people coming in for help who had as many of the ideal qualities as possible: articulate, intelligent, troubled but quite able to carry on a regular life, interesting to listen to, young, female. An example would be a college coed troubled by problems of intimacy with her boyfriend and her parents.

The desire to cure was also modified in significant ways. By the second year, residents had concluded: 1. that they could perhaps cure outpatients but not inpatients; 2. that improvement must be measured in months, not days; 3. that the healthiest patients are the most worthwhile patients to treat. Learning to sit with inpatients in the first year helped residents nurture enthusiasm for their work in future years. For if they could make it through the winter of the first year, they were able to see themselves as increasingly effective and their work as increasingly pleasant.

Finally, inpatients were the best patients to work with in order to learn a modified medical model. They came to regard "management" as secondary and less important than "therapy," even though management consisted of activities central to medical practice. Prescribing drugs, handling medical problems and other physiological practices became regarded as interfering with the "real business" to be done. Inpatients succeeded in discouraging those medically-oriented residents who tried to cure patients with drugs. To the extent that drugs "worked," residents were constantly told by their seniors that drugs and other such devices merely relieved symptoms. Even if the patient showed dramatic recovery and appeared to be "normal," he was not considered to be much improved, and a relapse was predicted. Until one had "worked through the dynamics," it was argued, substantial improvement was not possible.[10] Statistics did not bear out this ideology, but figures on symptom improvement were not relevant. The spirit was captured by another investigator who wrote, "I have heard therapists claim that, should even symptom relief achieved without insight prove to last the lifetime of the patient, they would still regard it as a transference cure and something less than desirable."[11] More generally, those activities which made up the administration and management of the patient's life received no serious attention. Despite a proud tradition in the hospital of "the therapeutic community," residents gave little attention to the ward as an organization or a milieu.

Working with inpatients in a hospital preserved the doctor-patient relation found in medicine, even as residents learn to transfer more and more responsibility for the patient's improvement from themselves to the patient. "Even if a patient denies his illness or dislikes his doctor, he must still concentrate upon the doctor because the hospital's organization forces him to deal with this authority."[12] This institutional power shores up the young psychiatrist's professional authority and helps to disguise his ignorance until he can acquire the language and knowledge that will allow him to assert his professional superiority over his patients.*

Ideological Closure[13]

It is not a foregone conclusion that starting with psychotic patients on hospital wards will have these effects. For example, the residents could learn from it, as they did in medicine, that behavioral symptoms are the measure of pathology, and that physiological forms of treatment are the best. In low-prestige residencies this is the emphasis, though as we saw before, the tendency to regard psychoanalytically oriented psychotherapy as the ideal treatment heavily pervades even these residencies in state mental hospitals, where the press of workloads makes it nearly impossible to do much of anything but treat behavioral symptoms with drugs and shock. Moreover, a few distinguished residencies have emphasized alternate models of mental disorders, and as work on genetic causes of schizophrenia and other biological research progress, this number will increase. But at the University Psychiatric Center in the late 1960s, electroshock therapy, though acknowledged as effective, was regarded as "revolting" and "barbaric"; behavioral therapy as showing "escape from personal involvement with your patients"; desire to cure as "rescue fantasies"; and an interest in community psychiatry as "acting out" and as being "superficial." At the same time, the program advertised itself as an eclectic integration of all the relevant approaches of the sixties. This gave the illusion of more choice than existed.

Jeff talked to a medical student interested in coming here as a resident. Only after the student asked did Jeff say that the program was

*By contrast, one-fourth of the residents began training in the Day Hospital, a facility for seriously disturbed patients who needed care every day but who went home every night. By definition, the care of these patients deeply involved their families, and residents in the Day Hospital had a different, more social-psychological view of care. The medical model was considerably weaker, because they had to work closely with relatives and social workers in order to treat the patients. The cases ranged over a wider variety of problems, and the thick texture of everyday life coursed through therapy more than it did with inpatients or with outpatients seen during disembodied hours of the week in a resident's office. Thus the structural distortions of starting with inpatients were considerably mollified in the Day Hospital.

heavily analytic. The rest of the time he emphasized that you could do anything you wanted—behavioral therapy, shock, drugs, anything.

The student asked why these things were not done, if residents are free? Jeff said he didn't know, except that the best people are all analytic.

Later in the conversation, Jeff said that for the first time, after the APA meetings, he had become aware of the alternatives for treating patients, and now he said he was questioning a lot more that goes on around here.

The student kept asking what theory do you learn here, because he said he wanted a broad exposure. He seemed to be thinking in terms of classes, readings, etc. Jeff said soberly that "here you read your patient." The student laughed.

The psychoanalytic bias permeated the program in a number of ways. First, nearly all of the supervisors were not only psychoanalytically inclined but also attached to the Psychoanalytic Institute, so that the chief source of models for socialization represented this one approach to psychiatry. Moreover, they focused on countertransference issues—a psychoanalytic theme—and moved residents toward having their own psychoanalysis. This is about as thorough an immersion into one ideology as one can have in a voluntary program.

Second, most of the alternate models were weak. The first-class minds were psychoanalysts, and the residents knew it. As one chief resident said, "The system is biased. All the senior men are analysts, and the representatives of other areas are slobs. And this leads you to say, 'I want to be smart. I want to get with it. So I'll go into analysis and it will make me smart.' " For example, the teacher of psychopharmacology was held in such low regard that attendance dropped at his seminars until he finally circulated a memo urging residents to attend. Everyone interpreted this memo as advertising for clients. The lone representative of behavioral therapy was described by unsympathetic residents as very junior, working with homosexuals and having his office in the dank bowels of the basement.

The ideological closure of a program provides a vocabulary and interpretive framework for residents to understand themselves and their patients. Interpretations from chiefs and supervisors never stop. One chief told his residents, "You find in the middle of your second year that the patients you still have or are still in the hospital [from the first year] are those who have the same problems you do." When a resident admired a visiting interviewer for her brilliance, a supervisor said, "Perhaps you like her because you want to avoid your feelings of despair." In time the residents found in this framework the solution to their professional crisis.

> . . . it was so convenient to be able to explain all observed behavior on the basis of psychoanalytic tenets. One can "explain" the most peculiar and complex interreactions and verbalizations with a fair knowledge of psychoanalytic theory, a thorough knowledge of its jargon and a bit of *sangfroid*. Every psychiatric resident in an analytically-oriented training program learns sooner or later with more or less awareness what a whore a psychodynamic formulation is. Anyone can use it for just about anything.[14]

Yet the ideology of eclecticism gave residents the sense of choice and made it more difficult for them to perceive the channeling of their preference and values toward psychoanalytic psychiatry. Rue Bucher found beneath the superficial eclecticism a deep monotheism at Michael Reese Hospital, and pointed out that only by virtue of dogged determination could residents get their own projects off the ground.[15] The tactic in both places was not to oppose independent projects (that would be antiintellectual and hard to defend) but to subtly discourage them as not the best use of one's time and to passively resist them by giving no support. The few residents who experienced this but went their own way during the study were interested in R. D. Laing, hypnosis, behavioral therapy, and Zen therapy. The subtle impact of repressive tolerance on other residents is seen in the conversation which ends this chapter.

The disinterest in community psychiatry at a time when it was all the vogue is more difficult to explain, because Distinguished Medical School had some of the best people in the country representing this approach. Yet with exceptions, residents acquired the psychoanalytic attitude toward community psychiatry—that it was largely irrelevant and stupid. The broader resistance to community psychiatry at the height of radical activism deserves reflection. At the time, the hospital had taken on responsibility for a catchment area; the residents reacted by whining all year about the so-called incontinent old people and inarticulate, lower-class blacks. Echoing the predominant opinion, one resident said, "This isn't what we came here for." Structurally, the residents of all three years worked together to get around the "disadvantages" of community psychiatry. The older residents became more sophisticated about how to "dump" such patients in other community facilities, such as various nursing homes and other state hospitals. Similar feelings of anger, disappointment and frustration have been reported from programs with more systematic training in community psychiatry.[16] These reactions seem to have two sources: an ideological preference for psychodynamic psychiatry and the failure of community psychiatry to develop clear professional roles or careers for physicians.[17]

Finally, the structure of careers seemed to the residents centered around psychoanalysis, because the leading figures and best jobs were held by or controlled by the psychoanalysts. Nationally, at that time, the professional market was changing quickly. Analysts were running short of patients, and positions in community psychiatry were opening up fast. But the ideal career for most of these residents centered on psychoanalytic psychotherapy, with a change of pace provided by supervising some residents, doing a bit of research, or perhaps helping out a community mental health center for a few hours a week.[18]

Intense Supervision

A third structural feature of the residency program in psychiatry was intense supervision. Not only did each resident have several supervisors, but in the first year he met for a feelings meeting with other residents on his service and attended a group dynamics seminar, which also met once a week. The overall tone was supportive and permissive. Insights were suggested and policies recommended. Supervisors were very circumspect in their criticisms.

Supervision—including these group experiences—was the major agent of socialization. Through the supervisor or group, the resident learned how to understand the psychiatric world by acquiring the right values and orientation. In supervision, the resident learned why his old practices and desires were not appropriate and what new ones were. By being so open and supportive, supervisors were able to effect internal change which orders and strict directives could not. Some senior staff call socialization a "collective search for reality." There is no evidence, however, that new residents have more fantasies than others. It is just that they have not been properly socialized, and the senior men have an edge in explaining away complaints.

In the critical first year, supervision was the structural counter-balance to treating inpatients in an acute hospital, for while the latter was designed to break down old ways and disorient the resident, the former supported and reoriented the resident toward new ways. In the varieties of supervision, the senior men used the same categories on residents that the residents learned to use on patients. Thus, super-vision reoriented the resident to *himself*.

The two group experiences were designed to be supportive during the residents' most difficult year, and to bring misery company. The small feelings meetings on each service seemed to be the most effec-tive two hours in the week for doing this. They were an important form of supervision. Yet many older residents advised me that it was the group dynamics seminars where the heart of psychiatric socialization took place. Unfortunately, they said, one could never get in to observe it. I did. The major theme of the group dynamics seminar, which was inwardly focused and self-conscious, was that residents had a hard time expressing how much they actually *liked* each other. The group leader, a senior analyst, raised this theme early in the year and con-tinued to suggest that getting close was "the hardest thing in the world." The analyst made this group a strained and artificial experi-ence as he emphasized any evidence showing how difficult it was to get close to one another and urged that residents try. But the effect, to this observer, was strained intimacy. Outside of the group, residents seemed to have no trouble making or keeping friends. There were no great obstacles to friendship, such as the fierce competition in premed years which can pit comrades against each other. Yet suddenly in this group, residents were struggling to get close—and trying to impress the senior analyst with their efforts. One can only conclude that if this was the heart of socialization in the first year, then the outcome was contrived neurosis.

Structurally, the tremendous amount of supervision had the effect of containing the anger, frustrations, and uncertainties generated by the program, so that this emotional energy could be molded to the shape the program desired. In so doing, it greatly increased the invest-ment and commitment of the residents to psychiatry; for that very pro-cess made the residents emotionally dependent on professional models. Moreover, unlike other kinds of training, psychiatric residency is designed to bring out fears, doubts and personal problems. This makes the socialization particularly thorough. Psychiatry is not interested in just a person's legal reasoning or executive talent or ability to perform surgery, but in the whole person back to early childhood.

While the program could draw out a resident's most personal and desperate feelings, it also exposed the resident to his own lunacy. Residents were encouraged to express their "crazy ideas" and their fantasies. All of these supervisory meetings were confidential, and the resident was assured that these expressions were natural. But supervision was the structural element which led the resident to see himself as a patient and in need of analysis. For with its emphasis on countertransference, supervision always contained the element of psychoanalysis.

That supervision was able to absorb anxiety and withstand criticism from residents did not mean that great answers were given to the troublesome questions which new residents asked. Rather, the resident passed through an emotional state of concern over an issue, such as the lack of evidence that psychiatry worked. Thus, when second-year residents heard that the first-year ones were feeling that psychiatry had no basis, they would reply that they too had gone "through a period like that." One passed on and continued. If pressed as to what answer they had found, they would say, "Some patients don't get better and some you can help, especially the healthier ones." This kind of self-fulfilling prophecy was also learned by residents to defend their personal shortcomings. If one were manipulative and ambitious, one simply said, "I'm a bit of a psychopath." Such a statement was admired, because it indicated that the speaker knew himself and had accepted his personality. In this culture, knowing and accepting one's limitations was much more important than overcoming them.

Supervision was the single most important source for professional models. Ironically, there were almost too many models, it seemed. Not only were residents exposed to seven supervisors and two groups, but also they attended diagnostics, case conferences and other activities where they watched senior psychiatrists. Some residents had in mind that they wanted their own personal analysis and used these occasions to review a parade of potential analysts. This variety, part of the structure of the program, served two purposes. Given that all of these models were members of the same analytic cluster, the numbers created the illusion of a variety in the face of uniformity. Indeed the structure worked; for the residents did not get bored with the analytic uniformity but learned to make refined distinctions within it. The variety of models allowed the resident to choose his own style but within one school of thought.

Reducing Peer Cohesion

One might wonder why the residents did not react collectively to the strains of residency. Had they pooled their disappointments and energies, they could probably have forced the program to take on new perspectives in patient care. Several structural features impeded peer cohesion. The residents were initially divided into four wards, around which their lives centered. The ward staff was a natural unit and residents' bonds across wards were weak, because so much of the day focused on the ward. Moreover, the main work of the psychiatric profession took place in private. Unlike training for internal medicine,[19] orthopedic surgery,[20] or medical school itself,[21] most professional work was not performed in the presence of others or openly discussed. As Rose Coser observed, the social arrangements were self-contained; a Calvinistic emphasis was placed on internal states and good faith.[22] Individual therapy occurred in isolation; no one else knew what happened. Mike said, "I felt great pressure when I came here to identify with my work, and that takes a lot of energy." A great proportion of a resident's energy, then, went into private therapy. Supervision of that therapy likewise occurred in private, and when a few residents had a supervisor together, they often came from different services. The most cohesive activities were the two group meetings. But here group feelings were turned back upon each individual, as in this exchange at the end of the first year.

> *Ned Reich:* I don't feel I've gotten to know people well this year. Compared to internship, I haven't had the time to kibbitz. I don't feel, as I did last [internship] year, I know how different doctors handle their patients.
>
> *Ken Reese:* I've felt this all year. In a way, we know each other well, but it's highly professionalized.
>
> *Ned Reich:* I have spent very little time over coffee, eating or walking home with someone.

Marc Raskin: It was looser, much looser, last year.

Ken Reese: I still have more going with friends from last year than ones I have gotten to know this year.

Ned Reich: I think it's the institution and how it's run. At [another hospital] they had two-hour coffee breaks in the day, when all the residents and staff got together. Very pleasant.

Carl Rabinovitz: I agree. . . . Yet I think you can get as close here as you want to someone.

Carl's last remark is a classic example of how residents learned to convert institutional forces to personal self-consciousness. This structure of divide and conquer increased in the second year, when residents worked even more on their own. Thus the structure of residency training, particularly the features highlighted here, greatly influences the values and practices of psychiatrists who go through it. Insofar as these professionals shape mental health services as leaders of the psychiatric domain, their values and practices influence the kinds of mental health care available in this country.

The Myth of Structureless Socialization

We have described the experience of going through residency, its social psychology, and how the structure underlying it embodies a theory of socialization in its organization and rules.[23] The purpose of socialization is to reproduce social life, to imbue a new generation with the customs, sanctions, and relationships that made a certain activity or group distinctive.[24] Symbolic interaction inadequately explains how this happens. Its proponents rightly argue that people must construct a definition of reality in order to cope with the demands of the situation they are in, and to allay their anxieties about how to respond to a new setting;[25] for rarely are recruits provided with prefabricated constructions or polished scripts that they can simply adopt. But the materials out of which residents or others construct their reality are not entirely random or personal; for any setting provides a limited number of resources, usually quite specific, and a limited number of ideas, rules, and organizational procedures. It provides a limited number of accounts—explanations of why things happen the way they do—and definitions of what is normal. Even deviations from what is normal must be fairly predictable, and there must be ways to normalize unexpected events such as suicide, described in chapter 9.[26] As a consequence of the need in practical work to normalize the unexpected, explanations must be tautologies, true by definition rather than by scientific proof. Thus socialization is organized and predictable, though the participants find it personal and idiosyncratic. Ideally, one should acquire a sense of authorship even though much of the material was provided.[27] This is why Anthony Giddens says that the essense of social action consists of the actor monitoring his or her own activities.[28] The professions in general and psychiatry in particular are so organized as to encourage authorship strongly.

Underlying the organization of reality a training program presents to its members is the power of those who define and run it.[29] They define both knowledge and the division of labor, what is known and authoritative as well as who is empowered to do what and how various people should be treated.[30] The structure of a program like psychiatric residency gives the institution and those in charge a moral authority and the means to control some of the uncertainties that inevitably arise in professional work.[31]

Structural Dimensions of Organizational Socialization

Beyond these general observations, it is instructive to examine the structure of psychiatric residency in light of attempts to identify the dimensions of organizational socialization. The well-known essay by Stanton Wheeler has been superseded by John Van Maanen, who identifies six organization features of socialization, though he chooses to call them strategies or tactics.[32] They are clear and need little comment:
    1. Collective vs. individual socialization processes.
    2. Formal vs. informal socialization processes.
    3. Sequential vs. random socialization processes.
    4. Fixed vs. variable socialization processes.
    5. Serial vs. disjunctive socialization processes.
    6. Investiture vs. divestiture socialization processes.
The program for training psychiatrists in this study had a clear, collective structure for processing residents through at least the first two years. Yet the importance of psychotherapy, which is not visible to

others, the emphasis on individual self-understanding, and the apprenticeship quality of supervision individualized the experience and undercut a strong collective conscience among fellow residents. Van Maanen and Schein predict that collective socialization will occur when people cross functional boundaries and learn new skills, while individual socialization will be more common when people are being prepared for promotion in the hierachy of the organization.[33] Residents, like many other professionals and skilled workers, are learning skills so they can move into higher positions, such as being staff psychiatrists. Thus in this case, the distinctions between a collective or an individual structure of socialization, or between functions and hierarchical dimensions of organization are heuristically valuable but blend in reality.

Psychiatric residency has formal elements in the sense that residents are set aside and processed through activities structured for them, but as working members of the hospital or clinic, much socialization is informal. Van Maanen and Schein believe that formal socialization is more intense the more concerned people are that trainees learn the right values. Strong examples, like Marine boot camp, support this view; but we have seen that an institution's values are deeply absorbed through immersion in its main work too. The authors point out that informal socialization gives trainees more opportunity to select their models; but if the models all represent certain values, one can control the choices without seeming to do so.

There is, in psychiatric residency, a rough sequence of training experience, but within this larger frame the sequence by which residents learn how to manage, prescribe, and do therapy varies with individual experiences. To call these variations "random" seems too strong; for close study will identify few if any cases of random socialization. The two words are almost contradictory. Van Maanen and Schein predict that sequential socialization will be more common when people are moving up the hierarchy, but sequence is very important for learning skills as well.[34] In psychiatry, the collective, formal part of the program is sequential, while the individual, informal parts vary somewhat from case to case.

By "fixed," Van Maanen means there is a timetable, which is indeed the case in psychiatric residency. There is some variability in the socialization process, but not much. Residency is also serial, that is, one cohort follows another. To some extent, upper classes serve as models for new residents; but to a significant degree, the emphasis on self-understanding, individual supervision, and private therapy adds an important disjunctive element to the socialization process. Residents in each year are quite segregated, except for carefully selected older residents whom the staff believe will make good role models.

Related to the dimension of continuity between cohorts is the continuity between what one was before entering the program and what one is to become. Van Maanen uses the term "investiture" to characterize organizations which build on the values and skills which recruits bring to the program; while divestiture indicates that the program tries to strip the person of old values, sever old ties, and put the recruit through an intense novitiate period during which a new self-image is built up. Again, psychiatric residency has both. As the stages of moral transition show, the training program divests residents of their old selves and infuses a new self. Yet that self builds on fundamental qualities which the residents bring to their training. First, residents are physicians, and while the socialization process tears down certain skills, values, and outlooks learned in medical training, it also builds on the status of the medical profession. In addition, the great emphasis on one's personality as a primary, therapeutic tool means that training builds heavily on the personality which the residents bring with them, all the while constructing a new language and a new framework for understanding it.

Thus psychiatric residency so intermingles the distinctions that constitute the best general theory we have on the structure of socialization that its usefulness is limited. Van Maanen and Schein predict that certain outcomes will result from a program falling on one side or the other of their dichotomies; but when they are blended, the contrasting outcomes cancel each other. Whether this would be the case in another setting, such as executive training in a corporation or socialization in a law firm, is hard to say, because the authors have not yet carried out research to test their theory. For the moment, this analysis suggests that it is most fruitful to analyze the structure of a socialization program in terms of its particular features, keeping the formal distinctions in mind to sensitize one's observations.

This study implicitly suggests there are other dimensions of socialization that need further examination. The extent to which socialization is *holistic* or *segmental* probably makes a significant difference in the process. Psychiatric residency is unusual in the degree to which one's whole personality, style, personal history, and future outlook are subject to intense scrutiny and recasting. This differs significantly from engineering school or from learning to be a meat packer. An allied distinction is role diffusion to the extent to which the socialization process is *role diffuse* or *role specific*. Some callings are a way of life; others merely get a job done.

The socialization process also varies in how *coercive* or *seductive* its techniques are for getting recruits to change in desired ways. Often they are mixed, with seduction up front and coercion backing it up, in case the trainee does not take the bait. This mixture often involves the distinction between minimal behavioral changes and changes in attitudes. If the trainee will not find a particular approach interesting and incorporate it into his or her viewpoint, at least appropriate behavior will be demanded.

Whether a socialization experience is *positive* or *negative*—that is, whether it principally aims to build an identity, as most programs do, or tear one down, as torture and concentration camps do—profoundly affects the impact of the experience on the individual. Finally, the degree to which the socialization processes are *intense* or *casual* will affect the pacing and relations which trainees have with their mentors. This psychiatric residency was basically holistic, diffuse, seductive, positive and intense, making for a deep, broad reshaping of professional identity. How these dimensions of organizational socialization affect other kinds of training will require further research.

Structural Links to Society

The influence of a program such as this one does not lie merely in its internal structure and socialization process but in its institutional relations with the outside world. In focusing on the internal social dynamics of the training process one can too easily overlook the simple fact that when trainees finish, they will be certified to the world.[35] In the case of a professional school like psychiatry, they will also be linked to a network of contacts, institutions, and clients that have built up around the program. Put another way, quite as important as training is certification. Beginning in the second year, residents start sensing the end of training and imagine they will soon be psychiatrists. (In four-year programs, I suspect this happens in the third year.) One can call this "anticipatory socialization," but the deeper point is the structural relations between the program and the rest of society that make such anticipation realistic.

Behind certification lies a set of powerful relationships that socialize as much as does training. Through its laws, society recognizes the merit of the training enterprise and imbues graduates with certain privileges, rights, status, and expectations. Viewed historically, the training group—here psychiatrists—has reshaped the organization of society to provide work for its graduates, to legitimate them with licenses, to bestow them with status, to provide a livelihood, and to institutionalize workshops (hospitals, clinics) that become part of the social fabric.[36] All of these arrangements make identification with the profession easier and deeper. First, one knows that one can fruitfully do this kind of work for the rest of one's life. Second, it is honorable work. Third, there is a network of colleagues and institutions for life-long support. Thus the central beliefs of the training program are prophecies fulfilled by its own structural arrangements with the rest of society. The idea that the program teaches critical skills is manifest in certification. The fact that some psychiatrists practice incompetently but remain licensed underlines the importance of these external arrangements. The idea that training makes graduates uniquely effective gets carried out in rules for hiring psychiatrists to dominant positions. In the case of a prestigious program, each of these elements receives added emphasis: the skills are presumed better, the network is more select and powerful, the rewards of professional work are greater, and so forth. Residents were acutely aware of all this, making socialization all the more complete.

Yet the very structural links to society which give professional socialization its ultimate power and make it consequential also release the trainee from having to observe lessons. Once graduated and certified, a professional has the autonomy to practice more or less as s/he pleases. This is not the bargain struck by society when it gives a profession a license; in return for autonomy it expects the profession to regulate itself and maintain high standards. But this *collective* autonomy, which implies individual obligation to the profession, is regarded by professionals as an *individual* right to practice as they see best, unregulated by their colleagues or anyone else. Although this attitude is now changing in response to external pressure, it may be one of the central but hidden lessons of medical training: get out from under and do as you please. How else is one to interpret the frequent observation that senior clinicians offer different, even contradictory, interpretations and recommend conflicting treatments of the same case? When a resident acts differently from his chief or supervisor, it is called an error, even an act of insubordination. When another psychiatrist acts differently, it is called a matter of style.[37] This argument, however, cannot be carried too far, because when the residents do attain individual autonomy, they still must diagnose, treat, and decide how to practice. Most likely, they will carry on as they did in residency.

13.

Training for Uncertainty and Control

Uncertainty pervades all social life, but it has particular significance for professionals because they depend on the public believing that they know what they are doing. Their license and mandate rest on the claim that they have mastered esoteric knowledge and can apply effective techniques. Yet uncertainties constantly arise in professional work, and professionals must learn to control them.

A peculiar and complex relationship exists between competence, uncertainty, and error.[1] Most clearly, any area of competence provides an occasion for error in the traditional sense of doing something wrong that could have been avoided. In gray areas of competence or knowledge, which are characterized by uncertainty, error is unclear. The practical pressures of time make these areas much larger than they are in theory; for most uncertainty arises from having to make a decision before all the facts are in. Yet paradoxically, professionals define the core of their work as making good decisions in the face of uncertainty. When their decision proves wrong, it may not be a mistake if it can be defended as reasonable.

In her classic essay, "Training for Uncertainty," Renée C. Fox insightfully described uncertainties of knowledge which medical students learn to address.[2] Yet a full portrait of how professionals are trained for uncertainty, one which describes the uncertainties not only of knowledge but of diagnosis, treatment, and interpersonal relations, has not been written.

Kinds of Uncertainty

Professional Knowledge

Early in professional training, students experience three kinds of uncertainty, which Renée Fox described so clearly. "The first results from incomplete or imperfect mastery of available knowledge."[3] Like medical students[4] and interns,[5] psychiatric residents are overwhelmed by what they have to learn. Then a second source of uncertainty emerges that cannot be mastered, the indeterminacy of the professional knowledge itself. In the final analysis, law students realize there is no such thing as "the law." Medical students discover that medicine is not a "science" but a series of observed relationships and probabilities with few laws. Psychiatry, on the other hand, seems to have plenty of theories or laws but few systematic observations to back them up. The student wonders: what knowledge is real or useful and what is conjecture?

This second source of uncertainty loops back on the first, to raise the question "Do I know the difference between where my knowledge is inadequate and where the field's knowledge is inadequate?" This is Fox's third kind of uncertainty: not being able to distinguish between imperfect mastery of available knowledge and imperfections in the knowledge itself.

These uncertainties reflect on professional knowledge in two senses: on the knowledge of the professional and on the knowledge of the profession. Later, in clinical training, they take on a different hue than they do in course work. One asks, "Do I know enough to treat this case?" "Does the field know enough to act effectively?" The concept of knowledge broadens beyond the thrust of Fox's essay to include experience and skill.

Uncertainties of Diagnosis

Besides Fox's three kinds of uncertainty that arise early in training, a new bundle of uncertainties becomes prominent as the young professional takes on actual cases. First, what is the problem? Often one is hard put to distinguish clearly what is the matter in a case. Evidence is often incomplete. The patient, moreover, may obscure it. The definition of the problem, or the diagnosis, depends heavily on the professional's model or theory of analysis, and it may be very difficult to translate the signs and language of the symptoms into the signs and language of the diagnostic model.

Two further uncertainties of diagnosis may confront the young professional: what are the causes of the problem and what will be its future course? Even if one achieves a lucid description of a case, one may remain uncertain of its origins or its future course. These uncertainties, like those professional knowledge, persist throughout a lifetime of professional work, but trainees feel them most acutely and must learn to cope with them.

Uncertainties of Procedure

The central uncertainty is not being sure which is the most effective procedure. Uncertainties of treatment become compounded with those of diagnosis. This is particularly true when disorders have multiple causes and the implications for treatment are unclear or conflicting. Inadequacies in one's own knowledge, limitations of the field, or uncertainties about the diagnosis, each contribute in turn to doubts about which course of action will be the most effective. Yet that is the primary reason why people seek professional help.

Even when a plan of action is clear, its outcome may remain in doubt. Often one is uncertain of how action will affect outcome. Medical students and residents soon find that bodies and psyches vary greatly in their response to a given treatment. Moreover, the treatment may affect the diagnosis, particularly in iatrogenic cases where the treatment itself produces new complications. One faces the risk of doing more harm than good or of helping one problem but creating new ones in the process.

Uncertainties of Collegial Relations

The uncertainties of collegial relations differ fundamentally from problems of knowledge, diagnosis, and procedure because they involve role relations among staff rather than aspects of the clinical case itself. When mistakes are made their nature differs too. As Charles Bosk has pointed out, technical and judgmental errors arise in diagnosis and treatment, while normative errors arise from not carrying out one's obligations conscientiously. Bosk argues they arise almost exclusively in subordinates' relations with superordinates, specifically by not doing things the way that superordinates want, and these errors are punished much more severely than errors of technique or judgment.[6] Yet as Bosk himself recognizes elsewhere, there are norms of relations with peers, nurses, and ward staff too,[7] and while their breach does not have dire consequences, they receive their share of concern.

However, it is not always clear who should be doing what or where each person's responsibility lies. This is particularly true in teamwork. A resident complained: "If you wanted to do something with the patient, you had to consult the team . . . which is helpful in some ways, particularly for the novice that I was—but after a while one felt as if one was not really treating the patient as completely as one would like."[8] Socialized to be in charge, teamwork not only frustrates residents but confuses them.

> . . . if you have a team, I would expect that each member of the team have some kind of specific function which they themselves offer to the team functioning, that no one else offers. And on the ward, I didn't know what the hell I was supposed to offer and I didn't really know what anyone else was offering. . . .[9]

Besides the uncertainties embedded in teamwork, residents experience the uncertainties of authority when they must learn from more seasoned subordinates. As we saw in chapter 6, nurses are the main teachers of management to residents; yet residents write their orders. Nurses get understandably annoyed at impractical or ill-considered orders, and they have much more experience on which to base their judgments. But as subordinates, they often seize upon the situation as an opportunity to safely deride their superiors and vent their own frustrations. "I found them [nurses] disrespectful. . . . They did not—or at least I did not feel like a doctor in front of them; they made certain remarks. . . ."[10] An important topic which we shall take up in the second half of this chapter is how professional trainees reduce uncertainties of collegial relations.

Uncertainties of Client Response

To some extent, one can distinguish between how the client's *problem* responds to treatment and how the *client* responds as a client. For example, fearing surgery is not part of diagnosing a toxic thyroid or deciding it should come out, or resistance to reducing is not part of diagnosing overweight.[11] But psychiatry differs from medicine in the way it incorporates client response into the diagnosis of the problem. For example, the patient who refused to be interviewed in public by a stranger in chapter 8 had her "resistance" incorporated into her diagnosis. Likewise, the difficulties of diagnosing become part of the analysis, as illustrated in the chapter on diagnosis. Yet the prevalence of such tautological procedures for normalizing the unexpected attest to the pervasiveness of uncertainties in diagnosis.

Training for Control

Although it is valuable to understand the faces of uncertainty in professional training, this study of residency puts into larger perspective Renée Fox's observation of medical school. *As clinical responsibilities grow, training for uncertainty becomes training for control,* a theme implicit in studies of internship and residency.[12] One finds evidence of this shift even in Fox's materials, as medical students take on more clinical work in their last two years. When entering a new residency program, however, the experience is much more intense. Physicians face not only the uncertainties of professional knowledge which Fox described but also the uncertainties of diagnosis, treatment, collegial relations and client response. The scramble for techniques of control is intense. Training for uncertainty means learning techniques of control.[13] A profession's raison d'être rests on the claim that it can handle other people's emergencies with routine control.[14] *Technically,* a profession's greatest need is for a better expertise in the form of knowledge and skills, but *sociologically,* a profession's greatest need is for control. Thus a major, implicit goal of training in psychiatry and in other professions is to learn how to control the uncertainties of the situation at hand. What follows are some of the techniques which trainees learn for controlling uncertainties.

Mastering Knowledge

Nothing quite so effectively allays doubts about whether one knows available knowledge as learning it. The problem is that one cannot learn everything, which leads students to other ways of gaining control over what they should know.[15] They learn what the situation calls for, which initially means what the course exam will test, and later means what the pathology of a case being discussed entails. Bone up on the problem at hand and move on to the next one. This approach is particularly emphasized in grand rounds and case conferences. Students also learn to work together, to share knowledge and to divide the work, with each becoming an expert in one area. This temporary arrangement then becomes permanent as young professionals specialize, a major way to control what one has to know, to more easily appreciate the limits of the field, and to recognize the difference between the two. Limiting what one knows and learning it well also help to control uncertainties of diagnosis, procedure, collegial relations, and clients.

Adopting a "School" of Professional Work

Most professional trainees soon find themselves being socialized into one or another school of thought. This happens even after one specializes, thus further delimiting and controlling uncertainties about what to know, how to diagnose and how to proceed with a case. As Everett C. Hughes once wrote, ". . . those who are subject to the same work risks will compose a collective rationale which they whistle to one another to keep up their courage, and . . . they will build collective defenses against the lay world."[16] Besides supplying defenses against the lay world, "schools" of professional work serve to provide "answers" to the gray areas of professional practice and knowledge.

Residency programs usually embody a dominant "school" or ideology, and if there are competing ones, there will be strong pressure to join one group or another.[17] They affect the structure of training, the kind of cases one treats, and one's career. But even in fields where a common body of technical knowledge has been built up, there are still schools or philosophies of professional work. For example, Knafl and Burkett studied a residency in orthopedic surgery and observed the following exchange:

In presenting the case, Dr. Lee quotes from a source in favor of such a procedure. Dr. Eddy, an attending physician, interrupts with, "I know that's what he says, but that's not the way we do it here." Another one of the attending men adds, "That's the way some of us do it!"[18]

Early in clinical training, professionals conclude that there is no such thing as a right way to treat a case, even in orthopedic surgery. But by the time they finish, this objective analysis, born of bewilderment, changes to a conviction that the "school" they have adopted is the right way. Most will end up talking like Drs. Lee, Eddy and the third attending physician. This study alone contains many examples of nar-

Figure 13.1   Kinds of Uncertainty and Their Control in Professional Training

KINDS OF UNCERTAINTY	FORMS OF CONTROL LEARNED

1. Of Professional Knowledge	*Mastering Knowledge*
	    Specializing
	        Adopting a "School" of Professional Work

2. Of Diagnosis	Mastering Knowledge
	    Specializing
	        Adopting a "School" of Professional Work
	Deferring to Clinical Experience

3. Of Procedure or Treatment	Mastering Knowledge
	    Specializing
	        Adopting a "School" of Professional Work
	Deferring to Clinical Experience
	Turning to Technique

4. Of Collegial Relations	Mastering Knowledge
	    Specializing
	        Adopting a "School" of Professional Work
	Deferring to Clinical Experience
	Turning to Technique
	Gaining Autonomy

5. Of Client Response	Mastering Knowledge
	    Specializing
	        Adopting a "School" of Professional Work
	Deferring to Clinical Experience
	Turning to Technique
	Gaining Autonomy
	Maintaining a Dominant Class Relationship
	    Institutionalizing Authority
	    Keeping Clients Ignorant

rowing the sphere of uncertainty by interpreting events in psychodynamic terms.

Adopting a school of thought raises the question of whether control of uncertainty is objective or subjective, and it shows how this distinction is ultimately impossible to make, because the resident's frame or criteria for deciding that a certain kind of control objectively reduced uncertainty and was not just in the eye of the beholder necessarily means that the resident has taken sides in deciding what is objective and what is subjective. Uncertainty and its control reside in the perception of the actor or group of actors, though to call this definition subjective merely reveals one's bias. F. R. Leavis echoes Wittgenstein when he observes that "Terms [such as 'control'] must be made means to the necessary precision by careful use in relation to the concrete; their use is justified insofar as it is shown to favor sensitive perception; and the precision in analysis aimed at is not to be attained by seeking formal definitions as its tools.[19]

Deferring to Clinical Experience

An important source of control over uncertainties of diagnosis and treatment comes from deferring to clinical experience. By this term is meant the ultimate respect given to judgment based on experience. During their training for control, physicians learn that technical knowledge is essential background for making a decision, but ultimately clinical judgment prevails. In orthopedic surgery, for example, two residents look at the X-ray of a man's foot and one, named Stevens, says, "Well, technically it doesn't meet the criteria for [cites a specific procedure], but clinically I think it's indicated, since he's had repeated sprains." Then the attending physician walks in and discusses the case with the resident. He disagrees, "saying how it's been his experience that what Stevens wants to do just doesn't work in practice. He suggests a more conservative treatment of injecting the foot with cortisone. After a bit more discussion, Stevens agrees with this and prepares the injection."[20]

This example illustrates the hierarchy of judgment based at least partially on experience. The resident's clinical judgment was based on what had happened to this particular patient before, not on experience with the procedure he wished to use. The attending physician, on the other hand, had worked with cases like this using the procedure and could say, as the resident could not, that it "just doesn't work in practice." In terms of training for control, this means that experience alone is considered to bring with it greater command over uncertainties which technical knowledge cannot provide. In psychiatric residency, it is the person in the room who has the most experience with the kind of case at hand whose opinion prevails, and that person is usually a senior clinician. Thus deferring to clinical experience clarifies collegial relations.

From observations and comments, it appears that the authority derived from clinical experience is more prominent in psychiatry than in many other parts of medicine, where more issues can be settled by lab reports and established research findings. The paradigm in psychiatry (especially in psychoanalysis) has rested heavily on clinical experience, while the paradigm in medicine has rested heavily on scientific discovery. If so, this form of control plays a more important role in psychiatry; for one can defer to clinical experience only to the degree that its authority is recognized. An emphasis on clinical experience naturally places greater authority and honor on senior staff, while science may honor the young.

For the profession as a whole, expertise based on clinical experience can lead to inbreeding, cliques centered on charismatic, senior figures, and a neglect of research. But for the individual resident, the deference to clinical experience guarantees his or her own growing authority through mere experience. Unlike research in the literature, it has no outside referent, and as residents begin to work with clients, it constitutes a body of wisdom over which they have complete control and which others must either respect or arbitrarily reject. Residents gain a sense of mastery by collecting success stories which show them that they are effective and by selectively drawing on their growing number of cases to make clinical judgments. Once this process occurs, they become almost completely immune from criticism. Reviewing a longitudinal study of training in three professions, Eliot Freidson writes, "Once those trainees learned to practice the basic skills for which they were being trained, and gained some personal 'sense of mastery' over them, they tended to become self-validating; they were no longer responsive to the evaluations, direction and criticism of others."[21] A study of psychiatrists practicing several years after residency confirms this pattern.[22] Thus initially the resident defers to the clinical experience of others; but later it provides him with a tool of control over patients and colleagues.

Focusing on Technique

A major way in which professionals learn how to control the uncertainties of treatment lies in the subtle shift from considering technique as a means to considering it an end. We have documented this shift as residents work clinically with patients (chapter 5). They become fascinated by ways of sitting, of opening and ending a session with a patient, of breaking down the defenses in a patient, and of effecting a transference in a patient. But the ultimate control attained through technique comes when one realizes that not only have the ends with all their uncertainties been diminished, but one can also choose from a variety of means and defend the choice as personal preference. (See, for example, page 200.) A focus on technique also defines more narrowly relations with colleagues and clients.

The point here is that by emphasizing technique one controls important sources of uncertainty in how patients or their bodies will respond. Quite simply, the outcome of treatment is more uncertain than the treatment itself. At the end of their careful study of professional socialization, Bucher and Stelling conclude: "Given the tenuous nature of much professional knowledge, it is perhaps not surprising that the trainees, in evaluating themselves and others, come to give greater emphasis to the actual process of doing their work than to the results of that process."[23] So long as one does the right thing, one is practicing competently.

The emphasis on technique in training for control also leads the young professional to redefine what is competence. It eliminates the layman's definition of competence—whether the patient gets better—and redefines it in terms of clinical procedures. This, of course, makes a great deal of sense; why should a psychiatrist be blamed for each patient who does not improve? But sociologically the point is that emphasizing technique does serve as a major form of control, particularly for residents who lack clinical experience.

Just as technique redefines what is competence, so it redefines the nature of mistakes in terms of procedure rather than outcome. In the professional world, one can make a mistake in technique without its affecting outcome, or one can have perfect technique with poor results. Only when poor results can be directly attributed to technique does outcome contribute to the definition of mistake, and often this is not the case. This is the most insightful way to understand what happened when two sociologists asked residents in psychiatry and internal medicine to define mistakes in their work.[24] The residents could not give clear answers, because the layman's idea of mistake had become foreign to them through their professional training. When something happens that might look like a serious mistake to the rest of the world, professionals enact specific rituals (like reviews of a death) which have their own language and features designed to deflect or mollify charges of bad practice.[25]

Gaining Autonomy

A major goal of aspiring professionals is to gain autonomy; for autonomy enables them to gain control over relations with others. They get out from under supervisory relationships so they can shape their relations as they wish. During training, residents struggle constantly to gain as much autonomy as possible, largely by moving away from visible settings and making their work as unobservable as possible. Once training is completed, the professional norms of autonomy protect them from many uncertainties by giving them the power to define reality as they see fit.[26] The unwritten law against criticizing a colleague, the tendency for like-minded professionals to seek each other out, and the institutionalizing of professional authority all reduce uncertainties. In circumstances where other professionals are participating in the case, the greater clinical experience of senior staff defers to the colleague in charge of the case, unless a serious error is about to be made.[27] When the attending in orthopedic surgery recommended another procedure to Stevens, it was *Stevens* who agreed, after discussing the matter. This is why Burkett and Knafl note that in discussing various treatments of a case during grand rounds, a final decision is rarely made. "In the end," one attending physician explained, "it has to be one man's decision. Sometimes there are a variety of procedures that are suitable and one has to choose the procedure that he's best at—that he's most comfortable with."[28]

Maintaining a Dominant Class Relationship

One fundamental way in which professionals control clients is by institutionalizing their authority. As Freidson has so clearly shown,[29] gaining legal and administrative monopoly forces the client to come to the professional for the services s/he needs. By controlling valued resources and powers, professionals increase the chances that clients will cooperate. The goal is to minimize the need for persuasion and replace it with residual coercion, forcing the client's choice by closing off alternatives. As they gain practical experience, trainees learn how to use the institutional resources available to them in managing cases. The administrative and legal privileges are assumed as natural tools in learning how to manage clients.

The relative ignorance of the client is a second basic form of control.[30] Residents learn the smokescreens and evasive replies that answer a patient's question in form but not in content. Rarely in psychiatry does the therapist tell the patient his or her diagnosis. Besides treating the patient as ignorant of his or her own condition and working to keep it that way, residents learn quickly that patients are to work for them in therapy, and if they do not respond to therapeutic efforts, they are defined as chronic and relegated to a custodial service. The ambiguities of this pattern emerge in the case conference on Mr. Downs.

These examples reflect the basic class differences between professional and client in the Marxian sense that they have different structural relationships to the means of production and to authority relations.[31] As a result, the dominant class of professionals has power over and can predict the behavior of the underclass of clients. Within this institutionalized inequality, professionals often satisfy clients' wishes in small, symbolic ways. A pervasive example in medicine is giving a patient a prescription even though none is needed, because the patient wants to feel that something is being done.

Professional mystique is also a part of controlling patient relations. Making the patient think you know more than you do, keeping the patient himself uncertain, and other devices are part of the impression management that many psychiatrists and other physicians cultivate. Thus there are two interrelated aspects of dominant relations: the objective powers of controlling valued resources and the mystique of impression management.

These forms of patient control have their price. Patients often feel alienated. They do not understand what is wrong with them or what their role is in treatment. They do not "comply" with doctor's orders. They do not use medical and psychiatric services in an optimal manner. For these reasons, a movement is growing to respond to the uncertainties of patients by making them partners in medical and psychiatric work. In psychiatric residency, we have seen how trainees learn to make the patient responsible for his or her progress in therapy, but this is done while maintaining all the vestments of dominance. It is a way of attributing to the patient one's own limited ability to be effective, instead of giving the patient the power and knowledge commensurate with the responsibility. In the movement toward self-doctoring and open medicine, power and knowledge accompany responsibility.

Paradigm Development and Training for Control

At the close of her essay, Renée Fox asked how training would be affected by the relative development of the field. "Are students made most aware of uncertainties when they are exposed to fields in which these uncertainties are greatest?"[32] The range of uncertainties in a field depends on its paradigm development and paradigm strength, two concepts derived from the work of Thomas Kuhn.[33] By paradigm development I mean the degree to which there is consensus among practitioners about the theory or paradigm underlying their work. By paradigm strength I mean its ability to explain well the phenomena it addresses. If a paradigm is undeveloped, it will compete with others, and uncertainties will arise from the ensuing confusion. If a paradigm is weak (even though it holds wide consensus), uncertainties will arise around the relations between diagnosis, treatment, and outcome.

The studies of residents in orthopedic surgery and psychiatry are particularly useful for looking at awareness of uncertainties, because the strength and, to a lesser degree, the development of their paradigms contrast so sharply. Psychiatry is widely regarded as having weak and competing paradigms to guide its diagnosis, treatment, and research; while orthopedic surgery has a strong paradigm with competing derivations. We would expect that residents in orthopedic surgery would perceive fewer uncertainties because it is one of the most clearly defined of specialties and technically quite mature.[34] On the other hand, we would expect residents in psychiatry to be aware of the more numerous uncertainties which pervade that field, where the relations between diagnosis, treatment, and outcome are often unclear. Yet the studies reveal a number of surprising similarities in the training process of both residencies.[35]

1. Residents in both specialties quickly learned from senior residents that theirs was one of the most ambiguous of specialties.

2. Despite the great difference in paradigm development and strength in the two fields, residents in both specialties spent a great deal of time overcoming feelings of inferiority and uncertainty.

3. In both residencies, the effort to evaluate oneself moved from an emphasis on supervisors' opinions to opinions about oneself, the shift occurring as one gained confidence and comfort.

4. In both programs, administrative duties, negotiations with hospital staff, and the hospital itself as an institution were seen as annoying impositions on autonomous professional judgment.

5. Regardless of the technical refinement of the field, trainees were urged to develop a clinical philosophy. For example, when asked to explain bone grafts, a resident in orthopedic surgery replied, "Well, I'm not really sure I *believe* in them. I mean I'm not sure I understand the *philosophy* behind them" (emphasis added).[36]

The key to understanding these similarities that transcend technical maturity and the amount of control which the field itself allows is clinical judgment. By definition, clinical judgment is demonstrated in ambiguous cases. If the case is "open and shut," the preestablished knowledge of the field makes understanding it a certainty. And in fact many cases are routine, but the point is that they receive little attention. This leads to the proposition that *regardless of how technically developed a professional field is, it will define the treatment of problematic cases as the true measure of its worth.*

Most people think of a competent professional as someone who knows his/her field and handles cases with dispatch. The essence of professional work is coping with clients' uncertainties and emergencies, by using expertise and clinical experience. But professionals have their own uncertainties, as described before, and mastering them is the mark of the "true professional." As a consequence, regardless of whether a field has a strong paradigm or a weak one, it will proclaim its heroes and define its essential work at the edge of competence, where problematic cases are successfully treated. Since this edge is always relative to both how much the field knows and how much the individual has mastered, issues of uncertainty and control loom as large for the student of a profession with a strong paradigm as for the student of a profession with a weak one.

Besides these similarities and a shared edge of competence, the precision and extent of knowledge produce differences as well. It is the clarity of *outcome,* not the clarity of *treatment,* that distinguishes a more mature profession.[37] The treatment decision in the case of orthopedics may be ambiguous, but its highly developed paradigm means that the criteria for evaluating the treatment are often unambiguous. In psychiatry, the outcome is often ambiguous, and psychiatrists often do not bother to learn about it. On the other hand, the treatment may be clearer than in orthopedics, because one holds a treatment ideology which simplifies decisions to habit and dogma.

> *Interviewer:* As you go through (psychiatric) residency, how will you know how well you are doing?
>
> *Resident:* That's a very anxiety-producing question (*laugh*). It's not like medicine where you can feel that, ah, your medical acumen is sharpening and, ah, whereas before you couldn't diagnose, uh, now you can do it, uh, because you have more experience and have had more patients with that disease. In psychiatry, it's just—the whole field is so vague. . . . So a lot of it is just your own evaluation of yourself and how you're doing and how you're affecting your patients.
>
> *Interviewer:* How do you know, as an orthopedic surgery resident, how do you know how well you're doing?
>
> *Resident:* Well, we have, you know, there's several things. First of all, you have the means that every doctor has at his disposal, and that's how well your cases are turning out.[38]

Thus, while trainees in both fields spend a great deal of time overcoming feelings of inferiority and uncertainty, the process differs significantly. Residents in orthopedic surgery know the outcomes of decisions and actions by themselves and others. Related to this is a second difference: mastering the technical literature is an essential prerequisite for discussing cases in orthopedic surgery, because the literature is precise. On the other hand, residents in psychiatry do not know the outcomes of decisions and actions by themselves or others. Concomitantly, reading is not an essential prerequisite. In fact, at University Psychiatric Center, one of the nation's leading residencies, the director of training actively discouraged reading in the first year as a form of escape from the primary task—learning to sit face to face with the pain of crazy people.

Organizational features of the two residencies reflect this basic difference in a number of ways. First, because the results of treatments were not clear, the teaching staff with a weak paradigm could not agree on what constituted "success," while the teaching staff with the strong paradigm could more precisely identify the results of treatment so that their disagreements covered a smaller range of debate.[39] Second, the trainees using a weak paradigm worked and learned their roles largely in private, while trainees using a strong paradigm worked and learned their roles in the presence of other residents, staff physicians and medical staff who could immediately evaluate their performance. A third, related, difference is that supervisors using a weak paradigm tend less to observe trainee performance directly, but rely on the trainee's description of what happened. These organizational features are generally assumed to be necessary for effective psychotherapy and not connected to the technical base of the field. Yet a causal relation seems plausible. The arrangement of private treatment and supervision based on what the trainee says is admirably suited to a profession whose subjectivity could lead to collegial embarrassment. It does, however, contribute to a fourth difference, that the trainee's role is less clearly defined than it is in a field with a strong paradigm.

If the relation between technical base and visibility exists, one would predict that psychopharmacology, which is technically sounder, would be practiced more in public. This is indeed the case. Residents prescribe drugs in the presence of teaching staff and nurses, and together discuss the choices, observe the results, and recommend changes, much as do residents in orthopedic surgery.

In sum, the weaker and less developed the paradigm(s) of a field, the greater the difficulty trainees have in evaluating their progress. Yet their need for control is as great as it is for any other professional group. Control can only be attained by reducing uncertainties, and therefore we would expect that fields in which uncertainties are greatest have ways of making their students less rather than more aware of them, as Fox suggested. *Elaborating institutional myths is a substitute for measurable productivity, with success getting measured in terms of agreement rather than results.*

The influence of ideology reflects the paradigm strength of a profession. For example, while there are schools of thought and philosophy in orthopedic surgery, their influence is restricted by extensive tools for diagnosis, numerous refined techniques whose uses depend heavily on diagnosis, and by fairly clear measures of outcome. Amidst all these uncertainties, one's point of view helps one cope with the remaining uncertainties of professional work.

In psychiatry, schools of thought *determine* thé categories and tools of diagnosis as well as techniques for treatment to such an extent that a person often uses one kind of therapy for a wide range of diagnoses. The resulting internal and circuitous consistency, which one could call ideology, greatly aids evaluation as it bypasses the need for objective measures of outcome. Psychiatric residents resolve difficulties of self-evaluation by incorporating an "approach," which then allows them to believe in themselves. Thus being comfortable and being effective become synonymous.[40]

Conclusion: The Danger of Overcontrol

In this chapter, we have defined the kinds of uncertainty and identified some of the major ways residents learn to control them. The nature of this training differs in some respects, according to the paradigm strength and development of the field. But there are an unexpected number of similarities as well. Residents initially share strong feelings of inferiority and uncertainty in a field they regard as ambiguous. In trying to overcome these feelings, they are taught to concentrate on clinical judgment and technique and to develop a treatment philosophy, while dispensing with administrative tasks as quickly as they can.

Clinical judgment and emphasizing technique are two major ways in which professionals control their work. They redefine competence and mistakes in terms of technique, bypassing the layman's concept of these terms. But good technique in turn rests with the clinical judgment of the professional, which is essentially individual judgment. Thus in gaining control over their work by acquiring a treatment philosophy and exercising individual judgment without question, residents run the danger of gaining too much control over the uncertainties of their work. Their emphasis on technique can make them oblivious to the needs of patients as patients define them; yet the patients' trust that professionals will solve their complex problems provides the foundation of professional power.

Renée Fox has written about *detached concern,* the human but professional balance between concern for the patient and scientific detachment.[41] The complementary ideal in professional work is *tempered control,* that is, sufficient control to overcome the uncertainties of practice so that decisions can be made, but tempered by the continued awareness of those uncertainties and one's own fallibility. Unfortunately, these ideals are not always attained. For example, by starting with the patients most likely to make intense, disturbing assaults on their concern for getting the patient better, psychiatric residents react in alternating waves of detached numbness and intense concern. Residents turn to technique on one hand and become preoccupied with their own psyche on the other. This can produce a twisted kind of detached concern—detachment from the patient and concern for one's self.

Likewise, in training for control, residents become immune to criticism once they become somewhat confident. A longitudinal study of training in both psychiatry and internal medicine found that by the second year, residents discounted even blunt criticism by a number of techniques which included disparaging the source of criticism, dismissing it as irrelevant or unimportant, and attributing it to a difference in approach.[42] This immunity to criticism has become a major social problem. To reduce it, educators will have to pay more attention to the unanticipated consequences of training programs, and administrators of professional facilities will have to change practice routines to minimize these dangers.

Acquiring immunities to criticism is part of a more profound tendency for all professional education to cover up uncertainties inherent in their work, through the techniques of control described in this chapter. Psychiatric residents quickly begin to absorb the dogma of the ideology prevalent in their program, just as in medical school they were forced to unquestioningly absorb thousands of facts and to accept the given interpretation of data as fact. Inquiry, systematic examination of medical data, and a tolerance for ambiguity are strangers in the halls of most medical schools or residency programs. As Harold Schoolman has written, "It is the physician's job to make decisions in situations that are uncomfortable. Thus, the indispensable role of the physician is that of decision maker, as the patient advocate, when such decisions are uncomfortable because of their uncertainty."[43] When they are certain, they can be made by a technician or a computer. But if a physician or psychiatrist has been trained to avoid the discomfort of uncertainty by emphasizing technique, giving ideological formulations, and keeping the patient ignorant, the patient and the quality of care suffer.

14.

Narcissism and Training for Omnipotence

Psychiatry, like other professions whose reach seems to exceed their grasp, seeks control over its environment and the uncertainties of its work in a way reminiscent of the omnipotent tendencies in certain narcissistic personalities. Although Susan Sontag has warned against using medical terms metaphorically, such as "the cancer of Vietnam," applying psychiatric terms to social institutions is of a different and more appropriate order.[1] To characterize corporations, professions, or social agencies as depressed or grandiose is not a metaphor but an analogy between single individuals and the collectivity of individuals that steer organizations. The strength of such analogies depends on how well they are developed, and the purpose here is to show that the psychoanalytic concept of narcissism, when properly adapted, provides sociological insight into professional behavior.

Narcissism, Omnipotence and the Professions

According to Otto Kernberg, one of the leading authorities on narcissism, its main characteristics are "grandiosity, extreme self-centeredness, and a remarkable absence of interest in and empathy for others in spite of the fact that they are so very eager to obtain admiration and approval from other people.''[2] Such individuals can be outstanding leaders and performers, and the reader can readily think of national leaders who fit this pattern. The narcissistic drive may lead to outstanding performance and leadership, marred by envy and manipulation of others.

Narcissism arises from a fusion of the ideal self, the actual self, and the ''ideal object,'' by which Kernberg means another person one would like to have an ideal relation with. By building up a self-image as great as one's ideal self-image and better than those idealized others whose love one wants, the narcissist is saying he does not need anyone else any more.[3] Remnants of unacceptable self-images ''are repressed and projected onto external objects, which are devaluated.''[4] The normal tension between who one is, what one should be, and relations with others is lost. Kernberg concludes, ''[narcissism] is extremely effective in perpetuating a vicious circle of self-admiration, depreciation of others, and the elimination of all actual dependency.''[5]

This syndrome is familiar to any student of the professions. As a group, they have worked to attain self-sufficiency by vigorously promoting a grandiose, idealized image of themselves and institutionalizing their power so that they no longer need to depend on others. They have tended to repress or deny unacceptable aspects of their behavior. They vigorously attack critics for malicious distortion and competitors for shoddy work. Their tendency to demand admiration while showing little genuine interest in others has been the source of much recent criticism by the public against lawyers, doctors and psychiatrists. Ironically, at the same time that such criticism against these professions has risen, the number who want to join their ranks has also risen. There is great attraction to people with power, to being autonomous and not bound by normal social bonds and restrictions.[6]

As with narcissistic individuals, there is always doubt and illusion among professionals about their omnipotent tendencies. Despite the genuine benefits that accrue from professional expertise, professions' claims usually exceed their accomplishments. It is difficult for both professionals and willing clients to accept evidence, for example, that clinical medicine has contributed little to improved health over the last century,[7] or that psychiatry has not been very effective.[8] The self-sufficiency of a profession is also illusory, because, like the narcissistic personality, its claims to omnipotence in its domain depend upon public belief and admiration. At root, any profession rests on a social contract that gives it authority over at least the technical if not the legal, social, and economic aspects of its work, in return for promises to treat the needs of its clients fairly and effectively.[9] If a profession starts to serve itself more than its clients, then its prerogatives will be challenged and its autonomy shaken. When this happens, as it has in recent years, professions work vigorously to regain public admiration, only to ignore it once assured.

Yet grandiose tendencies are built into the institutional arrangements that follow from a profession's social contract. Special laws are written to exempt it from many civic strictures; regulatory committees are composed of its own members or their friends. A profession protects its own esoteric body of knowledge and develops a language which serves as much to mystify as to delineate the technical aspects of its work. The social contract allows a profession to build institutions where it controls its work and accumulated economic power. While the ideal is for the professional to view all this with privileged humility, the temptation to regard it as one's birthright is great.

The Nature of Professional Authority

It is important to realize that were professional authority based exclusively on expertise, it would be precarious, a word which means not just dangerous but "dependent upon the will or favor of another person."[10] The only way in which an expert could get a client to follow his advice would be through persuasion—a risky process that makes the expert dependent on the client. The precarious authority of expertise in the presence of the nonexpert leads the professions to parley their expertise into other forms of authority, and it is this activity which can lead to abuses of professional power. The most solid form of authority is legal, which is why any occupation with expertise is eager to gain professional status in the eyes of the law. As Max Weber pointed out long ago, legal authority defines the holder of power, the sphere of power, and the sanctions in an impersonal, objective way.[11] Persuasion is reduced to a minimum. Only a doctor can prescribe a drug; only a pharmacist can fill it. The same firm, impersonal authority characterizes bureaucratic rule, which Weber called the purest form of legal authority.

In addition, professions greatly enhance their authority by institu-

tionalizing it. By translating their expertise into bureaucratic procedures which a client must follow to get what he or she wants, authority
is not only solidified but is made organizational, so that the individual
professional need not bother establishing it through persuasion. Moreover, the legal-bureaucratic authority of professions usually grants
them considerable latitude in which to exercise their expert judgment.
Because professionals are experts, and because only experts can specify what is to be done, professionals can gain legal and organizational
authority without being tied down.

Abuses can result. With much less need to persuade the client, his
needs and preferences as he sees them can be ignored. The organization of work reflects the concerns of the professional, not the client.
Writing of medical bureaucracies, David Mechanic argues that the
problem of patient abuse or neglect lies not in bureaucratic organization per se but in the fact that few medical centers are patient-cen-
tered.[12] While Mechanic is correct—a bureaucracy can be client-cen-
tered—this statement overlooks good sociological reasons for bad
patient care. Professional expertise becomes the taken-for-granted
basis for legal and bureaucratic forms of authority. These are used not
to regulated expertise but to protect it from outside scrutiny and to extend professional power beyond it—two tendencies of narcissistic omnipotence. Thus a malignant strain of professional superiority accompanies the effort to extend the basis for professional authority.

Finally, the acquisition of legal and bureaucratic authority gives a
profession a firm advantage over others working in the same field
without having to demonstrate that it is technically superior. One example has been psychiatry's ability until recently to keep clinical psychologists from being listed as legitimate therapists by insurance companies, so that patients could not be reimbursed for their services.
Another has been the struggle of chiropractors to get licensed. Like
narcissistic personalities, professions want their domain all to themselves.

Besides securing legal and bureaucratic authority, professions
work at acquiring what Weber identified as the two more ancient
source of authority, charismatic and traditional. While Weber limited
the idea of charismatic authority to the appeal of a person, its qualities
can characterize a group as well. ''The legitimacy of their rule rests on
the belief in and the devotion to the extraordinary, which is valued
because it goes beyond the normal human qualities, and which was

originally valued as supernatural."[13] Since professions have or claim
to have extraordinary powers, they are candidates for charisma. To the
extent that a profession can get its public to believe in the magic of its
expertise without persuasion in each case, it gains a third powerful
form of authority.

Although powerful, charisma is also precarious, for as soon as the
believers lose faith or no longer witness feats and miracles, the aura
vanishes. Of all the professions, medicine has been the most successful
in generating charismatic authority. The special awe and deference
which much of the population expresses in the presence of a doctor,
even if unknown as an individual, attests to the charismatic authority
of the medical profession. Other professions continually attempt to
transform expertise into charisma, and this is most easily done through
heroic feats of expertise. Since the public craves charisma, it eagerly
reads about the surgical miracles of a De Bakey, the powerful build-
ings of a Louis Kahn, the courtroom performance of a Melvin Belli, or
the heroic battles of a General MacArthur. These giants come to sym-
bolize the profession.

What are the relationships between charisma, the structure of the
profession and professional arrogance? First, charisma is latent in the
structural position of the profession as a group of people with extraordinary powers and status. It seems as if no profession can avoid acquiring some kind of magnetic attraction or repulsion or both. While
charisma centers most intensely around heroic or villainous individuals, it spreads out to large segments of the profession or to the profession as a whole. When charismatic authority is strong, the ideal posture of privileged humility is hard to sustain, and *hubris*—one of the
seven deadly sins—takes over. Moreover, forms of superiority which
would normally be offensive are allowed; for charismatic authority
gives its possessor the widest kind of mandate.

Professions also seek to establish themselves as the traditional authority in their sphere. They invoke a long and venerable heritage to
back up present authority. As quickly as possible, they act as if their
professional power were a timeless right granted by God and nature.

Besides converting expertise into the major social forms of authority, professions attain self-sufficiency and supremacy over their
domain by substituting ceremony and institutionalized myths for products.[14] This is particularly true for professions with weak technical
paradigms, such as psychiatry. Work is measured in terms of proce-

dure rather than in terms of results. "Goals are made ambiguous or vacuous, and categorical ends are substituted for technical ends. Hospitals treat, not cure, patients. Schools produce students, not learning. . . . Integration is avoided, program implementation is neglected, and inspection and evaluation are ceremonialized."[15] Confidence, good faith and observation of the ceremonies the profession itself has established create a semblance of accountability and inspire admiration, while allowing the profession as much self-sufficiency as any institution can have.

The individual professional embellishes the omnipotent tendencies already fixed in the structure of the profession. Arguing that his expertise gives no one else the right to judge his work, the professional strives for and usually obtains virtual autonomy from his profession. Thus, if the profession has nearly complete power over *its* domain, the professional has autonomous power over *his own* work. This is not, however, what the state intended and it constitutes the chief betrayal of the social contract by the profession. Personal autonomy also enables the individual to define the boundaries of his power. Kahn-Hut, for example, found that a selective sense of powerlessness allowed psychiatrists to excuse failures, yet take credit for successes.[16]

An important manifestation of individual autonomy is the cardinal rule of noninterference or criticism of others in the profession. This rule applies even when professionals are working together.[17] On the infrequent occasions when a colleague is ostracized, he simply goes somewhere else with those of similar standards and becomes even less observable.[18] When laymen try to monitor a professional's work through malpractice suits, it may actually increase his practice as sympathetic colleagues refer more patients than before.[19]

The ethos of expertise also includes an omnipotent view of the client as impotent: too ignorant to understand his case and too upset to use whatever information the professional might give him wisely. One consequence, Freidson argues, is that professions provide fewer rights or modes of appeal for the client than do bureaucracies.[20] Moreover, "To question one's doctor is to show lack of faith and is justifiable grounds for the doctor to threaten to withdraw his services. Such insistence on faith . . . neutralizes threat to status. The very special social position of institutionalized privilege that is the profession's is threatened as well as demeaned by the demand that advice and action be explained and justified to the layman." Thus, "in any profession one working definition of success is the attainment of such prestige that one need not deal with anyone who does not come in as a humble supplicant eager to obey.''[21]

Omnipotent Tendencies in Psychiatric Training

Enough has been said about psychiatry to make it apparent that all these patterns of narcissistic omnipotence exist in it to some degree. Moreover, the defensive origins of narcissistic omnipotence characterize psychiatry and provide insight into its peculiar mix of low self-esteem, arrogance and sensitivity to criticism. The origins of narcissism, to restate Freud's argument more broadly for our purposes, lie in vigorous attempts to recover an initial state of harmony with one's mother.[22] When this initial, ''primary narcissism'' is ruptured too severely, the person forms an ego ideal. This ''new ideal ego, . . . like the infantile ego, deems itself the possessor of all perfections,'' and protects the person from the fear of rejection by his parents and, later, by others. ''To this ideal ego is now directed the self-love which the real ego enjoyed in childhood.''[23]

This ideal self-image means that the quest for power is not merely compensation for deprivation, as Harold Lasswell argued in his famous book about politics, *Power and Personality,* or the Georges explained in their psychobiography of Woodrow Wilson.[24] It is doubtful, prima facie, that people with low self-esteem can become political activists or professionals. Paradoxically, high self-esteem must coexist with a sense of inferiority. This happens when the narcissistic defense is not so perfect, as Kernberg described above, and the person finds he does not measure up to his own idealized self-image. He turns on his actual, ''empirical'' self, condemning it almost as an alien betrayer. Thus, unnaturally high and low estimates of the self coexist, with an effort to repress the latter. As Karen Horney observed, the narcissist must ''inflate his feelings of significance and power. That is why a belief in his omnipotence is a never-failing component of the idealized image.''[25]

The specific source of psychiatry's defensive superiority lies in its ambivalent relation with medicine. From the beginning, psychiatrists were physicians who deviated enough from medicine to disrupt the protective, harmonious relationship of a specialty with its mother profession and to earn deep skepticism about their medical identity. In response, psychiatrists have developed an ideal image of themselves as more than physicians, as masters of both the body and the psyche. But much of the medical profession and the public have not been convinced, openly suggesting that psychiatry is less than the master of either. Thus the neurotic compulsion to prove its ideal self-image has led to the mixture of narcissistic omnipotence, with its eagerness for approval, low self-esteem, and sensitivity to criticism.

How persuasive this analogy has been between a certain personality pattern and the organizational behavior of a profession will depend on the biases and intellectual style of each reader. Our purpose here is to suggest the interplay between personality and social structure; for professions are made up of people. This is not to say that all psychiatrists or lawyers are grandiose and narcissistic. But we are proposing that the organization and prerogatives of a profession incline its members in this direction. It is also reasonable to speculate that young people with narcissistic personalities are intuitively attracted to those occupations which offer the conditions for acting out their neuroses.

Freud's student and biographer, Ernest Jones, wrote that people with a "God complex" have fantasies of omnipotence, "a colossal narcissism," and they tend to enter psychology or psychiatry.[26] The only evidence that such personalities go into psychiatry is supplied by E.S.C. Ford, who had his residents write autobiographies and keep journals during their training.[27] He found that a great proportion of the residents had once been close and secure with their mothers, whom they described as dominant, caring, strong and understanding. But rebuffs and separation created strong anxieties and led them to seek the lost intimacy by identifying with one idealized figure after another through the years. It was finally in psychiatry, the journals reveal, that residents found an ideal, omnipotent model who did not let them down, as had happened before. The residents identified with and "introjected" this model, reports Ford, thereby resolving both their professional identity crisis as psychiatrists and their personal quest for narcissistic omnipotence. Whether one considers this outcome a "resolution" or not, Ford's detailed biographical material is fascinating[28] and invites further investigation of how professional training builds on unresolved personal needs.

It would be worth investigating whether the structure of professional training and the socialization process work to promote the narcissistic syndrome in each new generation of professionals. This appears to be true for psychiatry. *The structure and dynamics of residency training echo the structure and dynamics of the narcissistic personality and therefore may heighten omnipotent tendencies in those who have them.* To briefly restate the theory underlying the moral career of the psychiatric resident, the training programs reviewed introduced residents into a situation which discredited old supports and competencies and created great anxiety at the same time that an ideal professional self-image was presented. This image has many omnipotent elements—high status, supreme power in its domain, great knowledge, wealth—which some trainees expect society to confer on them. As Gary Tischler also found, residents coped through regression to a medical approach that had once worked and through "therapeutic megalomania."[29] The structure of the program exacerbated the residents' need for a strong professional self-image to protect themselves from uncertainty and humiliation. It channelled the search toward a dominant professional model that was backed up by a network of contacts and opportunities for a successful career. In the most famous study of the quest for omnipotence in psychiatric training, Sharaf and Levinson described how residents then sought omnipotence by identifying with idealized supervisors, though the authors did not have much to say about what happens after that.[30] Our study indicates that residents assimilate or internalize these role models and professional values and make them compatible with their own style of working with patients. The striking deprivation, anxiety, and search that they go through increases the chances that they will be very protective of the professional prerogatives they inherit. At the same time, their ambivalent relation with medicine and the doubtful effectiveness of their techniques will lead some to vascillate between low self-esteem and grandiose behavior. Thus the structure of the training program and the nature of professional work stroke their narcissism and reinforce omnipotent tendencies in people who have them.

Relations with Clients

Omnipotence, paradoxically, depends on an audience. The audience may range from institutions to political bodies to individuals, but for simplicity we shall call them clients. Clients (or patients) have problems they are concerned about and which they have not been able to solve by other means. They turn to professionals for help and expect them to succeed where others have failed. They may attribute omnipotent powers to them, for the structural relation here parallels the one in early childhood, with the professional as the parent and the client as the child.

This relationship has its origins in psychiatric training. Rudolf Ekstein writes:

> The beginning resident frequently tries to meet the helplessness of his patient with an authoritative, directive, all-knowing, Godlike attitude; then, in turn, he brings to the supervisor his own helplessness and omni-impotentiality, a phase-specific attitude. The supervisor, in turn, may safeguard himself behind dogmatic, authoritative attitudes. . . ."[31]

The temptations to be godlike are great, and clients (whether patients or residents) play a vital role. In particular, patients provide a foundation for omnipotence in residents by expecting these still-shaky trainees to take command. This vital impetus helps residents in the last stage of weaning themselves from their mentors.[32] To become at last the source of power and love is very gratifying:

> In our own omnipotent-based guilt, we try not to see that while consciously we struggle to help the patient to mature and become well, unconsciously we have been struggling to make him become increasingly regressed, and thus to lend a Godlike status, and vicariously to fulfill, through his acting out, the various warded-off aspects of our self. I want to emphasize that we all do this, in my opinion, in our work with all our patients, in varying degrees.[33]

As the quote implies, the audience for omnipotence can become internalized so that one *assumes* that people see one as a god, or one treats them so they have little choice but to do so. Part of this is to sustain the patient's dependency as long as possible. In psychotherapy, one form this takes with psychiatrists and other therapists is to have sexual relations with patients, who may have their own need to identify as closely as possible with an omnipotent figure. According to a recent report, one out of every ten therapists admitted to erotic relations, usually with younger women, averaging twenty-nine women per therapist. Explaining why she allowed her therapist to seduce her, one woman said, "The fact that he had power . . . I had none."[34]

Making and keeping the patient dependent, exaggerating one's

powers, handling patients in a grandiose way, or institutionalizing omnipotence may in part be the unintended consequences of training programs in the profession. By structuring them so that trainees experience feelings of intense anxiety, ignorance, and dependence, such
programs may be teaching professionals to treat clients as they have
been treated. And by exaggerating their power or expertise, mentors
establish a model of omnipotence that their students are fated to repeat.
To the extent that laymen accept this mythology, omnipotent tendencies become reinforced in daily life. To the extent that they challenge
it, professionals like physicians or psychiatrists become embattled and
defensive.

15.

The Nature of Professional Socialization and Its Effects on Practice

Becoming a psychiatrist is a complex and deep process. It demands a transformation of self, even if this only means that the old elements get recast in a new guise and the old thoughts are expressed in a new rhetoric. It entails powerful forces outside the individual, not well understood yet incorporated in ways that endure. The going term for all this is "socialization," a word that offends the ear and turns the tongue into a drunkard's slur. A more serious intellectual problem is the static connotation built into the very construction of the word. At a time when everyone writing about the subject emphasizes its continuous dynamic nature, the word socialization, like its brethren computation and construction, implies a completed act and a static perspective. And while everyone emphasizes the active participation of the individuals being socialized, one is forced into phrases like "the individuals being socialized," whose very passive construction contradicts one's argument. What one needs is a word with the flexibility to be used for both the psychological and social aspects of the process, a word that conveys the participation of the subject but in the context of others, a word whose construction implies an ongoing process, a word we do not have.

Socialization as a Personal Construct

Regardless what term is used, however, there are certain aspects of the process as it pertains to professional training that need clarification, and observing psychiatric residency has helped to do that. One issue concerns how active people are in becoming psychiatrists, or soldiers, or any other calling. The critique of socialization theory, with its connotation of passivity, emerged in the 1960s and must be understood, like other shifts in social theory, as part of that era's culture. But just as a preoccupation with the activities of the socializer had neglected the various ways in which people negotiate their identities, so a celebration of the individual and the emergent quality of reality can overlook the prefabricated realities and selected resources that people in a program use to construct their identities. For example, John Van Maanen, one of the best writers in the field, states, "People are not mere puppets responding to the firm tug of social strings. Indeed, socialization settings do not have unambiguous, natural properties beyond those which individuals attribute to them."[1] Leaving "unambiguous" and "natural" aside, properties such as routines, roles, symbols, accounts and sanctions do exist beyond what trainees think. In fact, professional socialization centers on the discrepancy between the properties which recruits bring with them or attribute to the program and the properties of the setting which those in charge have organized. Whether it is Van Maanen's police department, this psychiatric residency, or the four professional programs studied by Bucher and Stelling, one is impressed with the influence of the mentors' beliefs and the program's structure even when these are played down.

There is no doubt that people are very actively participating in the construction of their identity, but they turn out surprisingly alike in those aspects which their mentors deem essential because they work with the same materials and with a lot of counsel (if not coercion). The main differences among programs are how many qualities are deemed essential and how much deviation will be tolerated. Such differences are crucial; for most programs include a variety of roles, accounts and rules. But this rarely means that recruits can assemble their own individual mix. Except for programs that lack coherence, this variety is clustered into competing approaches to work which offer alternative professional identities. Trainees find strong pressure to align themselves with one group or another, and even then what appear to be alternative models often share a common core. At University Psychiatric Center, for example, second-year residents came to perceive wide choice among models of psychiatry though in fact most were variations around a psychodynamic core.

Negotiated Order and the Structure of Power

These observations pertain to another concept, that socialization is a negotiated order. This view holds that subjects negotiate with others in the setting, but particularly with mentors, over how things will be organized, who will do what, and even what various activities mean. Again, there is no doubt that negotiations take place constantly, as materials in this study show; but the differences in power between the parties are considerable. Those in charge have far more knowledge, accounts, sanctions, and experience, so that negotiating often gives the novice a sense of personal power when the outcomes are predictable. The larger question is whether socialization ever occurs without power on one side and resistance on the other. Freud did not think so, and one might argue it is true by definition. When someone enters a group or setting to which s/he is fully acclimated, s/he is called "a natural" because no socialization is necessary. All that's needed is time to learn the skills and the details of style. What this argument implies is that *to be useful as a word, socialization should not be synonymous with learning*.

Although negotiation has been used to connote an emergent social order which parties work out in a dynamic, ongoing process, the concept need not be confined to unstable situations where one takes the subjective perspective, overlooks structural and historical influences, ignores power, focuses on cooperation, and assumes everything important can be negotiated.[2] There is good reason for Anselm Strauss to warn adherents of these dangers, but as he demonstrates, the concept is very useful.[3] One must delineate what is being negotiated, by whom, for what stakes, with what resources, in what structural context, with what options. In organized programs of socialization, the trainees constantly try to negotiate terms and activities that reconcile their sense of identity with the social order of the program. While these negotiations are new for the trainees, they are repeated for their mentors, who thereby have much more experience, not only with the symbols, skills, language, and beliefs of the profession, but also with the negotiating process itself. The stakes for each are different as well. The trainees' professional identity is the major stake, perhaps in balance with their standing in the program. At stake for the program is its success in turning out competent graduates who have become members of the profession. The material on psychiatric residents shows that the character of negotiation changes by stages from a preponderance of conflict to increasing cooperation and from more fundamental issues which question the foundations of the profession to refinements of style and technique. What this implies is that negotiating lies at the heart of socialization, not because trainees work out important arrangements and deals, but because the process of negotiating actively involves the trainee in his own transformation. To negotiate one must understand the terms of one's mentors, use the language, symbols, and paradigms of the profession. Then the process itself immerses one even more and teaches one the refinements, which in themselves already take for granted what was doubted or challenged before. Parents can also observe this process with their children, and one may call the result cooptation leading to false consciousness. But who is to say what is false, and by what criteria? In an organization, a small-scale society, where the definition of the situation rests with those in power, down to the vocabulary one uses to communicate and the accounts by which one understands one's actions, the answer is clear. Professional socialization is, to use Strauss's term, a *structural process,* where the process not only has its own structure but the larger structure of the profession is built into the process, which in turn recreates that structure, altering it as forces of change affect both.

Socialization vs. Role-Learning

The concept of socialization as role-learning prevails in sociology, and I should like to argue against it. Parsons used socialization, "to designate the learning of *any* orientations of functional significance to the operation of a system of complementary role-expectations."[4] But why be so vague? And since we have the term, role-learning, why make socialization synonymous with it? If one must choose, certainly role-learning is the more descriptive superior term. In *The Student-Physician,* Robert Merton wrote a well-known essay on professional socialization. It is, he says, "the process through which individuals are inducted into their culture. It involves the acquisition of attitudes and values, of skills and behavior patterns making up social roles established in the social structure."[5] Merton uses the passive voice to convey a passive individual being acted upon. The perspective is that of society. The second sentence provides an all-inclusive definition, which for reasons stated before is too vague. However, Merton goes on to emphasize that "Adult socialization includes more than what is ordinarily described as education and training."[6] He does not precisely say just what that "more" would be, but one gathers from the essay as a whole that he would emphasize values and attitudes to distinguish socialization from role-learning.[7]

Often, those who write about socialization as role-learning also write about developing a self. This leads to the basic question, "Is the self anything other than the sum of one's roles?"

Orville Brim, a leading role theorist of socialization, gives a strong answer. "In our view socialization is the process by which one learns to perform his various roles adequately, and our concern here is with the acquisition of social roles."[8] In another essay appropriately titled "Personality development as role-learning," Brim goes further. He states that "the learned repertoire of roles is the personality. There is nothing else. There is no 'core' personality underneath the behavior and feelings; there is no 'central' monolothic self which lies beneath its various external manifestations."[9] However, Brim's position is more assertion than argument. He makes little effort to grapple with major theorists who argue that the foundations of personality are laid in the early years. Nor does he confront the considerable accumulation of evidence showing that people exhibit continuity across roles and through the years.

The role theory of socialization has evident weaknesses, and as it became more dominant, it drew more criticism. In their study of student nurses, for example, Olesen and Whittaker portrayed the individuals implied by role theories of professional socialization as faceless and ahistorical. These theories assume that people start out with equal abilities and experiences, have no private interests or values, and are filled with perfect values, behaviors, and viewpoints for the roles they are to fill. Upon graduation, "like the dolls in nurse-doctor play kits,

young professionals move as equally substitutable units from the
school assembly line into a world where no further change can be
wrought upon or with them, they being now fully garbed with the in-
disputable trappings of the professional.''[10]

This intentional caricature differs from what many investigators,
including Olesen and Whittaker, have found. Students (and others)
shape their roles and participate in their own socialization. They work
out both individual and collective strategies. While Olesen and Whittaker accept role as a structural concept, they also emphasize that roles
are negotiated and involve new perspectives on one's self. The process
is problematic and varies from one person to another. With this critique, some people believe that Olesen and Whittaker have overthrown
the role theory of socialization and replaced it with another. More accurately, they have modified it by emphasizing the activity of the subjects. Inputs and outputs are still there, though more subtle and dif-
ferentiated.[11]

This approach is usually characterized as the active model, in
contrast to the passive subject in the role theories above. More accurate
than active-passive is the distinction between inner- and outer-directed
models; for the issue is not energy but susceptibility. All socialization
requires active, emotional involvement; even when molded, one is
engaged.[12] The passive person would be indifferent, apathetic. Thus
the important change which this critique makes of socialization is to
recognize that people come with an inner life which seriously affects
their socialization experience.

Yet the power—both personal and structural—of those in charge
is evident. For example, Robert MacKay observed adults and children
and found the children to have competent interpretations of what was
happening. But when they did not fit the adult's interpretation, they
were ignored or discredited and replaced by the adult one. Ironically,
the adult ''relies on the child's interpretive competencies to understand
the lesson but treats him throughout as incompetent (i.e., she creates or
gives the 'correct' answers).''[13] Any observant parent will recognize
this process, which occurs in a different manner in this and other training programs.

In conclusion, the concept of socialization as role-learning defines man, by logical extension, as nothing but the sum of his roles, a
definition which is empirically inaccurate and simplistic. The importance of interpretation and internal states indicates both that those

being socialized are more than a bundle of roles and that the essence of socialization lies in incorporating values and attitudes.

Later vs. Early Socialization

Having clarified the differences between role-learning and socialization, we turn to the question of how adult or professional socialization differs from socialization in childhood. No statement on this question is so widely cited, accepted and unchallenged as Orville Brim's "Socialization Through the Life Cycle." In it, Brim argues that adult socialization differs in seven ways from childhood socialization. "With respect to changes during the life cycle, the emphasis in socialization moves from motivation to ability and knowledge and from concern with values to a concern with behavior."[14] Third, one moves from acquiring new material to synthesizing old material. Fourth, later socialization is oriented toward realism rather than idealism. Fifth, adult socialization is role-specific rather than general. Sixth, it shifts from teaching expectations to teaching how to mediate conflicts. And finally, there are fewer "I-Me" relationships in adult socialization.

These distinctions are difficult to support in either direction. That is, the qualities which Brim attributes to adult socialization are equally prevalent and important in childhood, and the qualities which he attributes to early socialization are also important in later socialization. The detailed observations of Jean Piaget and others show the importance of knowledge (No. 1), behavior (No. 2), realism (No. 4), and increasing specificity (No. 5) in early socialization. Piaget, Freud and Erikson all give central attention to mediating conflicts (No. 6) and synthesizing old material (No. 3) in childhood.

Looking at the other side of the pairs, any example of adult socialization centers around learning new materials (No. 3). They are usually specific, but no more so than much childhood learning (No. 5). Idealism (No. 4) too is commonly found in cases of adult socialization. Values (No. 2), motives (No. 1), and expectations (No. 6) are central to all socialization, including experience in adult life. Likewise, all socialization involves I-Me relationships at its core (No. 7).

That Brim emphasizes these last four as attributes of early socialization tells us more about his view of adult socialization than it does about the process itself. For Brim's adult socialization is really

training—relatively impersonal, realistically centered, focused on acquiring knowledge for a certain role and not values that might affect
the person more broadly, low on expectations and idealism. His description of the setting and process of adult socialization also sounds
like training.

This problem in Brim's essay leads us to distinguish between
training and socialization; for many sociologists use an all-inclusive
definition of socialization to mean learning anything—knowledge,
skills, habits, values, attitudes. The trouble with so broad a definition
is that it becomes useless. The word no longer designates something
distinctive, so that theoretically one can say nothing clear about it.
Such breadth has been one cause of the vague, useless quality of much
writing about socialization. To avoid this, we shall define *training* as
learning certain skills or knowledge, and *socialization* as internalizing
values and attitudes. Quite often both happen together, and since all
values are a form of knowledge, socialization requires learning new
knowledge. But training which does not change one's personal or
social character does not involve socialization.

What, then, is *adult* socialization? If the seven distinctions do not
work, how shall we understand this phenomenon? First, we must abandon the term "adult" as analytically weak and talk of *secondary
socialization*. Adult is merely descriptive and raises the question of
when someone qualifies—at twenty? Eighteen? Sixteen? It is on a par
with "professional socialization" or "adolescent socialization." It
designates a time and perhaps a setting where the process takes place.
These terms are not very useful because they make no *conceptual* distinction between early and later experiences, while primary versus secondary socialization does.[15] The very phrase, secondary socialization,
implies that it happens later and is less profound. Thus, in keeping
with our critique of Brim, secondary socialization can and does occur
in childhood, while primary socialization can occur but rarely does in
later years. The distinction is one of degree and can only be worked out
in the context of human actions, but it does lead to some theoretical
distinctions that are more useful for research than adult vs. child socialization. First, secondary socialization builds on primary socialization.
One should observe how it elaborates or recasts what is already there,
rather than replacing it, as happens in some experiences of brainwashing, torture, or conversion that lead people to say "It completely
changed who I am." In addition, later experiences necessarily *de*socia-

lize as well as *re*socialize. Old assumptions and postures are questioned or simply shown to be inadequate to the new situation. The person struggles for a new understanding. The prominence of desocialization is what underlies Wilbert Moore's "punishment-centered theory of socialization" which stems from the prevalence of suffering one finds in "the training for all occupations that exhibit strong attention to standards of competence and performance and to identification with the occupation as a collectivity."[16] They isolate trainees, either physically or through "the sheer burden of work."[17] Despite student commitment, at least part of the work is unpleasant, even hazardous. While most succeed, failure is made to be felt a real possibility, and this continues even after one graduates and begins full practice. These trying experiences are shared with others, creating a "fellowship of suffering" that becomes a nostalgic bond over the years.

This theory of socialization is provocative because it is incomplete. Moore treats desocialization as if it were the entire process. One does not know why an occupation would organize its program this way, nor why tightly knit occupations with excellent standards should be more inclined to begin training this way than others. The argument makes an unexamined leap from various tortures to the final product without explaining how one progresses beyond suffering to become a full member of the occupation. By focusing on the process (and only on the first stages at that) without the goals, Moore leaves the impression that punishment is the goal of such programs as medical or law school, and that their graduates share little but fond memories of suffering and of their success at overcoming failure. He seems to forget his own criterion, that these be occupations which command high loyalty. Yet through exaggeration, Moore's punishment-centered theory of socialization highlights the importance of desocialization and power relations in secondary socialization.

Socialization as Situational Adjustment

A major question for this study is whether professional training has any enduring effect. This has been, in fact, the central issue in a debate between sociologists for over twenty years. One group of researchers, represented by Robert Merton and his students, believes that professional training is the crucible of professional identity.[18] The values and perceptions one incorporates are a major force throughout one's career. However, the Merton group has largely considered the influence of training on the individual rather than on politics and institutional organization. Another "school" of research on medical training and practice, led by Howard Becker, emphasizes the situational nature of socialization: the person being socialized takes on perspectives related to the problems and alternatives built into the structure of the situation at hand.[19] As a reaction against the Freudian view that one's personality is formed for life by the age of six, this view is understandable. But the Becker school of situational socialization, embraced recently by Miller and Freidson, goes too far.[20] This is not to deny that situational perspectives abound, but rather to add that enduring values and ways of acting are learned as well.

The Becker school actually distorts the more balanced findings of *Boys in White*. The book identifies numerous situational perspectives, but it also finds a few values like "clinical experience" and "medical responsibility," which are learned in school and endure. The distortion is Becker's fault, because he formulates his general argument around the fate of idealism. In distinguishing between "immediate and long-range perspectives" (p. 433), Becker and his colleagues argue that the basic idealism which is tempered by but endures the situational pressures of medical school is not learned there but is antecedent (pp. 420–33). The general conclusion is that "values learned in school persist only when the immediate situation makes their use appropriate" (p. 433). This may be true of idealism but is not true of clinical experience and medical responsibility, two "long-range perspectives" which carry on into internship and residency. There are similar problems between Freidson's situational argument and his recognition of underlying values.[21]

The logic of the argument creates a further problem: it cannot explain how long-range perspectives arise in the first place. On one hand, Becker writes, "The perspectives a person acquires as a result of situational adjustments are no more stable than the situation itself or his participation in it."[22] On the other hand, he assumes the existence of long-range perspectives without being able to explain them. Becker offers an apparent solution which ends in tautology. "In large part, cases in which it appears that people are not adjusting to situational pressures are cases in which closer analysis reveals that the situation is actually not the same for everyone involved in the institution."[23] Since this concept of situation is flexible, it can be adjusted to fit every case.

Another important concept in Becker's approach to secondary

socialization is *commitment*. He notes that many sociologists use it without formal analysis, to explain consistent lines of activity.[24] They assume its meaning is self-evident, and this results in tautological arguments that committed behavior can be explained by commitment.[25] To avoid this problem, Becker sets out to specify the independent qualities of commitment, a task highly relevant to the issue of socialization as situational adjustment.

> First, the individual is in a position in which his decision with regard to some particular line of action has consequences for other interests and activities not necessarily related to it. Second, he has placed himself in that position by his own prior actions. A third element is present, though so obvious as not to be apparent: the committed person must be aware that he has made the side bet and must recognize that his decision in this case will have ramifications beyond it.[26]

This theory of side bets, stated in the first sentence, is merely a rephrasing of an earlier argument by Abramson, et al. that "Committed lines are those lines of action the actor feels obligated to pursue by force of penalty. . . ."[27] He only seems to have restricted the concept by requiring that the person be aware of the side bet and its consequences. The portrait that emerges is that of the perpetual side-bettor, placing bits of himself on calculated odds whose direct and indirect consequences place him in the next situation, from which he makes further side bets.

Here is an extraordinary concept of commitment. Not "to give in trust or to pledge oneself" (as The Random House Dictionary defines the term),[28] but to make situational side bets. Becker's numerous examples accentuate this impoverished sense of commitment; for in each one the person acts consistently because the price to do otherwise is too high. Moreover, all of the examples are tautological; they do not explain the actions of those who made similar side bets but acted otherwise. That is, one knows that a person is "committed" only when one can see in retrospect that the side bets kept his actions consistent. Thus Becker solves none of the problems he found in others' treatment of commitment.

What emerges from Becker's ideas about socialization is an anti-utopian view of people. They are determined by their situation; adjustment is all. The only exception is the "clever and determined operator."[29] Daniel Levinson, in his important review of *Boys in White*, remarks, "To submit or to 'operate'—this is indeed a pathetic view of man's possibilities."[30] Becker's man is also purely utilitarian. Whatever suits the situation is his goal. Levinson notes that feelings are not important in Becker's work; beliefs and actions are "combined in the service of effective adaptation."[31] Kai Erikson notes the lack of persona. "I do not mind that Becker fails to talk about human motivation, but I am disturbed that his approach almost entirely rules it out as a relevant variable."[32]

In conclusion, the term socialization will have useful meaning only if reserved for enduring changes in the individual and not used to also mean situational adjustments. As Glen Elder writes, "socialization outcomes are more than simply response patterns in a situation— i.e., they are relatively enduring attributes of the person. . . .[33] Theoretically this means that the Becker school of adult socialization is not concerned with socialization but with situational controls that induce certain behaviors.[34]

The term "situational perspective" should be restricted to context-specific values and action patterns. The key dimension here is not duration but the relative dependence on situation. Underlying this distinction between "perspectives" and "socialization" is the one which Kelman made between identification and internalization.[35] Identification occurs when a person adopts behavior derived from a group or individual because it is associated with a satisfying relationship between the person and the other. Should that relationship weaken, identification and the behavior associated with it would also weaken. Internalization, on the other hand, implies that the adopted behavior has become incorporated into the person's value system and no longer depends upon external relationships which might once have been associated with it. Thus, if the pure social relativist wishes to say there are only situational perspectives, let him say there is no such thing as socialization.

Socialization and Practicing after Residency

A professional training program shapes the practice of its graduates both through the values, skills and folkways it transmits and through its structural links with the larger profession and the social institutions in which it works. The latter has been the focus of an intense debate in recent years, centering on whether publicly supported residents serve the public or go off to practice on private patients. This crude, political question has elicited crude, political research, showing that even the best trained and most respected research psychiatrists can easily be corrupted when the state threatens to cut funds. For example, faculty at University Psychiatric Center published research that "proved" to the state legislature that 240 of its 484 alumni surveyed had remained in the state and worked in public or private nonprofit facilities. But to be counted in the state, a psychiatrist had to have worked only one year in it; while to be counted out of state, he had to have worked elsewhere every year of his career. Likewise, to be counted in nonprofit service, a psychiatrist had to have worked only one year in it; while to be counted in private practice, one had to have worked every year in it. This article was published in the most prestigious, stringently reviewed journal in the psychiatric profession and was typical of numerous articles recently published on patterns of practice after residency.

It is clear from recent surveys that psychiatrists continue to work in a wide variety of settings, many of them public. This is particularly true of young psychiatrists, which has more to do with the informal network of the psychiatric profession, the difficulties of establishing a private practice, and especially with the changing structure of psychiatric work, than with the kind of training received. As noted in chapter 1, a great many jobs have opened up in general hospitals, community mental health centers and other public agencies. For example, 40 percent of the residents graduating from programs in the University Psychiatric Center area between 1953 and 1963 devoted 25 percent or more of their time to a public facility in 1963. In 1973, the comparable figure for 1967–73 graduates was about 75 percent. Whether the federal or state governments fund training or not, these major shifts in the job market result in figures that "prove" that recent residents who received those funds work for the public more than ever. But none of the studies look at a matched sample *not* receiving public funds. Moreover, to the extent that the informal network around a training center helps young graduates obtain jobs, it will be more influential in public circles.[36] For even if many of the supervisors or staff have private practices, they cannot "sponsor" a young psychiatrist into a practice. They can help him obtain a position at a private hospital or clinic, just as they can help him find a job in the public sector, but establishing a private practice is another matter. First, psychiatric work is sufficiently episodic and irregular and personal that a retiring psychiatrist cannot turn over his practice to a chosen successor, as can someone running a general practice, an insurance agency or a numbers racket. One does not have a large, regular population of clients whom one services. What a senior psychiatrist can do is refer extra patients to a young colleague, which over time can contribute to building a practice. Thus, the financially sensible road to private practice is to hold a regular job (public or private) and build up a practice on the side. Moreover, private patients are found through the job as well. This pattern is reflected in a national survey of 1968–72 graduates from residencies affiliated with teaching hospitals, which found that the percent in private practice rose steadily from 9 percent after one year out of residency to 37 percent after five years out.[37] The percentage in public service remained the same, about 27 percent, while the proportion in military service declined from 21 percent to 1 percent in the five years after graduation. But people in public service are probably not the same people over the entire five years. Rather, there is probably a circulation whereby some graduates in public service build up a side practice and then go private, while those discharged from the military fill their place. Since private practice is competitive, particularly with psychiatric social workers and psychologists of various persuasions siphoning off many clients, the public service jobs are usually filled. Moreover, jobs in the public service frequently allow the ideal balance of patient care, administration, research, and teaching that many psychiatrists seek, while private practice can be isolating. One has to develop these ties; they are not built into the job, as they often are in institutional positions.

Some of these observations about career structure were reflected in a study of 1967–73 graduates who were on state stipends in their third year, three-quarters of them from University Psychiatric Center. The impact of the local network is reflected in figures showing that 31 percent had resided in the state before residency, 42 percent had graduated from medical schools in the area, 100 percent had, naturally, graduated from residencies in the state, and 61 percent were presently working in the state. Again the authors found that a strong majority worked over half their time in a public institution but that this decreased as the years passed. Of relevance to the discussion above, 69 percent of those in the public sector participated in all three of the major activities surveyed—clinical, administrative, and academic work. Only 17 percent worked exclusively with patients. By contrast, only 29 percent of those in the private sector participated in all three areas, and 42 percent worked exclusively with patients.

More important, however, than the question of whether publicly funded or psychodynamically trained psychiatrists work more in public settings is how they organize their work and carry it out. Professionals have an advantage over many occupations in this regard, because they have more power to put the values, beliefs, and techniques they have learned into practice. This is exactly what Rachel Kahn-Hut found in her study of psychiatrists ten to fifteen years out of residencies in the Boston area.[38] The institutional setting where they worked did not affect their professional orientation, because the hospital-based psychiatrists set up the same conditions as did private practitioners, for office-based psychodynamic therapy within the hospital. Psychiatrists in various institutional settings, she found, continued to have the same professional orientation they had had at the end of residency. This finding is supported by a large, detailed study of psychotherapists in four major cities, which found that the structure and content of therapists' training programs affects the type of patients seen and kind of work done.[39] "Training systems thus contain within them an image of the fully formed professional and a model of the process of transformation required to realize that image. . . . In the context of this developmental process the striking thing about our findings is that they give little indication of subsequent modification of professional commitments during the course of the psychotherapist's organizational practice. . . ."[40]

Ironically, more subtle evidence indicates that the continuities between professional training and later practice include, not only elements of professional identity and approach to treatment, but also the unresolved problems and inherent difficulties of the field. The study by Kahn-Hut is important here, because she gathered subtle and detailed information about a sample of psychiatrists much like those in this study. She interviewed forty-eight psychiatrists at length on tape, all of them affiliated with an influential hospital in the Boston area.

Once out practicing in a private or hospital office, these psychiatrists reported old problems in new guises. So much of the work was boring as one listened hour after hour to the same obsession phrased in the same way, or to the same depression that would not move. Repetition and routine is something which psychiatrists share with other professionals, and they reported a sense of pent-up frustration. They felt they could not be creative; some felt their special talent and training going to waste. In addition, psychiatrists must bear the burden of silence. Although they went into a profession based on verbal skills, they found themselves listening for hours and hours, unable because of their ideology to respond very much even when they felt strongly. This ideology also induced self-estrangement; some saw themselves as a tool, scrutinizing their natural reactions with a critical eye.

Besides these problems of practice, psychiatrists reported to Kahn-Hut the lack of status in the eyes of physicians and the public; they felt that people were suspicious of psychiatry. Some also complained about their low salaries—when compared to other medical specialities, which was their reference group. Those in hospitals traded autonomy and prestige for variety. Yet autonomy had its price; the private practitioners found autonomy brought loneliness. These problems give us insight into the *structural* reasons why so many psychiatrists seek a mixture of private patients with research, work in a clinic, or supervision of trainees;[41] for these latter provide experiences of efficacy, variety, dialogue, and creativity.

While psychiatrists expressed one or another of these problems when asked about dissatisfactions, and while structurally psychiatric practice had the classic elements of alienation (anomie, isolation, lack of control, estrangement), in open-ended questions most expressed satisfaction with their work. The problem, argues Kahn-Hut, is to understand how psychiatrists transformed potentially alienating conditions into satisfying images of accomplishment. Her answer is that "a context so open that it might be meaningless and so isolated that it might be lonely can also be open enough to include any meaning one wishes to find there, and isolated enough so that no one else can question anyone's construction of a positive reality."[42] From her interviews she found that psychiatrists credited themselves with successful cases and blamed the discipline or the patient for failures. Is this so different from medicine and other professions?

However, psychiatrists did not deny the alienating conditions of their work. Instead Kahn-Hut found that they converted them into sources of satisfaction. For example, the lack of control that came from not being able to know just how one was affecting the patient provided an opportunity for creativity. Thus the scientific primitiveness of the field contributed to its creative potential. The sense of powerlessness derived from the limited effects of psychiatric techniques, she found, was used selectively to explain failures. Professional isolation (as opposed to physical isolation) stemmed partially from the doctrine of confidentiality, which gave the therapist control over the patient and the direction of the therapy without undesired criticism. Confidentiality, Kahn-Hut argues, may help establish trust with the client, but it also helps the psychiatrist construct his/her own reality without interference. Professional isolation also stems from rules of collegiality, which psychiatrists reported are very strong. One does not criticize a colleague. It is improper. It is dangerous too. In a field of low paradigm development, where there is little consensus and one's theories are not very powerful, criticism is likely to become personal. One psychiatrist said: "We don't get individually into comparing our work very often or in any depth because this kind of opens up a person to questioning. And . . . the questioning is likely to get devastatingly critical, so that there isn't that freedom to exchange [ideas]."[43] This limitation is compounded by psychiatry's tendency to interpret differences of opinion as a function of personality! Needless to say, Kahn-Hut found that psychiatrists minimize these problems by seeking the company of compatible colleagues, a form of professional isolation which Freidson found in the medical profession as well.[44]

While these observations are critical of psychiatry, they are also material for a sociological analysis of the profession. What Kahn-Hut and others are saying is that *estrangement from laymen, confidentiality, and the cardinal rule of collegiality are fundamental conditions for the survival of this and other professions in their present form.* To say that without these conditions professional work would be impossible is to play into the hands of apologists for present arrangements; one can only say that without them professional work would be different. An instructive example is medical work in China, where the three guiding principles are the opposite of those above: maximum involvement of the people served, sharing of professional information with the client and others, and mutual criticism for improving services. Most American physicians cannot imagine working under such circumstances; yet these principles have contributed significantly to accomplishments of Chinese medicine, which have never in the annals of medicine been realized so quickly.[45]

To summarize, it appears that the professional socialization we have described is crucial in providing definitions of one's work and one's professional stature, thereby influencing how services are organized and delivered. This fills a major gap in the sociology of mental health, which has focused on epidemiology and patient care without examining the people who define it and control its treatment. At the individual level, we have learned the importance of discontinuities between one's values or ideals and the circumstances of one's work. Although Kahn-Hut implies that most of her psychiatrists have resolved these problems, it is more likely that they will reappear. Periodically a sense of futility or of false practices returns to many professionals. Therefore it seems natural that Ingmar Bergman's film about a competent psychiatrist portrays her temporary break-down in terms very close to this study: "She and Dr. Wankel talk about the myth of 'curing' mentally disturbed patients, and about 'the bankruptcy of psychoanalysis.' More and more, nothing quite works, in spite of the heroine's surface of efficient good humor."[46]

Bergman's film explores what scattered evidence indicates is a second identity crisis for psychiatrists, some of which stems from the nature of professional work. After working hard through residency and further training, establishing himself in a career and attracting a circle of patients, the psychiatrist finds financial and career pressures lessening and his freedom increasing. He begins to think more about what he is doing for patients and realizes that many of them change little.[47] The profession has a large body of knowledge and experience, implying that therapy works, but improvements seem small. The doctrinal diversity of the field may also be disturbing; listening to colleagues with their spectrum of viewpoints, he wonders if anyone knows what he is doing. Meanwhile more and more people turn to him with their problems; the burden of helping grows, yet he has no one to turn to himself. This account, based on the work of Kenneth Fisher, leaves aside middle-age difficulties at home or in the life cycle that are widely shared by nonpsychiatrists. Recently a psychiatrist held a session at annual meetings for those interested in learning about group therapy. He reports that a number of colleagues unburdened themselves during the meetings.

> The dominant theme that emerged each year concerned the participants' oppressive feelings of being overwhelmed by the responsibilities of caring for psychiatric patients and their deep feelings of discouragement.
> One psychiatrist in his early 50s felt discouraged by what he was

able to do for his patients . . . he began to talk about his situation back home, where he had become a sort of father-confessor to almost everyone, it seemed. He spoke of his professional colleagues and their wives and families, all of whom came to him with urgent personal crises. Since he had assumed this role in the small community, he felt there was no one to whom *he* could go to talk about his feelings.[48]

Other cases follow, indicating that the initial questions of efficacy, relations with medicine, responsibilities with patients, and the extent of one's own neurosis are never quite resolved for at least a certain portion of the profession.[49] Answers are provided, and they are incorporated; techniques for controlling uncertainty are absorbed into one's daily habits of practice. Yet since the answers cover over as much as they resolve the problems, doubts arise from time to time. These observations and speculations about practice after residency are all that can be offered; for not much is known. They do suggest an interesting line of thought for personal reflection and future studies: that in training, professionals absorb the flaws and self-destructive aspects of professional identity as well as its strengths and self-renewing qualities.

In conclusion, socialization involves becoming the values, language, behavior patterns, and beliefs of a social group which have a relatively enduring impact on how a person conducts him- or herself. This definition builds on that put forward by Robert Merton in his classic essay on medical education, but it defines the term more sharply. Socialization differs from learning, whether one is learning knowledge, skills or roles, because it indicates a personal involvement and absorbtion that "learning" does not. Cognitive learning is necessary but not sufficient for socialization.

Situational adjustment is also different. The Becker school of socialization not only suffers from theoretical inconsistencies but is not borne out by the data presented here. At the same time, the Merton-Becker debate is based in part on a false dichotomy, because the power of professionals allows them to construct their work environment so that it is relatively consonant with the beliefs they hold. This sharpens Merton's observation that values and norms are "greatly reinforced by the social organization of medical practice."[50] Practice reinforces because much of its organization is designed by those who carry the values and beliefs. This situation contrasts with that of nurses, who constantly suffer from being socialized as professionals, but then work as subordinates. By contrast, medical or psychiatric beliefs embody a model of practice reflected in the structural relations between the training program and the larger profession. When major, external changes occur, the structure and beliefs of training adjust, but with a significant time lag. Thus future studies of professional socialization must examine not only the structure and process of training, but also the structural relations and problems between the program and the world of practice as well as its strengths and self-renewing qualities.

Professional socialization has more than a passing semblance to conversion, with all its blindnesses and convictions. We have argued that it is more than learning roles or situational adjustment. In professional socialization, certain aspects of a person's identity and life patterns are broken down (desocialized) so that a new identity can be built up. While the person actively participates in the process and to some degree negotiates the terms of his or her new identity, this activity serves more to coopt the person into using the concepts, values, and language of those in power. Conversion occurs through the stages of moral transformation which intensify trainees' commitment to the professional community.[51] As Rosabeth Kanter found, the greater the difficulties encountered, the greater the trials undergone, and the more active the commitment required, the more likely the new identity will be sustained.[52] But the price of this pervasive approach to professional training may be an insensitivity to patient needs, an intolerance of uncertainty, a false and unwarranted sense of conviction, and grandiose behavior that betrays the original mandate of the professions to serve the people.

16.

Professional Training and the Future of Psychiatry

Stepping back to view the relation of psychiatric education to the profession as a whole puts it in a different light. For ironically, this famous training program was setting its graduates on a trajectory that would be increasingly tangential to the profession and, more important, to the needs of society. These pages describe the end of an era, the final years of a great psychodynamically based program before it changed under pressure from the state and the profession. But it was not atypical in its values and techniques from the programs that trained the vast majority of psychiatrists in the profession today. Even at that time, one could see the signs of insularity from major shifts in mental health care: the disgust expressed at having to work with ordinary "cases" from the community—black, uneducated, old, or some combination thereof; the poor attendance at required drug seminars and the view of drugs as tools of management rather than therapy; the disengagement from medicine; and the almost exclusive preoccupation with the inner dynamics of a patient, leaving work with the family, employer, and social agencies to the social workers. How did this insularity come about?

Professions are not unitary but are made up of factions or segments with their own view of what work is essential, of what techniques are best, and of how care should be organized.[1] Psychoana-

328

lysis, and its broad, diluted form known as dynamic psychiatry, had been the dominant segment for so long that it regarded the development of new therapies as epiphenomena or as irrelevant. Moreover, dynamic psychiatry has the fatal qualities of low paradigm development already discussed: strong on theory or ideology but weak on evidence and research. One consequence is a hierarchy built on authoritative figures, a deference to senior figures and the lore that surrounds them rather than a deference to research and new knowledge. These qualities have often been noted. The enlightened analyst, Robert Wallerstein, for example, has deplored the ideological factions that build up around authority figures and has called for rigorous research that involves other disciplines in the university.[2] But the argument here is sociological, namely that a weak technological base leads to these structural and cultural characteristics that promote a certain arrogant insularity in major scientific advances.

One consequence of these qualities was that dynamic psychiatry never integrated well with the rest of medicine. Theoretical incompatibility was not the central problem. Nor was psychiatry shut out of the curriculum. In fact, under the grandiose name of behavioral science it has gained more and more time in medical education, from 112 hours on the average in 1940 to 458 hours in 1966.[3] And leading psychiatrists would insist that they use the medical model of diagnosis and treatment. Nevertheless, courses in psychiatry have been consistently looked down on with disdain, as described in chapter 2, and physicians in medicine have consistently regarded psychiatry with suspicion if not hostility. Besides the obstacles of clashing personalities and a certain queasiness around disturbed minds, the problem seems to lie in dynamic psychiatry's reliance on sages and insight rather than researchers and lab tests.

On the other side, dynamic psychiatry has done little until recently to bring about this integration. Residents at University Psychiatric Center and across the nation learned to dislike or belittle the most medical aspects of psychiatry. They learned that organic brain syndromes were not interesting because they were "cut-and-dried" and did not involve psychodynamics. Electroshock therapy repelled most of them. Despite its quick, dramatic results for certain disorders, it was the treatment of last resort. We have already mentioned the belittling of psychopharmacology. Residents even learned to abandon the physical exam. A recent study of young psychiatrists trained at the University

of California Medical Center found that none of the respondents performed a physical on outpatients and 85 percent did not do it on new
inpatients.[4] Yet psychiatrists are quick to emphasize their medical
affiliation as distinguishing them from other psychotherapists.

Besides keeping medicine in an ambivalent, arms-length position,
the inbred qualities of the psychodynamic segment have made psychiatry slow to respond to the changing needs of the population. Although
psychodynamic theory emphasizes the importance of the family, it was
clinicians in social work and segments of psychology that expanded
family therapy. The major cultural trends which have torn at the family
led to a great need for this work, but psychiatry entered the field late.
Group dynamics and group therapy were also picked up late, though
Freud had written brilliantly about them. As recently as 1977, a survey
by the American Psychiatric Association found that family and group
therapy were still little used by psychiatrists.[5] Sociologically, group
therapy was an important response to the widening demand for therapy
from people who could not afford it individually. Group techniques
were both developed and proliferated outside of psychiatry. As one observer put it, "psychiatry is losing its grip on the non-psychotic
world."[6] The reasons, again, do not seem to lie in the limits of psychodynamic theory but in professional habits, a fixation on individual
therapy.

Certain other kinds of therapy which would naturally seem to fall
within the purview of psychiatry have grown tremendously but have not
seemed quite proper or tasteful to most members of the profession.
Public concern over alcoholism and the large government programs
devoted to it reflect a major trend away from regarding it as a crime or
the result of bad character toward a therapeutic and medical approach
to the problem.[7] Naturally, psychiatrists work with alcoholics, but as
little as possible. Although alcoholism inherently combines medical
and psychological dimensions and therefore is an area in which psychiatry could have established a monopoly, it did not. A more recent field
of growing demand has been sex therapy of the Masters and Johnson
kind. Again, it combines physiological and psychological dimensions.
Although psychiatrists deal with sex problems all the time, they do it in
their own way and for the most part did not participate in developing
the new techniques based on careful medical research. To summarize,
the psychiatric profession and its association have passed up twenty
years of extraordinary opportunities and creative developments. It is

one of the few professions which, despite its prerogatives, lost ground in a period of expansion.

A preoccupation with the individual has contributed to psychiatry's unresponsiveness to the victims of discrimination. Therapists outside the profession were much quicker to understand the nature and pathologies of racism and sexism. Of course there were exceptions, both good and bad. In all of these areas, a certain number of psychiatrists pandered to social fads and another small number did pioneering work of enduring significance. But these exceptions are less important than the norms in training and practice.

An indication of psychiatry's insensitivity to social forces and cultural needs can be seen in how little it has done for blacks and women in its own training programs. A report commissioned by the American Psychiatric Association concluded: "The meaning of being a woman to the woman resident and her teachers, to the woman therapist and her patients . . . has received scant attention."[8] A recent survey reported in the study of residency training by the American Psychiatric Association that "approximately 71 percent of the programs acknowledged that they had no affirmative action programs specifying active efforts to recruit women residents . . . 48 percent of the programs did not consider the supervisor's sex important . . . 87 percent of the programs did not offer courses on the psychology or sociology of women."[9] The same study found only one recent article on the training of Afro-Americans and less than one hundred blacks in psychiatric residencies. Yet the APA study correctly anticipates a tremendous demand for therapeutic services among blacks. The survey found most of the residents critical of their program's understanding of racial issues. They felt that psychiatric theory had little to do with social problems and the needs of the patient population.[10] While psychiatry is certainly capable of addressing these needs, the residents are correct in their assessment of actual training and practice.

Similar qualities of the profession underlie the broken marriage between psychiatry and community mental health. The origins of this movement are complex.[11] They entail humanitarian, liberal politics both in psychiatry and in government, the hard politics of academic psychiatrists (who occupy key federal positions) wresting control of public psychiatry from the states and their mental hospitals by establishing a new institutional network to replace those hospitals, the advent of new drugs that could maintain hospitalized patients in the

community, and the desire to cut hospital costs by transferring patients
to programs of the welfare state.[12] The grandiosity of the project was
staggering. "The CMHC program would be one of the federal government's first attempts to raise national mental health by improving the
quality of general community life through expert knowledge, not
merely by more effective treatment for the already ill."[13]

There was "the fantasy of an omnipotent and omniscient mental
health technology that could thoroughly reform society. . . ."[14] Given
the difficulty psychiatry had in treating disturbed individuals, the assertion that it could also treat whole communities, carry out primary
prevention, and eradicate mental illness was extraordinary.

No one inside the profession or out has yet explained such arrogance except to dismiss it as "naive."[15] But since highly sophisticated
leaders of psychiatry, including the director of the University Psychiatric Center, promoted the idea, naiveté is too simple an answer. The
profession needs to take itself on as a patient; for never has a profession carried out so grandiose a scheme on so large a scale with such
widespread consequences. Part of the explanation lies in chapter 1.

We cannot digress to describe and explain the community mental
health movement. For interested readers, the two most balanced accounts are by Musto and by Bassuk and Gerson.[16] Our interest is to understand the lack of genuine support for this movement once it was
started and the consequences of the movement for the profession. For
community mental health was a Trojan horse. Once psychiatry let it
enter the city walls, thousands of its rivals poured forth from it. Over
the years, psychologists and psychiatric social workers have gained increasing control over community mental health centers (CMHCs) and
an increasing proportion of the professional positions, while the proportion and power of psychiatrists has steadily diminished. Specifically, in the six years from 1970 to 1976, the number of positions per
center on the average decreased by 35 percent for psychiatrists, increased by 77 percent for psychologists, and increased by 35 percent
for social workers.[17] The reasons are not hard to identify. First, community mental health further demedicalized "mental illness" so that
psychiatry's efforts to claim exclusive rights over it became nearly in-
defensible. Admonitions that psychiatrists should "diplomatically
point out that their rigorous medical and psychiatric training, extensive
leadership experience in patient management, and ultimate legal responsibility for patient care differentiate them from other clinicians"[18]

miss the point. These arguments have been made and other clinicians are not impressed. They feel that their training is just as rigorous, that medical expertise is usually not important, that they can manage patients as well or better than psychiatrists, and that "ultimate legal responsibility" is usually not involved. Thus they need psychiatrists as a part-time resource because of their legal-medical monopoly over prescriptions and hospitalization. And this is exactly what has happened in many centers. Being a costly drain on an inadequate budget, psychiatrists' time is cut back to the minimum needed to carry out these functions. Aside from their legal-medical monopoly, psychiatrists do not have a clearly defined role and offer no distinctive model of how to do community mental health.[19]

Thus the fundamental problem with community mental health is that it created a new system of service without a new paradigm of care underlying it. Thomas Kuhn has pointed out that the organization of activities in a science is paradigm-specific.[20] One cannot successfully change the organization of research without a change in the underlying paradigm. It is illuminating to extend this argument to the delivery of services based on scientific work. Without a technology and clear examples of how community mental health differed from previous clinical work, community mental health has devolved into an outpatient variant of custodial practices previously found in state mental hospitals. This is what underlies the thoughtful assessment by Bassuk and Gerson:

> The very nature of many conditions psychiatrists attempt to treat is still not well understood. In view of this lack of basic knowledge it is not surprising that there are no accepted guidelines for establishing comprehensive systems for the delivery of mental health care—notably systems for reaching disadvantaged people.[21]

Besides the demedicalizing of mental illness and the lack of a new paradigm for mental health care, community mental health work did not attract the commitment of psychiatrists. As a study in 1974 showed, only 4 percent of psychiatrists listed community or social psychiatry as their area of specialization, though over 25 percent of them worked in the centers.[22] Unlike psychologists and social workers, they also tended to work part-time. Put simply, it is difficult to maintain a preeminent position when one is working part-time at an institution where one's competitors are working full-time and run it. He cannot lead who dabbles. The ensuing hostilities, when combined with inadequate and unstable funding, poor work conditions, and "uninteresting" clientele, have left psychiatrists with alternatives to go elsewhere. Thus, a quarter of the profession worked in CMHCs in 1974 because the jobs were there for the young and/or less qualified. A downward drift has developed "in which only those psychiatrists least qualified to work in other modes of practice perform [the CMHC's] long-term service and leadership roles. . . ."[23]

The lack of commitment and techniques is reflected in the poor training which most psychiatrists practicing today have had for community work. Like all training, appropriate preparation begins with appropriate recruitment. In the major study of psychiatrists, social workers and psychologists, Henry, Sims, and Spray found once more that therapists choose patients like themselves, and the modal psychiatrist is middle-class, educated, verbal, Jewish, and white.[24] The authors imply that one will have to recruit from a wider range than this if we expect therapists to work with the spectrum of patients found in any community.

Psychodynamic training does nothing to overcome the social and cultural biases of psychiatrists' background. A recent national survey concluded that "To the extent that community mental health is rooted—in part, at least—in a sociogenic etiology and social remediation of mental disorders, then psychiatrists' unwillingness to assume any but the most modest of community activist stances may hinder the continued development and elaboration of the movement. . . ."[25] Psychiatrists were more likely than other staff to regard their community mental health center as a medical facility rather than as a social service facility, and they had been considerably less involved in community situations requiring them to be a change agent.

These findings stem from the psychoanalytically based training which so many psychiatrists receive and pursue. As usually taught, it is distinctly inappropriate for work in community mental health.[26] A number of books have appeared trying to show how they are compatible; but the diagnostic focus on unresolved tensions in early childhood; the slow, expensive, careful unravelling of these in treatment; and the trained inattention to physical surrounding, political manipulation, or economics is hardly what most CMHC clients want or what the centers can afford to give. No wonder residents disdained patients from the community when the challenges they presented differed so from those the staff at University Psychiatric Center emphasized.

A psychodynamic training is not only inappropriate; it can be dangerous. A recent, detailed study of staff relations at CMHC illustrated this when investigators found that such psychiatrists infused the rest of the staff with their professional biases.[27] The staff became stratified according to how trained they were to give dynamic psychotherapy, and the patients were stratified according to how eligible they were for such treatment. Thus the psychiatrists saved all the "interesting" (articulate, neurotic, middle-class) patients for themselves and saw a few patients often. At the other end of the scale, any patient speaking Spanish or considered undesirable for individual therapy was given to the essentially untrained community mental health workers, many of whom could not speak Spanish either. Worse, these workers saw themselves as "getting the dregs." In this grotesque distortion of a community service, psychiatrists work the system to fulfill their own professional self-image which they acquired in residency.

To summarize, even when the omnipotent fantasies of psychiatry's leaders became manifest in the community mental health movement, the profession's elitist insularity prevented members from meeting the challenge. Meanwhile, what had been envisioned as an expanded power base for psychiatry turned out to be a power base for psychology and social work, albeit underfunded and pedestrian. Psychiatry developed an identity crisis of immense proportions, became disillusioned with community mental health, proclaimed over and over that it was "dead" even as new centers were being rapidly built, and rediscovered its medical roots.

The Return to Medicine

In a prophetic article, Eugene Pumpian-Mindlin warned that if community psychiatry diverted the profession from the doctor-patient relationship by defining the community as the client, the identity of the profession would become dissipated. He warned the profession "not to be corrupted by the wealth which is pouring our way. . . ."[28] The problem, it turned out, was not only losing sight of the doctor-patient relationship, but having patients who did not respond to psychotherapeutic techniques. The identity confusion of working with an interprofessional team, yet seeing oneself as a "doctor" and therefore leader, has already been noted in the chapter on uncertainty. An early report on a residency in Cincinnati described many of the problems that appeared at other residencies and at University Psychiatric Center.[29] Residents considered their assignment in community psychiatry a drudge and disparagingly called the clinic in Cincinnati a "drug clinic," showing in the process the psychodynamic bias against drugs as significant therapeutic tools. By 1974, such reports were more common, one on Tufts describing the "anxiety, loneliness, anger and disappointment" residents expressed toward their community psychiatry training.[30] By 1975, Roy Grinker declared, ". . . our discipline has lost its boundaries."[31] He deplored the dichotomy of the medical vs. the social model as "one of the worst possible examples of dualistic thinking,"[32] but he called community and preventive psychiatry illusions, saying psychiatrists cannot be social engineers and change socioeconomic predispositions. Looking back in 1977, Francis Braceland concluded, "We wandered too far afield in the 1960s, and some colleagues took on a sociologic cast of character that almost split our speciality in two."[33]

The return to medicine became a broad movement in 1974. While just the year before, sessions at the annual meetings of the American Psychiatric Association on training were filled with educators openly expressing their confusion about what psychiatrists should learn, in 1974 the same sessions were filled with assertions about the importance of medicine in psychiatry, the tremendous gains in biopsychiatric research and the value of going through internship. Community psychiatry had confronted the profession with the inability of its own psychodynamic paradigm to consider extrapsychic forces, and it had admitted nonmedical competitors in a flush of egalitarianism.

The timing of this professional shift could not have been better. Both the public and leaders of the medical profession were pursuing primary care medicine. Family practice had finally become a specialty with its own residency and board exams. Federal funds were prompting medical schools everywhere to establish primary care programs, and the major specialties of internal medicine, pediatrics, and surgery were all designing primary care tracks. Given how common emotional problems are in any primary care practice, and considering the psychiatric dimensions of most serious medical procedures, psychiatry reaffirmed its medical roots at a time when the previous prejudices which specialists had had were breaking down. There was in this an historical symmetry. After World War II, medicine carried its obsession with specialty research and training to its practical conclusion—80 percent became specialists when only 10 percent of all medical problems needed specialty care. During the same period, psychiatry was carried away from medicine by its psychoanalytic preoccupation. Now both sides were correcting and finding their common ground; therefore psychiatry could become full partner with the other major specialities in a new era of primary care and family medicine. It has not happened. In most schools, faculty in the other major specialities have not found their department of psychiatry very helpful or very willing to help. They feel perfectly capable of teaching psychiatry to their students themselves. An exception is "liaison psychiatry," a most interesting term, because it indicates that the profession had to have specialists to make itself useful and comprehensible to other physicians. A liaison psychiatrist recently wrote:

> The problem, then, is two-fold. We must persuade those in charge of psychiatric residency training of the need to inculcate candidates with the knowledge of the normal and abnormal psychological reactions to medical illness, including knowledge of recent findings derived from psychobiological research, and of the need to transmit this knowledge to the medical caretaker. At the same time we must persuade medical caretakers of the need for the liaison psychiatrist's clinical and educational services.[34]

But why has this not been a central part of training for *all* psychiatrists long before liaison psychiatry became fashionable? In short, through its pride and inflexibility, psychiatry succeeded in most medical schools during the seventies to make itself irrelevant even to its own parent profession. Not surprisingly, recruitment declined as those medical students more interested in people than organ systems found more versatile and expanding opportunities in family medicine or one of the primary care specialities.

Paradigm Shift: The Rise of Biopsychiatry

During the past thirty years, research in biochemistry and psychopharmacology has steadily grown and produced important drugs that are universally used. What the predominantly psychodynamic profession did not seem to realize as it used these drugs along with psychotherapy was that they contained a fundamentally different paradigm of psychiatry. The etiology of disorders, the process of diagnosis, the kind of training, the nature of research, and the course of treatment implied by biopsychiatry are all different. Ultimately they are reconcilable—Freud recognized that—but they are strikingly different as presently practiced. Everyone in town knew about this work in the late sixties, when this study was done. Some of the most important work was going on down the street. But so long as this work did not constitute a major power base in the profession, most psychiatrists could ignore its journal articles full of strange hieroglyphics and they could innocently reap the fruits of its research.

However, academic centers shape the future direction of a profession, and large grants for biochemical research gave biopsychiatrists power. This same pattern was dramatically illustrated in medical schools, where Flexner's choice of the Johns Hopkins model for training put researchers in charge of education. As Rosemary Stevens has traced so well, the Johns Hopkins academic model steadily altered the entire character and politics of the medical profession.[35] In many ways, the Association of American Medical Colleges is today more influential than the AMA in policies affecting the profession. Starting in the late 1960s, the same process began in psychiatry. Behavioral scientists and community psychiatrists were replaced by biochemical researchers. Department after major department replaced a chairman trained in psychoanalysis with a biopsychiatrist. One such chairman, who replaced a famous social psychiatrist, ordered that everyone start wearing white coats. At first, the staff joked about it: "Oh, I see you're wearing your white coat today!" But soon the joking stopped.

Biopsychiatry now has control of major power centers in academic psychiatry. Its proponents are rewriting the Diagnostic Statistical Manual to emphasize the biomedical etiology of mental disorders. Students who cut up in class, alcoholics, "antisocial" individuals, criminals, homosexuals, political dissidents, chain smokers, obese people, to mention a few, are increasingly seen to have biochemical imbalances, if not genetic defects. Like any social movement, it is rewriting history to show that before 1955 there was nothing but darkness and misery.

> Pessimism about psychiatric disorders was widespread, admissions increased, and discharges remained low.
>
> Living areas in public mental hospitals were poorly furnished and crowded. Hallucinating patients paced the floor, or rocked in chairs, and

talked to their "voices"; paranoid patients scanned the rooms, ever vigilant and ever fearful. . . .

The physicians responsible for the treatment of patients in public mental hospitals were poorly equipped for the task . . . [because] neither neurological diagnosis nor psychoanalysis had much to offer patients in public mental institutions.[36]

This account, in its exclusive focus on public mental hospitals as if their reality were the whole, glosses over so many issues irrelevant to physicians' techniques, and so ignores successful treatments without drugs, that only ideological distortion remains. Biopsychiatry now takes full credit for the community mental health movement; for it would not have been possible without the miraculous drugs it provided.[37] As Andrew Scull has shown, deinstitutionalization had less to do with new drugs than with saving money under the guise of humanitarianism.[38] And community mental health was hardly a movement which advocated proliferating the drugs of biopsychiatry to the underprivileged. To the extent that this has nevertheless happened, it has raised grave doubts about community psychiatry. While it began as a powerful humanitarian movement to break down class barriers in psychotherapy, to bring well-trained clinicians into close contact with the suffering of underprivileged people, to work jointly with ordinary citizens in campaigns against oppressive and dehumanizing forces from which they suffered, in fact community psychiatry has become a large set of underfunded centers that dispense drugs to large volumes of disturbed patients. It is estimated that the use of neuroleptics on patients in the community is 85 percent, at least as high as it was among hospitalized patients.[39] It is probably higher, because communities are less tolerant of deviant behavior than hospital staff, and life in a community requires more control.[40] Among discharged schizophrenics it reaches 95 percent.[41] The effects of these drugs extend beyond the individual to alter relations with his or her social network, reducing and distorting interaction in a variety of ways.[42] In California at least, most of the discharged patients have not returned to their families or communities of origin; so that patients do not have well-established social bonds with which to carry out the original ideals of community health work. On the contrary, many towns succeed in keeping state mental hospitals from discharging patients into their communities, so that large numbers of them are channelled into specific center-city areas.[43] These conditions further increase the dependence on drugs. The overall effect on health care is to medicalize it and play down educational, therapeutic, or rehabilitative alternatives.

As has been the case with previous new "cures," interesting doubts are being raised about how effective various drugs really are. Even lithium, "the first specific treatment for major affective disorders,"[44] may turn out to be effective only on the subsample of people it is purported to "cure." In his review of psychotropic drugs, Thomas Scheff puts "the phenothiazines (in the treatment of acute psychosis) and lithium carbonate closer to the positive value end of the continuum, the anti-depressants of lesser value, and the phenothiazines in the treatment of chronic psychosis and the anti-anxiety drugs, worse than useless."[45] Since even small doses of Thorazine decrease social communication, the sociological side effects may be significant.[46] The antianxiety drugs have a short but ominous history. Miltown, after being used by millions, was found ineffective and removed from the market, to be replaced by Valium and Librium, which now appear ineffective and also addictive.[47] But these problems are unlikely to slow down biopsychiatrists in their increasing influence over psychiatric practice. The technology of neuroleptics is increasingly imbedded in the social organization of care, subsuming more and more problems under its medical paradigm. Soon a complex division of labor may arise. In the model outlined by Fieve, one would have specialized clinics staffed largely by paramedics using routinized diagnostic tools, with a psychiatrist or two acting as supervisor and manager.[48]

Yesterday's Training—Tomorrow's Practice

This portrait of the profession makes clear how most psychiatrists practicing today were trained with skills and professional values that have made them marginal to the paradigm shift in the profession and to the widening needs of society. Psychiatry today seems as confused about how to train its members and about their roles relative to physicians, paraprofessionals, and nonmedical therapists as ever. The confusion is less obvious, because spokesmen keep uttering to each other reassuring phrases about "medical psychiatry." As always, there are individuals who have thought through the issues and know what they are doing, but viewing the profession as a whole reveals confusion and unresolved questions around the classic fault lines in the profession.

One of those concerns the relation between body and mind, between psychiatry and internal medicine, and a number of residencies seem to handle the internship year over which they now have control by asking themselves if residents should spend half or three-quarters of the first year "on the wards." It is, of course, the wrong question; for it barely addresses the integration of medicine with psychiatry or the future roles to be played by trainees in medicine.

Moreover, this study indicates that two years sufficed for training when three years were required. This had been true at least since the early 1950s, when residents at the Menninger School of Psychiatry were carefully tested after their first week, first year, second year and third year on their knowledge of psychodynamics, ward management, psychopathology, clinical judgment, neurology, psychotherapy, and history.[49] Alumni, senior and junior staff were also tested. In every category, scores improved markedly during the first year, slightly or not at all in the second year, and slightly or not at all in the third year. One should note that all groups—even alumni—did quite poorly on this painstakingly constructed test, with the *best* score in each category having about one-third of the answers wrong. The authors conclude that "there is no statistically significant advantage of third over first-year men in any tested area."[50]

This argument does not imply that the third year is worthless. Defenders could give powerful illustrations of how important the third year had been to individual residents. But they could just as easily defend the fourth, fifth, sixth and seventh years. The point is that formal, supported training should be the minimum necessary for a professional to begin practice in a limited way, analogous to the way a new associate practices the law. The sociological calendar (chapter 5) indicates that socialization is largely complete by the middle of the second year, and there is yet no evidence elsewhere that substantial new knowledge is acquired in the third year.

Whether training today requires three or even four years (which is in fact its actual length now) has not been determined. But until psychiatry straightens out its own house and is training physicians in useful techniques which could not reasonably be taught to less expensive personnel, it does not deserve public support. Why should taxpayers give their money to support such a program for people already trained in the best-paying profession in society?[51]

The garbled thinking which continues to plague the profession is found in the recent, major study of psychiatric education by the American Psychiatric Association. One section asks, "What is a psychiatrist?" On the one hand, it admits that any physician can limit his/her practice to psychiatry without any training. On the other hand, psychologists, social workers and nurses "contributed to the advancement of psychiatry."[52] The board of trustees held an official discussion about the resulting problem of defining a psychiatrist. The report concludes that

> the psychiatrist is characterized by the medical assets he brings to the treatment of his patients. His distinct training includes patient responsibility, knowledge of psychodynamics, a cultivated sense of human growth and development, a heightened awareness of interpersonal process, professional objectivity, expert interviewing techniques and experience in negotiating counter-transference phenomena.

Hence it may be said that a psychiatrist can be defined as someone who has the knowledge and skills indicated as minimally necessary to function in order to cure and prevent mental illness. The complete psychiatrist exhibits these qualities to such an extent that as a result of his training (and lifelong education) he brings to his performance the highest degrees of patient responsibility, knowledge of psychodynamics, sensitivity about growth and development, compassionate objectivity, interviewing expertise and awareness of countertransference.[53] Besides the embarrassment of redundancy, vague terms and ideological bias, these medical assets are not medical at all. In a similar vein, the commission concludes with criteria for being declared a psychiatrist. They are amazing for their lack of substance and for tautological dependence on the professional monopoly they already hold. The first five criteria, for example, are: 1. has completed medical training; 2. could be employed as a psychiatrist; 3. could be given a title which indicated psychiatric training; 4. defines himself/herself as a psychiatrist; 5. can meet requirements to join recognized professional societies.[54]

Such confusion is not new. In the good old days of the mid-fifties, when psychoanalysis was king and there was little psychopharmacology or behavioral therapy or community psychiatry to bewilder the mind, the confusion was just as great. So reliable an observer as Herbert C. Modlin wrote in 1955 of "the present unsettled state of psychiatric education"[55] and naively hoped that adequate evaluation would help establish standards for training. He naturally assumed that the profession would emulate the high quality of evaluation he himself had set when in fact there has been almost no systematic evaluation. A principal reason, of course, is one recognized by everyone from Modlin to the new APA Report: you cannot evaluate if there are no standards by which to measure.

If psychiatry did not know how to train its own members in the mid-1950s and continues not to know how to do so today, there is less chance than before that it will know how in the future. For the mental health scene is far more complex than it was after World War II. We have moved from the expensive, leisurely therapy of psychoanalysis for comfortable Victorians, to behavior modification and other short-term therapies for hard-working Americans in a hurry, to therapeutic games for today's people, who think mainly about themselves and want to feel good.[56] While it is politically shrewd for the profession to resolve its identity crisis by strengthening its ideological and organizational ties with medicine, this will not clarify how psychiatrists should be trained. Meanwhile, the problems people bring today for therapy are less and less medical; thus the conservative retreat to medical ties will simply make psychiatry more and more irrelevant and unable to reconcile its ideological convictions with community psychiatry or with the needs of contemporary patients.

The basic problem with psychiatric training today is that it finds itself encumbered with years of medical school and decades of ideological bias, so that the profession is full of self-preservation, defensive thinking, and inhouse fighting. Psychodynamic psychiatry, as portrayed in this study, served a great purpose. It brought a level of human treatment and innovative study that the field had never seen before. But in the last fifteen years vested interests have entrenched themselves, and the profession has shown a remarkable inability to incorporate new developments, because the psychodynamic segment became too ingrown. Fresh thinking is needed such as is shown in an article by two professors of psychiatry at the University of Wisconsin. "A New Mental Health Profession," by Drs. Gene Abroms and Norman Greenfield, starts from scratch and builds up a persuasive case for a shorter, yet more effective training program.[57]

The situation today in some respects resembles the state of medicine around 1910, when Flexner issued his famous report. A large number of general psychiatrists, trained in programs of widely differing quality which admitted nearly anyone willing to apply, is treating patients with few specific remedies and little technology. But science has provided the basis for a new breed of psychiatrist, highly skilled and conversant with the expanding armature of drugs and medical technology. How practitioners assimilate this new technology will depend on the politics of legislation and the use of continuing education. But as in 1910, the new mandarins are narrowly focused on what their technology can do, not what it leaves out. The chance for the integration of biopsychosocial knowledge, which is so badly needed in medicine and psychiatry, is at present not great. People may have bodies, psyches, and live in a social world, but psychiatric paradigms do not.

To conclude, the economic, cultural and scientific opportunities for psychiatry are so great that it is bound to grow in the future. There will be an increasing demand for therapeutic services as better insurance gives all social classes the power to purchase services, as the population gets older and more educated, and as the expectations for a happy life rise.[58] At a deeper level, this is the age of therapy, of narcissistic self-nurturance in the face of a transient, fast-paced world that fragments time and community. The underlying forces of technology and industrial economy have led to each individual occupying several "roles," each outside the true self and yet leaving that self vaguely defined. Modern psychiatry arose to bridge this gap, to nurture the private self.[59] Yet its growth will be troubled by such confusion and ambivalence that neither psychodynamic therapy nor community mental health nor psychiatry in primary care nor biopsychiatry will develop in a constructive, cohesive way. Some of the obstacles have their origins in the kind of training described in this study. Some of them stem from the limited, self-preoccupied way in which psychiatry has medicalized itself. Others result from competition rather than enlightened cooperation with other mental health professions. Only a united effort between social scientists, psychiatrists, and other physicians could develop the integrated biopsychosocial model that all of medicine needs, but at present such an effort seems unlikely.

Appendices

Appendix I.

Tables and Figures for "The Psychiatric Domain"

TABLE I   Midtown Manhattan Cohort's Distributions on CMHR Six-grade* Continuum, 1954 and 1974

Continuum Grade	In 1954 (20–59 years old)	In 1974 (40–79 years old)
N	695	695
% Base	100.0%	100.0%
1. "Well"	19.1%	21.3%
2. "Mild"	41.2%	42.9%
3. "Moderate"	21.3%	19.6%
4. "Marked"	10.6%	10.2%
5. "Severe"	6.2%	4.6%
6. "Incapacitated"	1.6%	1.4%
4–6. "Impaired" ("Marked," "Severe," "Incapacitated")	18.4%	16.2%

Source: Leo Srole, "Measurement and Classification in Socio-Psychiatric Epidemiology," *Journal of Health and Social Behavior* (June 1976), vol. 17, no. 2, p. 192.

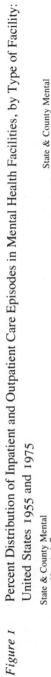

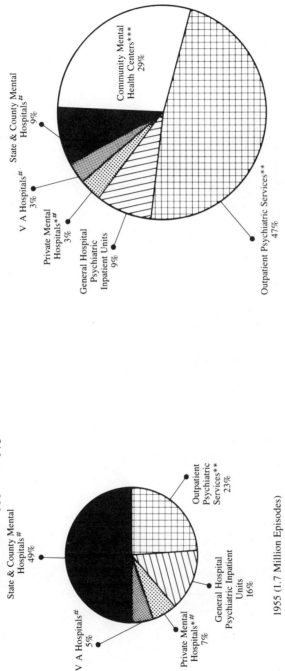

Figure 1 Percent Distribution of Inpatient and Outpatient Care Episodes in Mental Health Facilities, by Type of Facility: United States 1955 and 1975

State & County Mental Hospitals#
9%

Community Mental Health Centers***
29%

V A Hospitals#
3%

Private Mental Hospitals*#
3%

General Hospital Psychiatric Inpatient Units
9%

Outpatient Psychiatric Services**
47%

1975 (6.4 Million Episodes)

State & County Mental Hospitals#
49%

Outpatient Psychiatric Services**
23%

V A Hospitals#
5%

Private Mental Hospitals*#
7%

General Hospital Psychiatric Inpatient Units
16%

1955 (1.7 Million Episodes)

* Includes residential treatment centers for emotionally disturbed children

\# Inpatient services only

** Includes free-standing outpatient services as well as those affiliated with psychiatric and general hospitals

*** Includes inpatient and outpatient services of federally funded CMHC's

Source: Mental Health Statistical Note no. 139 (Washington, D.C.: NIMH, 1977), chart 2.

347

TABLE 2   Number and Percent Distribution and Rate per 100,000 Population of Inpatient and Outpatient Care Episodes,[1] in Selected Mental Health Facilities, by Type of Facility: United States, 1955, 1965, 1971 and 1075 (Provisional).

Year	Total all facilities[1]	INPATIENT SERVICES OF:						OUTPATIENT PSYCHIATRIC SERVICES OF:		
		All inpatient services	State & county mental hospitals	Private mental hospitals[2]	Gen. hosp. psychiatric service (non-VA)	VA psychiatric inpatient services	Federally assisted comm.men. health cen.	All outpatient services	Federally assisted comm.men. health cen.	Other
		Number of patient care episodes								
1975	6,409,447	1,791,171	598,993	165,327	565,696	214,264	246,891	4,618,276	1,584,968	3,033,308
1971	4,038,143	1,721,389	745,259	126,600	542,642	176,800	130,088	2,316,754	622,906	1,693,848
1965	2,636,525	1,565,525	804,926	125,428	519,328	115,843	—	1,071,000	—	1,071,000
1955	1,675,352	1,296,352	818,832	123,231	265,934	88,355	—	379,000	—	379,000
		Percent distribution								
1975	100.0	27.9	9.3	2.6	8.8	3.3	3.9	72.1	24.7	47.4
1971	100.0	42.6	18.5	3.1	13.4	4.4	3.2	57.4	15.4	42.0
1965	100.0	59.4	30.5	4.8	19.7	4.4	—	40.6	—	40.6
1955	100.0	77.4	48.9	7.3	15.9	5.3	—	22.6	—	22.6

Rate per 100,000 population

1975	3033	847	283	78	268	101	117	2185	750	1435
1971	1977	843	365	62	266	87	64	1134	305	829
1965	1376	817	420	65	271	60	—	559	—	559
1955	1028	795	502	76	163	54	—	233	—	233

[1] In order to present trends on the same set of facilities over this interval, it has been necessary to exclude from this table the following: private psychiatric office practice; psychiatric service modes of all types in hospitals or outpatient clinics of Federal agencies other than the VA (e.g., Public Health Service, Indian Health Service, Department of Defense Bureau of Prisons, etc.); inpatient service modes of multiservice facilities not shown in this table; all partial care episodes, and outpatient episodes of VA hospitals.

[2] Includes estimates of episodes of care in residential treatment centers for emotionally disturbed children.

Source (All years except 1975): The National Institute of Mental Health, *Utilization of Mental Health Facilities*, 1971, Series B, No. 5, January 1974. Table 22

Source (1975): Unpublished provisional data from the National Institute of Mental Health

Source: *Mental Health Statistical Note no. 139* (Washington, D.C.:1 N.I.M.H., August 1977).

Figure 2   Estimated Percent Distribution of Persons with Mental Disorder, by Treatment Setting, United States, 1975

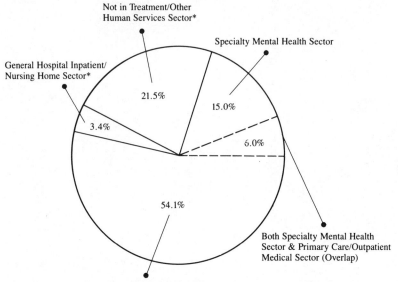

Not in Treatment/Other
Human Services Sector*

Specialty Mental Health Sector

General Hospital Inpatient/
Nursing Home Sector*

21.5%

15.0%

3.4%

5.0%

54.1%

Both Specialty Mental Health
Sector & Primary Care/Outpatient
Medical Sector (Overlap)

Primary Care/Outpatient Medical Sector

Note: Data relating to sectors other than the specialty mental health sector reflect the number of patients with mental disorder seen in those sectors without regard to the amount or adequacy of treatment provided.

*Excludes overlap of an unknown percent of persons also seen in other sectors.

Source: Regier, Goldberg and Taube, ''The De Facto Mental Health Services System,'' *Archives of General Psychiatry,* vol. 35 (June 1978), 690

TABLE 3
Estimated Number and Percent Distribution of Persons With
Mental Disorder, and Percent of Total Population, by Type of
Treatment Setting: United States, 1975

TREATMENT SECTOR AND SETTING	ESTIMATE OF PERSONS WITH MENTAL DISORDER		% of Total US Population
	No.	% of Total	
Total	31,955,000	100	15.0
SPECIALTY MENTAL HEALTH SECTOR			
State and county mental hospitals	789,000		
VA— psychiatric units of general and neuropsychiatric hospitals	351,000		
Private mental hospitals and residential treatment centers	233,000		
Nonfederal general hospitals with psychiatric units	927,000		
Community mental health centers	1,627,000		
Freestanding outpatient and multiservice clinics	1,763,000		
Halfway house for the mentally ill	7,000		
College campus mental health clinics	131,000		
Offfice-based private practice psychiatrists	854,000		
Private practice psychologists	425,000		
Subtotal	7,107,000		
Unduplicated sector total	6,698,000	21.0	3.1
GENERAL HOSPITAL INPATIENT NURSING HOME SECTOR			
General hospital inpatient facilities			
Nonfederal general hospitals without separate psychiatric units	812,000		
Federal general hospitals (excludes psychiatric units of VA hospitals)	59,000		
Nursing homes	207,000		
Nonpsychiatric specialty hospitals	22,000		
Unduplicated sector total	1,100,000	3.4	0.5

PRIMARY CARE/OUTPATIENT MEDICAL SECTOR

Office-based primary care physicians	10,710,000		
Other office-based nonprimary care physicians	2,337,000		
Community (neighborhood health centers)	314,000		
Industrial health facilities	314,000		
Health department clinics	941,000		
General hospital outpatient and emergency rooms	6,391,000		
Subtotal	21,007,000		
Unduplicated sector total	19,218,000	60.1	9.0

UNDUPLICATED SUBTOTAL ACROSS
SPECIALTY MENTAL HEALTH AND

GENERAL MEDICAL SECTORS	25,094,000	78.5	11.8

NOT IN TREATMENT/OTHER HUMAN
SERVICES SECTOR

Unduplicated sector total	6,861,000	21.5	3.2

Source: Darrell A. Regier, Irving D. Goldberg & Carl A. Taube, "The De Facto US Mental Health Services System," *Archives of General Psychiatry,* vol. 35 (June 1978), p. 688. For details of how these numbers were arrived at, see the article.

TABLE 4   Number and percent distribution of positions by status and full-time equivalent positions by discipline, mental health facilities, United States 1976

DISCIPLINE	Total (%)	Full-time (%)	Part-time (%)	Trainee (%)	Full-time equivalent staff (%)
Total all staff	100.0	100.0	100.0	100.0	100.0
Psychiatrists	4.9	1.9	14.5	25.8	3.6
Other physicians	1.1	0.6	3.4	3.3	0.8
Psychologists total	4.3	3.1	7.3	15.1	3.6
Psychologists MA & above	3.7	2.8	6.6	10.4	3.2
Other psychologists	0.6	0.3	0.7	4.7	0.4
Social workers, total	6.5	5.8	7.4	15.6	6.1
Social workers—MSW (or MA) & above	4.7	4.3	6.3	7.7	4.5
Other social workers	1.8	1.5	1.1	7.9	1.6
Registered nurses	9.4	9.0	9.4	15.5	9.3
Licensed practical or vocational nurses	3.4	3.7	2.1	2.1	3.6
Other MH professionals—BA & above (e.g., voc. rehab. counselors, occupational therapists, teachers)	8.3	8.0	9.9	8.5	8.1
Mental health workers (less than BA)	29.0	32.4	16.2	9.3	30.7
Physical health prof. & asst. (e.g., dentists, dental technicians, pharmacists, dieticians, etc.)	2.4	2.2	4.0	1.8	2.3
Total patient care staff	69.3	66.7	74.2	97.0	68.1
Total professional patient care staff	36.9	30.6	55.9	85.7	33.8
Administrative & other prof. (nonhealth) staff (e.g., accountants, business administrators, etc.)	2.7	2.8	3.0	0.5	2.7
All other staff (clerical, maintenance, etc.)	28.0	30.5	22.8	2.5	29.2

Source: Marilyn J. Rosenstein & Carl A. Taube, ''Staffing of Mental Health Facilities, United States, 1976'' (Washington, D.C.: NIMH, 1977), table 1.

TABLE 5   Percent of Psychiatrists by Status and Facility, 1976, U.S.A.*

MENTAL HEALTH FACILITY

	Total (23,390)	Full-time (7,549)	Part-time (9,210)	Residents (6,631)
All Facilities	100.0%	100.0%	100.0%	100.0%
Psychiatric Services in non-federal general hospitals	26.3	14.8	25.0	41.5
State & County Hospitals	21.3	39.5	7.3	20.0
Community Mental Health Centers	16.0	16.3	20.1	9.9
Freestanding Outpatient Clinics	16.0	7.2	27.8	9.7
Private Hospitals	8.2	8.1	7.5	9.3
V.A. Services Units	8.0	10.8	5.8	7.8
Residential Treatment Centers for Children	2.0	0.6	4.2	0.4
Other	2.2	2.7	2.3	1.4

*Adapted from table 4b in Marilyn Rosenstein and Carl A. Taube, "Staffing of Mental Health Facilities, United States, 1976" (Washington D.C.: National Institute of Mental Health Series B, No. 14, 1977).

Thanks to Peter O'Neill.

Appendix II.

Methods

To read the leading journals of sociology today, one would gather that there is no advantage to studying the internal complexities of one situation. Yet among the works that have contributed the most to the discipline and that make up the classic literature in the field, one will find a large number of case studies using participant observation.

Not many sociologists study social life by directly observing it, though observation is the essential technique of scientific inquiry. Most sociologists analyze questions which they ask people, or questions other people have asked, thereby obtaining what is called "hard data," on which they perform statistical operations. The advantages of a good sample are great, but equally great are the dangers of assuming that one's hard data from questionnaires and interviews capture what people do and feel. Usually they contain the indices of the codes of what people say they do, or claim to think about what they do, when responding to a stranger or a sheet of paper. Such were my observations of survey research as I learned it at the University of Chicago. The more adept I became at "manipulating data" (a telling phrase that was frequently used around the National Opinion Research Center) on social phenomena which I had never observed, the more suspicious I became of the artificial quality of the data and its analysis. The typical survey began with a group of experts in a room figuring out what ques-

355

tions to ask a sample of people they did not know and second-guessing what answers they would give. The product was "field tested," largely for technical matters such as whether the questions or instructions to the interviewer were clear, whether the ordering of questions worked smoothly, and whether the categories of answers were usable. Much later in the analysis, survey projects which did not turn up tables with significant differences would fish for them, ordering hundreds of tables to inspect. I knew that survey research need not be done this way, but this was the way some of the best people in the country were doing it.

Martin Trow once cogently argued that "the problem under investigation properly dictates the methods of investigation."[1] This is not what was happening at the University of Chicago, where the survey method was used almost exclusively for an extraordinarily wide range of problems. Personally, I began by wishing to learn other methods, and to explore close up the problems of information loss, so apparent in questionnaire data, by doing a field study. Thus I sought a sociological problem that would justify the method so I could expand my understanding of sociological research. The initiation of residents into psychiatry seemed admirably suited.

Field studies are usually considered as preliminary to large-sample, systematic studies which can test their findings. They are seen as exploratory, unsystematic and seriously limited by the small range of cases that any one field worker can encompass. This argument assumes that sociology is a cumulative science, which is not usually the case. It also assumes that at no time would the method of investigation for a problem be participant-observation. Martin Trow, for example, did not indicate what kinds of problems might dictate participant observation above all other methods. But in a major essay, Robert Weiss distinguished between problems calling for analytic methods and those calling for holistic methods.[2] Analytic methods lend themselves to examining properties of objects and relations between properties, while holistic methods lend themselves to studying complex situations with simultaneously interrelated activities.

> In the analytic approach the investigator . . . takes as his task the isolating of elements from each other, or, perhaps, the identification of a small number of linked relationships.
> In the holistic approach the investigator sees a complex situation as containing within itself, perhaps hidden from view by the action of extraneous variables, a system of interrelated elements constituting its un-

derlying structure, in terms of which the phenomena of the situation are to be understood. He is concerned with identifying the nature of the system rather than with focusing on particular independent-dependent variables relations. . . . His chief interest might be phrased as, "Taking it all together, how does the whole thing work?"[3]

This argument is important for field studies, because Weiss shows how their goals and data are different from, rather than preliminary to, analytic methods like survey research. The argument is particularly relevant to my study of psychiatric residency, because it clarifies why previous efforts to study psychiatric socialization through analytic methods of scaling isolated elements had failed.[4] A talented team had studied the residency at the University Psychiatric Center this way without much success, except for one seminal paper, and that paper was based on participant observation. Finally, Weiss and others clarify why studies using participant observation have contributed disporportionately to the theory and substance of sociology. In struggling to understand the structure of complex situations, investigators have made basic contributions in areas ranging from large organizations to interpersonal encounters.

Field studies usually employ a number of methods—techniques for observing, interviewing informants, analyzing documents, interviewing respondents, and varieties of participation.[5] Of particular importance is observation, not only for its own sake, but also for providing a basis on which to test the validity of information from interviews and documents.[6] Systematic comparisons between events people experience and their recollections of them indicate that people's account of them is markedly unreliable.[7] This advantage is particularly important in a study of self-transformation during which the individuals in the program alter their language and perceptual framework. Observation of events as they occur is more precise and more reliable than any other technique.

The importance of time in a study of training adds weight to the value of observation, because an observer can more accurately order the sequence of events than can an interviewer. The interconnections between multiple events and dimensions of a complex setting are observed more quickly and more accurately than by trying to reconstruct them through interviews. On the other hand, learning how participants reconstruct events can tell one much about their world view; but to properly assess them one needs independent observations as well.

Certain kinds of behavior are most readily documented through observation. These include social interaction among people being studied, comparing attitudes against what people do, nonverbal behavior, natural language behavior, crowd behavior, collective crises, and ecological settings.

Observation has various sources of error. One is the distorting effect of people knowing they are being observed. This can be minimized by making the act of observing less intrusive. Most important in a study of any length is the obverse; one is so fully integrated as the observer that people go about their business in full view of the observer. It is important not to assume that awareness of being observed necessarily leads people to change their ways. Equally important, most people, particularly in complex settings, cannot change things very much even if they wish to. Habits, structural constraints, rules, language, and personality are all well-established; so the degree of distortion possible may be quite low. A serious source of error is sampling bias, either at the level of studying a unique case but considering it representative, or at the level of observing only certain aspects of the complex setting. One must look out for these problems, compare one's data with data from other cases, and critically examine how one's role keeps one from observing certain kinds of events.

The actual process by which one can discover the interrelated elements of a complex situation is described by Glaser and Strauss in a book which crystalized the way many good participant-observers carry out their work.[8] It also describes the procedures of this study, to develop theory grounded in the data through an ongoing process of hypothesis formation, data collection to test it, refinement of the hypothesis, and further collection of data. I used the constant comparative method, wherein one is constantly comparing present to past incidents that illustrate a particular pattern of behavior as a way to substantiate it and/or refine it. Within the residency program, I increasingly used theoretical samples, as I moved from open observing and listening to more focused observing and interviewing. I would choose residents and activities that promised to maximize differences between groups, particularly between cohorts, because time was a central variable in this study of socialization. Observation, coding, and analyzing went on simultaneously, and I spent several hours each week thinking about patterns in the data. From this process emerged many of the concepts and typologies in the study, such as the four systems of diagnosis, the types of case conferences, the basic dimensions of socialization, and the structural features underlying the socialization process. At the same time, I wanted to build on previous grounded theory by testing it with new data and developing it further. For example, Goffman's concept of a moral career emerged from his observations of mental patients but did not have well-developed conceptual stages. The stages in that chapter fit both his data and mine. Renée Fox, whose ideas about uncertainty grew out of student diaries and her own observations, stimulated me to extend her analysis through residency. This was an example of theory developed after leaving the field and reviewing data which I did not fully understand at the time. One of the advantages of participant-observation is that data are collected on many more aspects of the project than preconceived notions would dictate, and some of this material later contributes new insights. Finally, Sharaf and Levinson's theory of the quest for omnipotence was grounded in their field research and developed further here. On the other hand, much of the theory of "adult socialization" is not grounded theory, and as I indicated by my analysis of it, much of it is unrealistic.

The limitations of a case study and of participant-observation, then, were compensated in a number of ways. In data collection and analysis, the constant comparative method and theoretical sampling were used to seek out negative cases, a stringent criterion for testing ideas. Studies of other programs were used extensively to gain a larger, comparative perspective on this one case. Validity was also gained by the fact that one can interpret particular data with full knowledge of its context and the persons involved, an advantage usually impossible to gain through interviews or questionnaries. One also saw the same people over time in a variety of situations, greatly decreasing the possibility that they could mislead or that one could interview a biased sample of subjects.[9] Both their biases and one's own become known. One comes to realize that although the data collected in participant observation are much "harder" than in questionnaire or interview, one is always interpreting most survey data because they more precisely measure actual human behavior and social action. It is important to realize that most of the "problems" which occupy the literature on participant observation—observer bias, comprehensive note taking, forms of distortion, and the like—do not even come up or are glossed over in other forms of social research.

In this study, the method was to listen, watch, feel, get into every corner and odd moment of residency culture, to interview, to collect and examine documents, to raise skeptical questions, to sympathize, and finally to develop theories about what was happening which one tested, retested, revised and tested again in a continuing dialogue between theory and the people being studied. Understanding socialization is the study of meaning, and that meaning is shared. The idea that meaning is private has been thoroughly attacked by Wittgenstein and the language philosophers, though psychiatry itself is still unclear on the matter. Psychiatrists base their work on the assumption that personal miseries have understandable meanings which they are experts at deciphering: yet psychiatrists resist applying this to themselves. They feel their own experience is just as private as does anyone else who has not thought carefully about the matter. Thus one finds psychiatrists surprisingly obtuse at times about the psychological dynamics of what they are doing or what is happening right in front of them, as we have seen in these pages. This seems to stem from learning to think in psychiatric terms as if they were private, when by definition they are cultural and therefore public. There appears to be a trained incapacity to perceive cultural and social dimensions. Most studies offer one interpretation, giving one meaning to what they find as if it were the whole truth. Often their theoretical premise is that true meaning can be found exclusively in functionalism, symbolic interaction, or conflict. But the significance of acts cannot be found in any one of these alone. One needs thick description and thick interpretation. Therefore the experience of becoming a psychiatrist has been analyzed from several points of view, each interpretation putting events and feelings in a somewhat different light. These chapters have argued that the concept of moral career illuminates some aspects of becoming a professional, certain structural features of residency training shape the personal experiences of residency training, uncertainty and its control is a valuable theme for interpreting professional education, and omnipotence is a danger built into the structure of professional training. None of these provides *the* theory of professional socialization, but each makes its own contribution and enhances the others. It is important that these explanations arise not from abstract chains of propositions but from a dialogue with long-term, fine-combed observation of social life. Thus the ultimate object of the study is not the residency, not this case, but the interaction of certain structures with the people who find meaning in them. "Our double task," as Clifford Geertz has put it, "is to uncover

the conceptual structures that inform our subjects' acts, the 'said' of
social discourse, and to construct a system of analysis in whose terms
what is generic to those structures, what belongs to them because they
are what they are, will stand out against the other determinants of
human behavior.''[10]

This study began when I was at the University of Chicago and met
a person knowledgeable in both survey research and participant observation who was willing to talk about how a researcher could best capture social reality. Larry Rosenberg had been hired as Chicago's token
field worker, but soon found the position untenable. He and I were
both seeking the old Chicago School of Sociology that had produced so
many insightful monographs of social observation. Before coming to
Chicago, Larry had applied to study psychiatric residents at the University Psychiatric Center. The project had been cleared by the Committee on Research at the medical school before Larry had been invited
to join the faculty at Chicago. He invited me to work with him on the
project, which seemed ideal for my purposes. Not only did the delicate, complex nature of the subject call for participant-observation, but
the subject of psychiatry interested me personally. However, Larry's
interests turned elsewhere, and I found myself in charge of the project
rather than assisting in it. Organizationally, the project fell under an
experienced and wise researcher who directed an institute at University
Psychiatric Center. All of these formal circumstances were most fortunate, because they gave me access to the entire training program with
official approval from the highest sources; so that later, when some
junior staff wanted to check me out, they found I was properly cleared
for the intimate settings in which I worked.

The research director gave me perspective when I most needed it
and steered me from a number of pitfalls. Yet he hardly interfered at
all, believing that young researchers grow most in freedom. He provided me with an office and typewriter, a place to assemble data and to
retreat. We debated on whether my office should be in the main hospital, where residents work, or in his adjacent building. If the office were
in the hospital, residents might drop by and it might become a hangout;
on the other hand, he suggested I might want to get away from my field
of observation to write and think. My intuition chose the latter argument. Already I had begun to define my role as participant-observer.

The chain of introduction is important in field work, and mine
began again with the research director. In June, at the end of a resident

year, he introduced me to the new chief on the service where he taught. Clearly he and the chief, Adam Cohn, had talked about my project beforehand, and it probably helped greatly that the research director was admired for his rounds; even with his help, Dr. Cohn treated me with extreme caution and circumspection. Dr. Cohn and I agreed that I could watch what I wanted of a public nature on the ward. As for other activities, such as supervision, it would be up to the residents to decide. This was his general, democratic rule, which worked to great advantage in time. I asked about the residents' Saturday morning Feelings Meeting, which I had heard from older residents was the most important meeting of the first year. Dr. Cohn doubted I could attend. His feelings at this time were easily understood: he was a new chief and he did not want any trouble. In particular, the Saturday meeting was his time to be with his residents. It was precious, and he did not want to tamper with it. At this moment and at other such moments of entry throughout the year, I did something I found invaluable: I deflected the issue, postponing the decision with a "Well, we can talk about that later."

On the ward during the first day, Dr. Cohn introduced me to one or two residents as the occasion arose, but to no one else. The introductions had ended. I was on my own.

The short chain of introductions and the vagueness of domain contributed immensely to the thoroughness of this study; for it allowed me to enter many more settings than an administrator would have allowed at the outset. This is especially true for an intimate profession such as psychiatry. Other investigators have negotiated domain of entry with a director prior to entering the field and have been closed off from what the residents regard as the most important experience. In this study, the senior men essentially said, "Go where you will, so long as you do not interfere, or act unbecomingly." Therefore, the rest of the field work developed informally. For example, on the first day a resident I met offered to show me around. He asked if I had seen supervision. I said I had not. "Well, I've got a supervision in an hour. Why don't you come along?"

As residents began to show me around and bring me into their work, I established precedents which I used in more touchy situations.[11] The most important example was that the old first-year residents in June let me into their Saturday meeting. By July, when the new group came, I was part of the Saturday meeting in Dr. Cohn's mind, and he comfortably said to them, "Don's been sitting in on these meetings, and if you don't object, he'll stay with us."

As I look back, the most important decision made was to begin in June *before* the new group of residents arrived. Originally, the decision was made off-hand. "Why don't you come for a few weeks in June to get a feel for the place?" the research director had suggested. Many other factors made the early start important. In June, the chief is new and nervous; the residents are finishing and feel relaxed. The residents were generous, expansive hosts, telling me what I should look for in the first year, giving their insights as they themselves were reflecting about the year gone by, introducing me to the program. This made the chief more relaxed about me, and in that time he got to know me. (We met every week, at least, and at this time I sought his counsel and shared my problems.) The chief, on the other hand, did not care too much about these old residents; they were not his. He did not worry, for example, about my being at the Saturday meetings of the old residents; the "real" meetings would begin in July. By July, however, he felt comfortable with me. Beginning in June, he also familiarized me with the routine, and when the new residents arrived, I could be helpful in little ways that mollified their extreme nervousness and defensive guard at the start.

Beginning in June also meant I got to know the people who were about to be second-year residents at their most relaxed and confident period. Knowing them allowed me to enter second-year settings easily. Through the chiefs, like Adam Cohn, I got to know third-year residents.

The informal style of entering a highly structured community worked well, because I liked most of the residents, and I think almost all of them found me tolerable to be with, or even enjoyable.[12] A few objected to my role. One said, "I like to talk to you, but you are objectifying us and this is immoral."[13] (As if he were not learning to do the same to patients!) In background, it probably helped that I was like them in many ways. I was about the same age (twenty-six) and had an equal education. I could talk to any resident about almost any topic that might come up, except medical technology. I dressed the same way that they did, in suits or dark slacks with conservative sports jackets. The range of resident dress is very narrow.[14] The residents were entering a professional milieu in which I had been raised. If anything distinguished me, it was my Yankee appearance, but this never seemed to interfere with relations except with one of the few *non*-Jewish residents in the program. From the first we had a hard time talking. To me he seemed a Western caricature of a Yankee, taciturn, formal in the most informal settings, socially so overcorrect as to be incorrect, placid, professionally principled. Many members of the staff found him inaccessible and coldly unresponsive when they needed emotional support. He remained so much this way that to this day we have never discussed our relationship. Nevertheless, I suspect he felt some WASP competition, and I think his ambition-driven awareness of status marked me as irrelevant. His superiors found him more accessible.

Compared to the description by Stanton and Schwartz of the first many months of field work, I experienced very little resistance.[15] To the patients, my presence was, I believe, never an issue. Had it been, I am sure the residents or chief would have told me. I became friends with a number of patients, especially those whose progress I was following along with that of their residents. Rarely did patients make me feel uneasy, including my friend Joe the murderer. I had no connection with the hospital and no activities in it, a distinct advantage, I think. Therefore, issues of spying did not arise. Tension and suspicion might have been greater had I imposed myself, but even at the beginning there was enough to do so that I was content to wait for a self-conscious resident to relax, before asking him about something close to his work. Nevertheless, with some residents a personal rapport would grow, only to have sudden reversals come when they became self-conscious.

More profound is the problem of closely examining the practices of friends.[16] The residents who knew my role clearly and accepted me in it, such as Adam, Ned, and Jeff, were most comfortable. Reversals came from residents who tried to separate me from my being an observer, like Carl. Marc saw my role clearly and rejected it, feeling that it is immoral to observe other human beings and to implicitly objectify them. At the other extreme were residents who so much saw me as a friend that it became uncomfortable to be an observer. Friendship can sometimes be a way of covering up the observer-observed relationship.

Most important for field work is that the person feel relaxed and enjoy his work. I found my work fascinating and enjoyable, more so than I expected. The routine required that I get up about 6:30 A.M., and sometimes I truly hated the project by the time I had arrived at the hospital. But after ten minutes on a ward, I found myself relaxed and eager to do more.[17]

Observation basically took place in three settings, meetings of various sizes, interviews, and just hanging around.[18] Few descriptions of field work describe the crucial aspect of note taking; so I shall try to give a full portrait of how this was done. Morris and Charlotte Schwartz have given us a fine description of the mental intricacies that go into registering, interpreting and recording an event.[19] Because of the complexities and dangers of distortion involved in observation, I tried increasingly to jot down notes as close to the event as possible. One should realize that here we are talking about problems of precision and refinement that do not even arise in the much coarser techniques of sociology, such as survey research.

At a meeting I would always take notes throughout the occasion on a three-by-five-inch pad of plain white paper which I carried in my jacket pocket. In general, I would find a back chair, preferably with others sitting in front of me. My rule was that while others knew I took notes and while I did not hide that fact, I took them as inconspicuously as possible, so that no one would feel embarrassed or self-conscious.[20] At meetings with only residents, I would sit with them, and since they could see me writing, I learned a number of leg positions which made it least apparent that I was writing, like crossing my leg at the ankle and writing on the uncrossed leg. As measured by the paucity of questions and glances from residents, these practices worked very well.

The most difficult meeting for note taking was the Saturday Feeling Meeting. For a few months, I never took notes in the meeting. It is considered so special, and note taking would be so obvious with only eight men in a horseshoe, that I did not try. One day I began writing and no one seemed to notice. What drove me to take notes was a desire for details of the conversations, which were so rich and were a microcosm of the residency experience. Several months later, off-hand remarks were made about my note taking on Saturday. One resident said something emphatic, adding, "Be sure to get that in your notes." I smiled and nodded.

At the beginning of field work, Adam Cohn urged me to speak up at meetings. He seemed more nervous at the idea of a silent observer than a participating one. During June I did speak and even asked questions of the guest psychiatrist at case conferences. This also made me more comfortable. By July, I spoke very little publicly. However, when directly addressed I did not pretend to be dumb.

After an interview, lunch, or a meeting where no notes were taken, I would immediately disappear and jot down key words, quotes and passages, enough to bring back to memory the order of events, the different levels of response to an event, and other dimensions of what happened. These I would write in a dozen corners of the hospital, empty offices, toilets, over in the research building. I learned, as most field workers do, to memorize whole conversations, sequences of topics, nonverbal aspects, and the like. One problem with taking notes during an event is that one misses the action as one looks at the note pad. This dilemma—to look or to write—is partially solved by learning to write without looking.

From these notes and recent memory, I typed my field notes in an office located across the street from the hospital within hours of taking them. They were typed in triplicate, because Erving Goffman, on a visit, said I would want to cut up one or two sets into categories and would want one set intact and choronological. I also left a large left margin and no right margin, one large margin being more practical for cross-referencing, indexing, and other uses.

The notes, single-spaced, had two parts, those in parentheses and those out of parentheses. As Morris and Charlotte Schwartz indicate, the field worker constantly evaluates what he observes. I would describe the event or conversation as it occurred from the point of view of the actors or from a flat descriptive point of view, with my own responses, reactions, evaluations, and biases in parentheses. In retrospect, I find this method admirable, because it retains the flavor of the event and also the flavor of my experience, keeping them as separate as possible.[21] One advantage is that this method of noting makes one immediately and continuously self-conscious of one's biases. For example, I found that I would judge what the residents did or failed to do, competing with them in my notes even if I did not in the field. A second advantage is that I captured many valuable insights or analytic thoughts I had after some occasions which otherwise might have been lost. Most field workers I know take straight notes instead and then later pull together related ideas about some part of their work in a separate set of reflective notes. This method implies that the ''straight'' notes lack bias, and if they have bias it is so intermingled that it cannot be later separated. It also assumes that the field worker will retain a string of related insights in his head until he puts them down. I would imagine that some of the pearls fall off the string.

A full day of work would begin with the morning report of 8:30 A.M., continue with the morning's case conference, followed by lunch with some residents. The afternoon would hold one seminar and a supervision, plus informal visits with patients, nurses, or others. Such a day would produce about twenty pages of scratch notes on my little pad, which would in turn produce about ten to fifteen typed pages of final notes.[22] That is a *long* day.

The typing took a long time, several hours. Almost every day I typed the day's notes on that day; one has to be religious. Many asked me if I did not tire of typing; usually I did not, because of the satisfaction of seeing the day finally portrayed. One must enjoy the doing of one's craft.

Some field workers talk into a tape recorder after some period of observation. Given that those words will in the end be typed, the tape recorder does not allow for the subtleties of asides, dashes, and parentheses which typing allows. Since speaking is less disciplined and careful as communication, one's personality is more likely to enter the material in an unexamined way. Also, I find that if I am trying to remember ten items (try it), I am more likely to succeed if I write them down as I recall them than if I have to retain in my head the previous eight as I am trying to recall the ninth. It is hard to imagine that one would not forget more when using a tape recorder. Another part of this difficulty is that if one has an outline such as my scratch notes provided, one can fully immerse oneself in one event, portraying all its refinements and at the same time forgetting all else that happened, because one can return both to the next scratch notes and to what one has already written before writing further.

Returning to the observations themselves, I set for myself a quite narrow range of hospital life, the experiences of the psychiatric residents. I learned about other aspects of the hospital through them. Even so, there are areas which I did not cover, and this study omits many activities which I did study in detail. A notable example of the former is electroshock therapy. Very early I knew that pairs of residents were assigned to help the neurologist perform electro-shock therapy (EST) before morning report throughout the year, but I did not attend. Some of the residents close to me had duty, but they did not mention it, and almost no references were made at any time by any residents about their experiences when on EST duty. A few times in the year a resident might allude to it. "Come over tonight." "No, I've got to get up early for EST," followed by more talk. Larry Rosenberg, who read my field notes, noticed that I had not attended EST and asked me if I too were "ignoring" it. I replied that getting up at 6:30 was early enough, or some other partial excuse. For three months he kept nudging me.

One day I rose early and arrived in time for EST. I had made precautionary arrangements, which I always did when I entered a new setting, calling the neurologist and residents on duty to ask if I could come. Three patients, two of whom I knew through residents, stumbled in bleary from sleep, lay down on three fresh beds with wheels, received shots to put them to sleep and relax their muscles in order to reduce danger from the spasms, and were rolled one by one to the EST machine. Briefly, I stood to the side and the residents hovered near the neurologist, the job being so simple that no more than two could do it. He explained every step, calmly and clearly. Conductive grease was applied to spots about the temples on the skull over each eye, the two electric nodes were pressed and held on the spots, and the machine was turned on. Nothing really happened. The machine made no sound; the neurologist continued without interruption, now explaining the size and frequency of the shocks, now pointing to the very slight twitches of the fingers and toes. All else was still. I felt faint. Colored dots danced before my eyes and the patient on the bed swayed gently like a Chagall lover, floating in colors. The nurse, a friend, asked, "Are you all right?" I said I was and stood my ground, but she knew better, suggesting I sit on a low stool nearby. I did. The neurologist included me in his commentary, saying that sometimes that happens to people new to EST. The residents smiled sympathetically. It all passed in a minute or two.

Given that I have never fainted, and have felt faint only a few times in my life, I was surprised by my strong reaction. Emotionally or viscerally I felt very little. What sticks in my mind are those twitching fingers and toes. I do not know if I would have reacted so strongly to a fully convulsing body without the relaxant, but I think I was overwhelmed by the antiseptic quality. There stood the nurse and residents, crisply dressed and still; the little machine was silent; the neurologist quietly described for the thousandth time what was happening. Then those twitches began, belying the tranquility and limp body which was filled with what I imagined to be a roaring, pulsating current.

I did not return. The experience led me to actively ask residents how they felt when they had been on EST duty. My hypothesis was that more were perturbed than let on, because it is unmanly and unprofessional to feel upset. If, however, I could coax them into the open by sharing my own experience, they might be more frank. Despite these efforts, few residents would say more than a few sentences. They usually replied, ''I was bothered a little at first, but you get used to it.'' About a third said it was a repulsive business. At the end of the year, the neurologist said he would no longer continue administering EST, in part, he said, because it was distasteful.

The year of field work divided into several parts. The first, pre-July period has been described. During the next, summer period, I worked six days a week and got to know the new residents. When school began in the fall, my routine changed to Monday, Wednesday, Friday, and Saturday morning, still, I thought, a heavy schedule. Within a week, residents began to ask, ''Where have you been?'' And Adam said, ''We miss you.''

Loosening old bonds and founding new ones required the greatest delicacy. When, in the winter, I decided to move to another service to test some hypotheses generated on the first one, I found the human adjustments infinitely complex. To come on to another ward, even when I knew all its residents, created great anxiety for the chief and superchief. They examined me in great and hostile detail, checked out my credentials, and finally gave approval. Why? I had visited the service often. In part, I broke my rule of informal entry and asked the chief if I could work consistently on the ward. In part the service was self-conscious about being judged because it was in trouble. But part of the problem was that I did not fit organically. If a student nurse comes for a few months of practice in the middle of the year, everyone knows how to handle her and how to regard her. She has access to some of the culture, but not to the intimate parts. No one will invest in her heavily, except perhaps some patients. I, on the other hand, wanted acceptance without having been part of the ward culture. The chief, superchief, and older nurses felt this most acutely; most of the residents did not seem bothered by my arrival one way or the other.

The other half of this story is that as soon as I changed services, the residents on the first service thought I had disappeared completely. Although I was around the building all the time, they asked if I had left the hospital. This illustrated to me the extreme insularity of the wards and of the residents' lives, despite the smallness of the building. Even chiefs, I learned, who met daily to discuss (among other things) problems and who met weekly for a bull session, did not know how the others had solved problems they all faced.

Relations with the people one is studying are the most complex and challenging part of participant-observation. Other field workers emphasize the importance of how one defines one's role. When asked, I explained that I wanted to learn how psychiatrists are trained. This definition justified my being just about anywhere, and it was a subject of personal interest to most of the residents as well. Further into the year, residents would ask me what I had found, and I would tell them something they had recently said or heard themselves. Since I got to know some of their patients well, they would also ask me about what was "really" happening with their patients, and I would point out that I held patients' conversations in confidence, just as I held theirs. My goal was to be the confidential stranger that Georg Simmel had described. Boundary issues arose in a number of dramatic ways—in coping with homosexual advances, in feigning schizophrenia on a dare and being taken seriously (that was foolish), in handling pressures from residents or patients to act as a go-between, and in deciding once to secretly alter a patient's treatment because the patient's life was at stake—stories that will have to await another occasion.

In all these episodes and other experiences parallels arose between field work and psychotherapy. As the residents were struggling with the moral dilemmas of how much to intervene in a patient's life or how to strike the balance of detached concern with a manipulating patient, so I was learning similar lessons. The tension between intimacy and impartiality is as great for psychiatric residents as it is for the participant-observer. In both lines of work, learning how to use one's own feelings as indicators of what is happening plays a central role.[23] At certain times, when I noticed work was dull, I suddenly realized that the residents were finding their work tedious. The field work literature correctly talks of empathy: "He takes the role of all the other people in the situation and tries to evoke in himself the feelings and thoughts and actions they experience at the time the event occurred."[24] The challenge is the same for residents. Field workers advise colleagues to contend with their feelings as part of the data. Residents are constantly told about countertransference. Thus the methodological concerns of the investigator ultimately resonate with the substantive concerns of those being investigated.

Appendix III ∎

The Problem of
Typing Residents by
Ideology

The first serious effort to differentiate between types of psychiatric residents was done by Myron Sharaf and Daniel Levinson in 1957.[1] They devised a bipolar attitude scale of Psycho-Sociotherapeutic Ideology consisting of specific items which measured the extent to which a resident was psychoanalytically oriented and the extent to which he favored more social approaches, such as group therapy, use of a therapeutic team, structuring the patients' milieu, and the like. Items also probed for the residents' inclination toward somatic types of therapies.

Several years later, Strauss and his colleagues[2] pointed out that the PSI Scale *assumes* the sociotherapeutic orientation to be the opposite of the psychoanalytic one, and that it *assumes* an orientation toward somatic therapies to be part of the sociotherapeutic perspective. To test these assumptions, they designed three separate scales and found a) that the first two orientations are not opposites but quite independent, and b) that a somatic ideology correlates negatively with psychoanalytic beliefs and is independent of a sociotherapeutic orientation. One might summarize these results by saying that the psychoanalytic and somatic ideologies are opposites along a psychological-physiological axis, and that the sociotherapeutic ideology is independent of the other two. However, there was a flaw: the sociotherapeutic ideology was not clearly formed in respondents who leaned in this direction, and so this important type was not well defined.

The political character of this approach to classifying residents is not hard to detect. The three ideologies reflect factions in the profession as a whole, not in new residents, who generally have only vague ideas about psychiatry.[3] *This approach of trying to create scales which slice up the resident's reality according to the ideologies of the day appears to be the central flaw in efforts so far to find out what kinds of residents enter psychiatry.* For these are not *their* terms but perspectives brought to them by the researcher. Thus we should not be surprised that neither effort at ideological scaling produced clear results.[4]

The very construction of these scales for distinguishing between types of residents also highlights the dangers of being taken in by the profession's ideologies. A good example is Strauss's point that Sharaf and Levinson's PSI Scale assumes the sociotherapeutic outlook to be opposite to the psychoanalytic one. So far as we know, this was the view which prevailed among the heavily psychoanalytic staff at University Psychiatric Center, where Sharaf and Levinson tested their scale. Moreover, the sociotherapeutic end of their scale was a catch-all for anyone *not* strongly committed to psychoanalysis.[5] Without realizing it, perhaps, they constructed an instrument which reflected the strong psychoanalytic orientation of the residency where they worked.

Strauss and his colleagues ran into the same problem, suggesting another pattern of interest—neither team in the late 1950s and early 1960s could find a clear pattern of the social approach to psychiatry. In sampling both an elite and a state hospital (where staff with a social approach was expected to be found), the Strauss group turned up so few people with either a sociotherapeutic or a somatic viewpoint that they had to draw special, biased samples just to test their instruments. This probably reflects the extent to which the psychoanalytic view held sway throughout psychiatry after World War II. Even people using shock therapy and caring for hundreds of patients at a state mental hospital believed in psychoanalytic values and psychotherapeutic approaches. At the same time, psychoanalytic principles became so diffuse (as do the core principles of any group that acquires a wide following) that greatly divergent practices became legitimated in psychoanalytic terms. One might say that psychoanalysis had become, as in *The Structure of Scientific Revolutions,*[6] the new paradigm of psychiatry. Today it is yielding to a chemical, physiological paradigm.

To summarize, the ideological scales used to characterize residents were a researcher's artifact that did not reflect residents' views. Moreover, the effect of such views on practice are not clear. For these reasons, I decided to observe how residents worked with patients and identify different work styles among them, as described on pages 52 to 56.

Notes

Preface

1. A. Strauss, L. Schatzman, R. Bucher, et al.: *Psychiatric Ideologies and Institutions* (Glencoe, Ill.: Free Press, 1964), chap. 4.
2. Ibid.

1. The Psychiatric Domain

1. Leonard Schatzman and Anselm Strauss, "A Sociology of Psychiatry: A Perspective and Some Organizing Foci," pp. 128–44 (esp. p. 129), in Eliot Freidson and Judith Lorber, eds., *Medical Men and Their Work* (New York: Aldine/Atherton, 1972). See also Park Elliott Dietz, "Social Discrediting of Psychiatry: The Protasis of Legal Disenfranchisement," *American Journal of Psychiatry* 143:12 (December 1977), 1356–60.
2. Thomas S. Szasz, *The Myth of Mental Illness* (New York: Harper & Row, 1961).
3. Andrew T. Scull, *Museums of Madness: The Social Origins of Insanity in Nineteenth-Century England* (London: Allan Lane, 1979), chap. 2.
4. Ibid., chaps. 3–4.
5. Gerald N. Grob, *Mental Institutions in America* (New York: Free Press, 1973), p. 132.
6. Ibid., chap. 4 (esp. p. 158).
7. Ibid., p. 141.
8. Ibid., p. 219, and more generally chap. 5.
9. G. Tourney, "Psychiatric Therapies: 1800–1968," in T. Rothman, ed., *Changing Patterns of Psychiatric Care* (New York: Crown, 1970).

375

10. This argument is based on Peter L. Berger, "Towards A Sociological Understanding of Psychoanalysis," *Social Research*, vol. 32 (Spring 1965), 26–41.

11. See *The Nation's Psychiatrists*, National Institute of Mental Health Publication No. 1855, 1969.

12. This paragraph is based on *The Nation's Psychiatrists* and on Arnold A. Rogow, *The Psychiatrists* (New York: Putnam, 1970).

13. Rogow, *The Psychiatrists*, p. 187.

14. Leo Srole, "Measurement and Classification in Socio-Psychiatric Epidemiology: Midtown Manhattan Study (1954) and Midtown Manhattan Restudy (1974)," *Journal of Health and Social Behavior*, vol. 16, no. 4 (December 1975), 347–64 (esp. 350–53). See also Bruce P. Dohrenwend, "Sociocultural and Social-Psychological Factors in the Genesis of Mental Disorders," *Journal of Health and Social Behavior*, vol. 16, no. 4 (December 1975), 365–92 (esp. 368).

15. Robert A. Scott, *The Making of Blind Men* (New York: The Russell Sage Foundation, 1969).

16. Dohrenwend, "Sociocultural Factors," p. 367.

17. See Daniel S. Levine and Dianne R. Levine, *The Cost of Mental Illness—1971* (Washington, D.C.: DHEW Publication No. [ADM] 76–265, 1975); Ronald W. Conley et al., "The Cost of Mental Illness, 1968," *Statistical Note 30* (Survey and Reports Section, Biometry Branch, N.I.M.H., 1970); and Daniel Levine and Shirley G. Willner, "The Cost of Mental Illness, 1974," *Mental Health Statistical Note No. 125* (Washington, D.C.: DHEW Publication No. [ADM] 76–158, 1976).

18. Ellen L. Bassuk and Samuel Gerson, "Deinstitutionalization and Mental Health Services," *Scientific American*, vol. 238, no. 2 (February 1978), 46–53 (esp. 51).

19. *Provisional Data on Federally Funded Community Mental Health Centers, 1975–76* (Washington, D.C.: N.I.M.H., April 1977), table 9.

20. Philip Berger, Beatrix Hamburg and David Hamburg, "Mental Health: Progress and Problems," in *Doing Better and Feeling Worse: Health in the United States* (*Daedalus*, Winter 1977), p. 261.

21. Andrew Scull, *Decarceration* (Englewood Cliffs, N.J.: Prentice-Hall, 1976). See also tables in *Task Panel Reports Submitted to the President's Commission on Mental Health, 1978* (Washington, D.C.: Government Printing Office). For example, table 3 on page 94 shows that the decline in patient population for state and county was very gradual from 1955 to 1965. Meanwhile, admissions to these hospitals rose rapidly after 1956. Table 6 on page 97 shows that first admissions did not decrease until after 1969, fourteen years after the first drugs were widely used.

22. *Task Panel Reports*, p. 362.

23. See Scull, *Decarceration*.

24. Earl S. Pollack, "Length of Stay in State and County Psychiatric Hospitals During 1975," *Memorandum*, August 26, 1977 (Washington, D.C.: N.I.M.H.). This figure is falling steadily; in 1972 it was forty-four days.

25. N.I.M.H., *Provisional Data on Federally Funded Mental Health Centers, 1976–1977*, Division of Biometry, May 1978. Also, N.I.M.H., *Community Mental Health Centers*, no date (1978?), typed.

26. Darrell A. Regier, Irving D. Goldberg, and Carl A. Taube, "The De Facto

Mental Health Services System," *Archives of General Psychiatry* 35 (June 1978), 685–93.

27. National Institute of Mental Health Work Group on National Health Insurance, *Draft Report: The Financing, Utilization and Quality of Mental Health Care in the United States, April 1976* (Washington, D.C.: Office of Program Development and Analysis, 1976), mimeographed, 27–28. See also the provocative article by Steven Sharfstein and Irving D. Goldberg, "Private Psychiatry and Accountability: A Response to the APA Task Force Report on Private Practice," *American Journal of Psychiatry* 132:1 (January 1975), 43–47.

28. Donald G. Langsley, "Psychiatric and Mental Health Manpower," report on a survey to the Task Panel on Manpower for the American Psychiatric Association (December 1977), p. i. Unless otherwise noted, this overview comes from Langsley.

29. Ibid.

30. See *Draft Report,* pp. 39–43. See also *The Nation's Psychiatrists.* On the similarity between therapists and their patients, see W. E. Henry, John H. Sims, and S. Lee Spray, *Public & Private Lives of Psychotherapists,* (San Francisco: Jossey-Bass, 1973), chap. 4.

31. Rogow, *The Psychiatrists,* chaps. 1, 5, 6. Politically liberal academicians are the same. See my monograph with Lorna Marsden and Tom Corl, *The Impact of the Academic Revolution or Faculty Careers* (Washington, D.C.: American Association for Higher Education, 1972).

32. Table 5 in Harold M. Visotsky, Everett C. Simmons, and Carol Nadelson, "The Development and Assessment of Faculty," pp. 75–113 of the Conference on Education of Psychiatrists, *Report of Commission IV* (Washington, D.C.: The American Psychiatric Association), mimeographed, no date, about 1976.

33. See E. M. Lemert, *Human Deviance, Social Problems and Social Control* (Englewood Cliffs, N.J.: Prentice-Hall, 1967) and Edwin Shur, *Labeling Deviant Behavior: Its Sociological Implications* (New York: Harper & Row, 1971).

34. See Thomas J. Scheff, *Being Mentally Ill: A Sociological Theory* (Chicago: Aldine 1966); T. J. Scheff, "The Labeling Theory of Mental Illness," *American Sociological Review,* vol. 39 (June 1974), 444–52, and the studies cited therein, and see the ensuing debate in the *A.S.R.,* vol. 40 (April 1975), 242–57.

35. Richard D. Lyons, "Psychiatrists, in a Shift, Declare Homosexuality No Mental Illness," *The New York Times* (December 12, 1973), pp. 1, 25.

36. See, for example, J. K. Myers and L. L. Bean, *A Decade Later: A Follow-up of Social Class and Mental Illness* (New York: Wiley, 1968); Scheff, *Being Mentally Ill;* M. Harvey Brenner, *Mental Illness and the Economy* (Cambridge: Harvard University Press, 1973).

37. D. Rosenhan, "On Being Sane in Insane Places," *Science* 179 (1973), 250–58.

38. See W. W. Michaux et al., *The First Year Out: Mental Patients After Hospitalization* (Baltimore: Johns Hopkins Press, 1969); G. A. Brown et al., *Schizophrenia and Social Care* (London: Oxford University Press, 1960); and G. Saenger, "Patterns of Change Among 'Treated' and 'Untreated' Patients Seen in Psychiatric Community Mental Health Clinics," *The Journal of Nervous and Mental Disease,* 150 (1970), 37–50.

39. Bruce J. Ennis, *Prisoners of Psychiatry* (New York: Harcourt Brace Jovano-vich, 1972), pp. 86–87.

40. Harold M. Schmeck, Jr., "Suit Asks Department of Labor to Halt Alleged Peonage in Mental Institutions," *The New York Times* (March 14, 1973), p. 21.

41. Dr. Paul Caron, voicing the opinion of others, believes that involuntary com-mitment is incompatible with treatment. "We admit patients to mental hospitals under legal custody, and then become upset when the hospital fulfills its legally mandated custodial function. . . . We demand that the doors be unlocked, but are not prepared to allow patients to pass through the open doors. We insist on forcing unwilling patients into treatment, and then we are dismayed when we discover that the use of force required by this policy is not very pleasant. We demand that mental hospitals set aside their traditional paternalism and grant patients self-determination but are not prepared to accept the consequences when the patients elect not only to be left alone, but also to leave the hospital. We criticize the emphasis on physical therapies, without realizing that non-physical therapies cannot be imposed on unwilling subjects. . . ." Quoted in "Forcible Commitment Called Incompatible with Treatment," *Psychiatric News* (No-vember 15, 1972), p. 13.

42. See references in footnote 38.

43. Nancy E. Waxler, "Culture and Mental Illness: A Social Labeling Perspec-tive," *The Journal of Nervous and Mental Disease,* vol. 159-6 (1974), 379–95; G. A. German, "Aspects of Clinical Psychiatry in Sub-Saharan Africa," *British Jour-nal of Psychiatry,* 121 (1972), 461–79.

44. Nancy E. Waxler, "Maintaining the Sick Role: Studies in Social Response," typed, Harvard Medical School (1974), p. 2.

45. R. L. Spitzer and P. T. Wilson, "Nosology and the Official Psychiatric Nomenclature," in A. M. Freedman, H. I. Kaplan, and B. J. Sadock, eds., *Compre-hensive Textbook in Psychiatry* II, vol. I (Baltimore: Williams & Wilkins, 1975), pp. 831–35.

46. Thomas J. Scheff, "On Reason and Sanity: Some Political Implications of Psychiatric Thought," in Hans Peter Dreitzel, ed., *The Social Organization of Health* (New York: Macmillan, 1971), pp. 291–301 (esp. p. 293).

47. See John S. Strauss et al., "Do Psychiatric Patients Fit Their Diagnoses?" Paper presented to the 130th Annual Meeting of the American Psychiatric Association, Toronto, Canada, May 2, 1977.

48. Spitzer and Wilson, "Nosology"; Donald Conover, "Psychiatric Distinc-tions: New and Old Approaches," *Journal of Health and Social Behavior,* 13 (June 1972), 167–80; Robert B. Edgerton, "On the 'Recognition' of Mental Illness," in Stanley C. Plog and Robert B. Edgerton, eds., *Changing Perspectives in Mental Illness* (New York: Holt, Rinehart & Winston, 1969), pp. 49–71; D. Bannister, P. Salmon and D. M. Leiberman, "Diagnosis-Treatment Relations in Psychiatry," *British Journal of Psychiatry,* vol. 110 (1964), 726–32; P. Ash, "Reliability of Psychiatric Diagnosis," *Journal of Abnormal and Social Psychology,* vol. 44 (1949), 272–77; Helen Nakagawa, Oliver H. Osborne and Kathleen Hartmann, "Fallacies in Schizo-phrenia," typed, (1975); S. B. Sells, ed., *The Definition and Measurement of Mental Health* (Washington, D.C.: National Center for Health Statistics, 1968); Bruce P. Dohrenwend and Barbara Snell Dohrenwend, *Social Status and Psychological Disorder* (New York: Wiley, 1969).

49. Henry Steadman and Joseph Cocozza, *Careers of the Criminally Insane,* (Lexington, Mass.: Lexington Books, 1974); Steadman and Cocozza, "Psychiatry, Dangerousness and the Repetitively Violent Offender," *The Journal of Criminal Law and Criminology* (1978), vol. 69, no. 2; Cocozza and Steadman, "Prediction in Psychiatry," *Social Problems* 25:3 (February 1978), 265–76.

50. Ennis, *Prisoners of Psychiatry.*

51. Michael A. Peszke and Ronald M. Wintrob, "Emergency Commitment—A Transcultural Study," typed paper presented at the annual meetings of the American Psychiatric Association, May 1973.

52. Ibid., p. 8.

53. Cited in ibid., p. 14.

54. David Bazelon, "The Perils of Wizardry," *American Journal of Psychiatry,* vol. 131, no. 12 (1974), 1317–22 (esp. 1319).

55. Scheff, *Being Mentally Ill;* Ennis, *Prisoners of Psychiatry;* D. Miller and M. Schwartz, "County Lunacy Commission Hearings: Some Observations of Commitments to a State Mental Hospital," *Social Problems* 14 (1966), 26–35; R. Maisel, "Decision-Making in a Commitment Court," *Psychiatry* 33 (3) (1970), 352–61.

56. Arlene K. Daniels, "Normal Mental Illness and Understandable Excuses," *American Behavioral Scientist* 14 (December 1970), 167–84 (esp. 175).

57. Ibid., p. 172.

58. Annette Ehrlich and Fred Abraham-Magdamo, "Caution: Mental Health May Be Hazardous," *Human Behavior* (September 1974), 64–70.

59. Helen Nakagawa, Oliver H. Osborne and Kathleen Hartmann, "Negotiated Images: Contributions to the Study of Symptom Pattern Change," typed paper presented at the VIIIth World Congress of Sociology, August 1974.

60. Dohrenwend, "Sociocultural and Social-Psychological Factors," 368.

61. I. K. Zola, "Medicine as an Institution of Social Control," in C. Cox and A. Mead, eds., *A Sociology of Medical Practice* (London: Collier-Macmillan, 1975), chap. 10, p. 170.

62. Scott, *The Making of Blind Men.*

63. Daniel Goleman, "Who's Mentally Ill?" *Psychology Today,* 11–8 (January 1978), 34–41. Quote from p. 41.

64. Robert L. Spitzer, Jean Endicott, Eli Robins, "Research Diagnostic Criteria," *Archives of General Psychiatry,* vol. 35 (June 1978), 773–82.

65. *Task Panel Reports Submitted to the President's Commission on Mental Health,* p. 14.

66. Allen E. Bergin, "The Evaluation of Therapeutic Outcomes," in Bergin and Sol. L. Garfield, eds., *Handbook of Psycho-Therapy and Behavioral Change: An Empirical Analysis* (New York: Wiley, 1971), p. 24.

67. Lester Luborsky et al., "Factors Influencing the Outcome of Psychotherapy: A Review of Quantitative Research," *Psychological Bulletin,* vol. 75 (March 1971), 145–185 (esp. p. 160).

68. Bergin, "The Evaluation," p. 242.

69. On the evidence for iatrogenic diseases, see Ivan Illich, *Medical Nemesis* (New York: Pantheon, 1977).

70. See Peter Schrag, *Mind Control* (New York: Pantheon, 1978); Dan Rather,

"Fifty Minutes" in *60 Minutes* (CBS News, February 19, 1978); Erving Goffman, *Asylums* (New York: Doubleday, 1961); Thomas Szasz, *The Manufacture of Madness* (New York: Harper & Row, 1970).

71. Bergin, "The Evaluation," p. 246.

72. Visotsky et al., "Development of Faculty," pp. 76–77.

73. David R. Hawkins et al., *Conference on the Education of Psychiatrists Preparatory Commission III: The Resident* (Mimeo, no date, about 1976), p. 22.

74. Ibid., p. 44.

75. See James S. Eaton, Jr. et al., "Psychiatric Education: State of the Art," *Psychiatry* 134 (March 1977): 2–6; Robert S. Daniels et al., "Characteristics of Psychiatric Residency Programs and Quality of Education," *American Journal of Psychiatry* 134 (March 1977): 7–10.

2. Getting into Psychiatry

1. Unless otherwise marked, quotes come from my field notes of conversations with residents and staff. This resident was echoing a famous line by Karl Menninger.

2. See the excellent discussion of socialization by Daniel J. Levinson in "Medical Education and the Theory of Adult Socialization," *Journal of Health and Social Behavior*, vol. 8 (December 1967), 253–65.

3. Throughout the text I will use the word patient rather than client or person, because psychiatrists use it and because it reflects the thinking of an important part of the psychiatric profession. Nevertheless, there are a number of psychiatrists, not necessarily young or radical, who find the term offensive and who publicly criticize their colleagues for using it.

4. About 90 percent of all psychiatrists are male.

5. This section appeared in a similar form as an article entitled "The Impact of Medical School on Future Psychiatrists," *American Journal of Psychiatry*, 132:6 (June 1975), 607–10.

6. Cited in LeRoy P. Levitt, "The Personality of the Medical Student," *Chicago Medical School Quarterly*, vol. 25, no. 4 (Winter 1966), 202.

7. D. Atchely, "The Physician as Scholar and Humorist," cited in Levitt, "Medical Student," p. 203.

8. Harrison G. Gough, "Some Predictive Implications of Premedical Scientific Competence and Preferences," *Journal of Medical Education* 53:4 (April 1978), 291.

9. Myron R. Sharaf, Patricia Schneider, and David Kantor, "Psychiatric Interest and Its Correlates Among Medical Students," *Psychiatry*, vol. 31 (May 1968), 150–60.

10. Levitt, "Medical Student," p. 204.

11. Ibid., p. 206.

12. Levitt, "Medical Student," p. 206; and Leonard Eron, "The Effect of Medical Education on Medical Students' Attitudes," *Journal of Medical Education*, vol. 30 (October 1955), 559–66.

13. Levitt, "Medical Student," p. 210.

14. This work began with Eron, "Effects of Medical Education," and his subsequent article, "The Effect of Medical Education on Attitudes: A Follow-up Study," *Journal of Medical Education,* vol. 33 (1958), 25–33. John G. Bruhn and Oscar A. Parsons continued the work in "Medical Student Attitudes toward Four Medical Specialties," *Journal of Medical Education,* vol. 39 (January 1964), 40–49. More recently, see Donald F. Kausch, "Medical Students' Attitudes toward the Mental Health Field: A Longitudical Study," *Journal of Medical Education,* vol. 44 (November 1969), 1051–55.

15. See Howard S. Becker and Blanche Geer, "The Fate of Idealism in Medical School," *American Sociological Review,* vol. 23 (1958), 50–56.

16. See Eron, "Effects of Medical Education."

17. Quoted in Levitt, "Medical Student," p. 204.

18. Adina Reinhardt and Robert Gray show that cynicism goes down in specialities characterized by higher patient-physician interaction, in "A Social Psychological Study of Attitude Change in Physicians," *Journal of Medical Education,* vol. 47 (February 1972), 112–17.

19. Robert E. Coker, Jr., Kurt W. Back, Thomas G. Donnelly, and Norman Miller, "Patterns of Influence: Medical School Faculty Members and the Values and Specialty Interests of Medical Students," *Journal of Medical Education,* vol. 35 (June 1960), 518–27.

Medical faculty's views of students are interesting. Besides neglecting relations with patients, students were "overly concerned that specific medical actions should lead to desired results, and placed too much importance on prestige among their colleagues, on income, and on manageable working hours. Faculty members also felt that students cared too little about making a contribution to knowledge, dealing with problems which require exacting analysis, or increasing their understanding of basic processes" (Coker et. al., "Patterns of Influence," p. 521). On the other hand, when students rated various medical values, the top five were: 1. having the chance to help people; 2. having the chance to continually increase understanding of basic processes; 3. developing warm personal relationships with patients; 4. having the greatest scope possible for independent action; 5. being virtually certain that specific medical actions will lead to the desired results (Coker et. al., "Patterns of Influence," table 4).

20. The ranking was (from top to bottom) basic science, internal medicine, pathology, pediatrics, surgery, obstetrics, public health, and psychiatry. The rank order correlation coefficient was .79.

21. For example, David Caplovitz, "Value Orientations and Faculty Members," cited in Coker et. al., "Patterns of Influence"; Richard Christie and Robert K. Merton, "Procedures for the Sociological Study of the Values Climate of Medical Schools," *Journal of Medical Education,* vol. 33, pt. II (October 1958), 125–53; and the general project which produced *The Student Physician,* Robert K. Merton, George Reader and Patricia L. Kendall, eds. (Cambridge, Mass.: Harvard University Press, 1957).

22. Henry H. Work, M.D., Director of Professional Affairs, American Psychiatric Association, personal correspondence, April 16, 1974, p. 2.

23. I am grateful to James S. Eaton, Jr., chief of the Psychiatric Education Branch at N.I.M.H., for this general description, given in 1978.

24. Bernard H. Hall, "Early Development of the Psychiatrist," *Journal of the American Medical Association*, 153 (October 17, 1953): 615–20 (esp. 615–16).

25. Bonnie Markham, "Second Year Medical Students' Views of Patients and Psychiatrists: 'Not Like Me'," mimeographed, 1975, Rutgers Medical School.

26. *American Journal of Psychiatry*, vol. 124 (January 1968), 990–91.

27. Pietro Castelnuovo-Tedesco, "How Much Psychiatry Are Medical Students Really Learning?" *Archives of General Psychiatry*, vol. 16 (June 1967), 668–75. This first belief is also an enduring myth among psychiatrists. See my paper, "Psychiatry and Suicide: The Making of a Mistake," *American Journal of Sociology*, vol. 77 (March 1972), 821–38.

28. Castelnuovo-Tedesco, "How Much Psychiatry," p. 669.

29. Surgery is the other. See Coker et. al., "Patterns of Influence," and Castelnuovo-Tedesco, "How Much Psychiatry." The following material comes from the latter's study.

30. This message comes through not only in Castelnuovo-Tedesco's article, but also in one by G. J. Tucker and R. E. Reinhardt, who write that the current vogue to teach psychiatry as an interdisciplinary science "may be more of a self-conscious attempt to *achieve among our medical colleagues a desired 'scientific' status which already seems to be present.* The emphasis on such basic science disciplines can often serve . . . as a source of further distancing maneuvers from patients." In "Psychiatric Attitudes of Young Physicians: Implications for Teaching," *American Journal of Psychiatry*, vol. 124 (January 1968), 988. Support for teaching psychiatry clinically in medical school also comes from the study of Rudolf H. Moos and Irvin D. Yalom, "Medical Students' Attitudes toward Psychiatry and Psychiatrists," *Mental Hygiene*, vol. 50 (April 1966), 246–56.

31. These conclusions are based on Moos and Yalom, "Medical Students' Attitudes"; Robert K. Merton, S. Bloom and N. Rogoff, "Studies in the Sociology of Medical Education," *Journal of Medical Education*, vol. 31 (1956), 552–65; Seymour Parker, "Personality Factors among Medical Students as Related to Their Predisposition to View the Patient as a 'Whole Man'," *Journal of Medical Education*, vol. 33 (1958), 736–44; Peter Livingston and Carl N. Zimet, "Death Anxiety, Authoritarianism and Choice of Specialty in Medical Students," *Journal of Nervous and Mental Diseases*, vol. 140 (1965), 222–30.

32. Moos and Yalom, "Medical Students' Attitudes," p. 251.

33. Kausch, "Mental Health Field."

34. Bruhn and Parsons, "Four Medical Specialties."

35. Ibid. See also Brian M. Davies and R. M. Mowbray, "Medical Students: Personality and Academic Achievement," *British Journal of Medical Education*, vol. 2 (1968), 195–99.

36. Bruhn and Parsons, "Four Medical Specialties." However, Sharaf et. al., "Psychiatric Interest," were surprised to find no relation with "intraceptive values" because in a previous study psychiatric students had scored higher on them than students heading for surgery.

37. See Sharaf et. al., "Psychiatric Interest"; Davies and Mowbray, "Academic Achievement"; and Eron, "Effects of Medical Education."

38. This argument is supported by Paul Nemetz and Herbert Weiner, "Some Fac-

tors in the Choice of Psychicatry as a Career," *Archives of General Psychiatry,* vol. 13 (October 1965), 299–303.

39. Sharaf et. al., "Psychiatric Interest"; Howard S. Becker et. al., *Boys in White* (Chicago: University of Chicago Press, 1961), p. 416.

40. See Robert R. Holt and Lester Luborsky, *Personality Patterns of Psychiatrists* (New York: Basic Books, 1958), vol. I, chap. 13; Arnold Rogow, *The Psychiatrists* (New York: Putnam, 1970); Livingston and Zimet, "Death Anxiety." The following correlates of authoritarianism come mainly from Parker, "Personality Factors."

41. William Martin, "Preferences for Types of Patients," pp. 189–205 in Merton et. al., *The Student Physician.*

42. See Holt and Luborsky, *Personality Patterns;* Livingston and Zimet, "Death Anxiety"; Rogow, *The Psychiatrists.*

43. Billy E. Jones, Orlando B. Lightfoot, Don Palmer, Raymond G. Wilkerson, and Donald H. Williams, "Problems of Black Psychiatric Residents in White Training Institutes," *American Journal of Psychiatry,* vol. 127 (December 1970), 798–803. Both quotes come from page 799.

44. See also Melvin Sabshin, Herman Diesehaus, and Raymond Wilkerson, "Dimensions of Institutional Racism in Psychiatry," *American Journal of Psychiatry,* vol. 127 (December 1970), 787–93.

45. Presumably the low scores mean that psychiatrists will not take advantages of these institutional features and use them against certain clients. Holt describes well the potential power given a physician in his 1959 essay cited before.

46. See summary of research in chap. 3 of George Domino, *Personality Patterns and Choice of Medical Specialty,* doctoral dissertation in psychology (University of California, Berkeley, 1967).

47. From a nonrandom survey of 2630 students at eight medical schools by John Kosa, "Religion and the Medical Student." Paper presented at the American Sociological Association's meetings, August 1968.

48. Livingston and Zimet, "Death Anxiety," p. 229.

49. Ibid., p. 224.

50. Arthur Elstein writes, "Thus, after a period of rapid biomedical advance, medicine finds it necessary to reemphasize its ancient pastoral functions and seeks to do this on a more 'scientific' basis than was possible before the social sciences had been developed. In the light of these pastoral functions, the recruitment, selection, and education of medical students are not merely a problem of personnel selection and training but rather one of determining . . . who has a true vocation and, therefore, merits training in the arts of the profession. . . . The psychosocial development and training of the physician—the personal changes he undergoes and the knowledge of others he is to acquire—is thus a matter of enormous importance." *Journal of Medical Education,* vol. 47 (April 1972), 310.

51. Lillian Kaufman Cartwright, "Personality Differences in Male and Female Medical Students," *Psychiatry in Medicine,* vol. 3 (1972), 213–18.

52. The segment is well-characterized by Rue Bucher in "The Psychiatric Residency and Professional Socialization," *Journal of Health and Human Behavior,* vol. 6 (Winter 1965), 197–206. See also A. Strauss, L. Schatzman, R. Bucher, D. Ehrlich

and M. Sabshin, *Psychiatric Institutions and Ideologies*, (Glencoe, Ill.: Free Press, 1964).

53. Holt and Luborsky, *Personality Patterns*.

54. While University Psychiatric Center allowed me to watch residents in more settings than any other researcher and to participate in many parts of the program, they would not let me see the files of the same residents or of residents I did not know from previous years. For over five years I persistently requested information on the selection process, often with backing from senior faculty, but to no avail. Finally, in the fifth year, I was allowed to go through a file of small index cards which noted the college, medical school and internship of residents.

55. Rue Bucher, Joan Stelling, Paul Dommermuth, "Implications of Prior Socialization for Residency Programs in Psychiatry," *Archives of General Psychiatry*, vol. 20 (April 1969), 397.

56. At the time these were Boston Psychopathic Hospital, Brooklyn State Hospital, Elgin State Hospital, Institute of the Pennsylvania Hospital, Langley Porter Clinic, Menninger Foundation, Michael Reese Hospital, New York Hospital, New York State Psychiatric Institute, Norristown State Hospital, North Little Rock V.A. Hospital, University of Cincinnati, University of Colorado, University of Michigan, University of Minnesota, University of Texas, and Washington University, St. Louis.

57. See Bucher, "Psychiatric Residency"; *Group for the Advancement of Psychiatry*, "Trends and Issues in Psychiatric Residency Programs," Report no. 31 (1955), 1–17.

58. Theodora M. Abel, Sadi Oppenheim, Clifford J. Sager, "Screening Applicants for Training in Psychoanalytically Oriented Psychotherapy," *American Journal of Psychotherapy*, vol. 10 (1956), 34.

59. Holt and Luborsky, *Personality Patterns*, vol. II, pp. 333–34. This shift is normal as a profession gets more established.

60. Ibid., vol. I, p. 262. See discussion pp. 262–65 and tables I-15.1, 15.2.

61. Managerial and therapeutic work-styles are two which are developed in Appendix III and pp. 52 to 56.

62. Holt and Luborsky, *Personality Patterns*, vol. I, pp. 264–65.

63. Menninger, Karl A., "What Are the Goals of Psychiatric Education?" *Bulletin of the Menninger Clinic*, vol. 16 (1952), pp. 153, 156.

64. In New Jersey, for example, two-thirds of the places go empty. See *A Descriptive Directory of Psychiatric Training Programs in the United States*, 1978–79, Lee Gurel, ed. (Washington, D.C.: American Psychiatric Association, 1979).

65. Bernard Riess, "The Selection and Supervision of Psychotherapists," p. 108, in *The Training of Psychotherapists*, Nicholas P. Dellis and Herbert Stone, eds., (Baton Rogue: Louisiana State University Press, 1960).

66. Reported in Holt and Luborsky, *Personality Patterns*, vol. I, pp. 5–6.

67. Ibid., vol. I, p. 129; vol. II, p. 119.

68. Bucher et al., "Implications of Prior Socialization." See also Holt and Luborsky, *Personality Patterns*, vol. I, p. 128.

69. Robert Plutchik, Hope Conte, and Henry Kandler, "Variables Related to the Selection of Psychiatric Residents," *American Journal of Psychiatry*, vol. 127 (May 1971), 1503–08.

70. Ibid., 1505.

71. Ibid., 1506–07.

72. Domino, "Choice of Medical Specialty," p. 55.

73. Ibid., p. 96.

74. William E. Henry, John H. Sims and S. Lee Spray, *The Fifth Profession.* (San Francisco: Jossey-Bass, 1971).

75. American Psychiatric Association, Conference on the Education of Psychiatrists: *Preparatory Commission III: The Resident,* David Hawkins, ed.; (typed, 1975). The material which follows is from pp. 22–23 of this report. The study cited is by A. T. Russell, R. O. Pasnau, Z. T. Taintor, "Emotional Problems of Residents in Psychiatry," *American Journal of Psychiatry,* 132:3 (March 1975), 263–67.

76. F. K. Garetz, O. N. Raths, R. H. Morse, "The Disturbed and the Disturbing Psychiatric Resident," *Archives of General Psychiatry,* 33 (April 1976) 446–47.

77. E. M. Waring, "Psychiatric Illness in Physicians: A Review," *Comprehensive Psychiatry* 15 (November/December 1974).

78. Holt and Luborsky, *Personality Pattern,* vol. I, p. 130.

79. Harold Garfinkel has long made the point that there is often more to be learned about social reality in the procedures and research "problems" of a study than in the final "results," which often obscure the ways in which "problems" were solved by making the data fit particular behaviors or attitudes fit an analytic model.

80. Holt and Luborsky, *Personality Patterns,* vol. II, p. 142.

81. Ibid., vol. I, pp. 150–51.

82. Ibid., vol. II, p. 150.

83. This argument would not be true for heterogeneous residencies. See Holt and Luborsky, ibid., vol. II, p. 84.

84. Ibid., vol. I, pp. 216–22.

85. Ibid., vol. II, p. 269.

86. Ibid., vol. I, pp. 220, 218 respectively.

3. Graduate Training in Psychiatry

1. Quoted in Rosemary Stevens, *American Medicine and the Public Interest* (New Haven: Yale University Press, 1971), p. 118. The following history is based on chaps 6, 15, and 17 of Stevens.

2. See Stevens's book, chap. 17, and pp. 71–74 of Howard B. Waitzkin and Barbara Waterman, *The Exploitation of Illness in Capitalist Society* (New York: Bobbs-Merrill, 1974). Harry Perlstadt found that the strongest correlations with choosing a straight versus rotating internship were percent of basic science faculty totally supported by federal grants and the ratio of full-time basic science faculty to first- and second-year students. "Internship Placements and Faculty Influence," *Journal of Medical Education* 47 (1972): 862–68.

3. This history and interpretation are based on a number of conversations with staff at the American Board of Psychiatry and Neurology, the American Psychiatric Association, and NIMH in February 1978.

4. American Board of Psychiatry and Neurology, *Information for Applicants* (Chicago, 1975), 8.

5. Stephen J. Miller, *Prescription for Leadership: Training for the Medical Elite* (Chicago: Aldine, 1970), chap. 5.

6. Ibid., p. 193.

7. For a critique and reanalysis of Miller's study, see my article, "The Sociological Calendar: An Analytic Tool for Fieldwork Applied to Medical and Psychiatric Training," *American Journal of Sociology*, 80 (March 1975).

8. Miller, p. 199.

9. Ibid., ch. 7.

10. Ibid., p. 79.

11. This analysis is based on Emily Mumford, *Interns: From Students to Physicians* (Cambridge, Mass.: Harvard University Press, 1970), chaps. 3, 5 and 8.

12. See Oswald Hall, "The Stages of a Medical Career," *American Journal of Sociology* 53 (March 1948), 327–36.

13. For an analysis of this research and full presentation of this trypology, see Appendix III and my article, "Work Styles Among American Psychiatric Residents," in Joseph Westermeyer, ed., *Anthropology and Mental Health: Setting a New Course* (The Hague: Mouton, 1976).

14. Paul Nemetz and Herbert Weiner, "Some Factors in the Choice of Psychiatry as a Career," *Archives of General Psychiatry*, 13: 299–303 (October 1965).

15. Ibid., 301.

16. Ibid., 301.

17. Ibid., 301.

18. Ibid., 302.

19. M. R. Sharaf et. al., "Psychiatric Interest and Its Correlates Among Medical Students," *Psychiatry*, 31 (May 1968), 150–60, esp. p. 160.

20. Nemetz and Weiner, 302. The Sharaf study also identified this type.

21. M. R. Sharaf and D. J. Levinson, "The Quest for Omnipotence in Professional Training," *Psychiatry* 27 (1964), 135–49.

22. Daniel H. Funkenstein, "Failure to Graduate from Medical School," *Journal of Medical Education* 37:6 (June 1962), 588–603.

23. Mark S. Plovnick, "Primary Care Career Choices and Medical Student Learning Styles," *Journal of Medical Education* 50 (September 1975), 849–55.

24. Harrison G. Gough, "Some Predictive Implications of Premedical Scientific Competence and Preferences," *Journal of Medical Education* 53:4 (April 1978), 291 ff.

25. Robert K. Merton, *Sociological Ambivalence and Other Essays*, (New York: Free Press, 1976).

26. Prestige comes from *praestigium*, meaning a juggler's trick. Ironically, social scientists, as well as psychiatrists since Hollingshead and Redlich, have assumed that affluent patients were being treated better because they received psychotherapy more often than poor patients. In fact, the research on the effectiveness of different therapies favors somatic treatments.

27. The term comes from Miller, op. cit., p. 65.

28. National Institute of Mental Health, *The Nation's Psychiatrists* (Washington, D.C.: Public Health Service Publication No. 1885, 1969).

29. Victor and Ruth Sidel, *Serve the People: Observations on Medicine in the People's Republic of China,* (Boston: Beacon Press, 1973).

30. Lee Gurel, "Some Characteristics of Psychiatric Residency Training Programs," *American Journal of Psychiatry* 132:4 (April 1975), 363–72.

31. Based on conversation with educators from various residencies, 1973–75.

32. The average medical school program had 26 residents, while the one at University Psychiatric Center had over 75. Programs at nonacademic mental hospitals averaged only 13 residents. Gurel, "Some Characteristics," p. 365.

33. Ibid., p. 368.

34. Ibid., p. 369.

35. Ibid., p. 369.

4. Experiencing the First Year

1. Accurate descriptions have been given by others of how new doctors are anticipated by all members of a ward or service in a mental hospital. See *Community as Doctor,* Robert N. Rapoport (London: Tavistock, 1960), chap. 5. *Psychiatric Ideologies and Institutions,* by Anselm Strauss et. al. (New York: Free Press, 1964), especially chaps. 7 and 13.

2. Definite patterns of naming for reference (as opposed to address) exist in the resident culture. "Doctor" implies distance of rank or unfamiliarity or both to the residents. The surname alone implies higher rank and familiarity. Referring by first and last name implies more equal rank but unfamiliarity of the listener with the person alluded to. If the person referred to is about of equal rank and is familiar to both parties talking, the first name is sufficient reference. These patterns exist when a resident is speaking to another resident about another doctor, that is, reference among professionals about professionals.

3. The terms and phrases in quotation are the precise words used and convey the flavor of the meeting as well as the culture into which the residents have just entered.

4. These terms are quite formal compared to those used by the chief after a few weeks.

5. Theoretically, the T-A (therapist-administrator) split should be ideal; the therapist need not confound the therapeutic relationship with issues of administration. In reality, both members of each T-A team usually complain, the therapist because he cannot control drugs and restrictions as tightly as if it were his own case, the administrator because he feels out of touch with the patient's therapy or because he thinks the therapist is mishandling the case.

6. This quotation illustrates a basic problem in diagnosing and treating patients. Patients participate in a great deal of role playing; they have all day to think of manipulations they can perform. Under these circumstances, crazy behavior becomes dubious. See chap. 3 of *Being Mentally Ill* by Thomas J. Scheff (Chicago: Aldine, 1966), especially the similar examples on pp. 61–62.

7. Throughout the text direct quotations will be used when the exact words are known. Often the observer's notes are very close to what the residents said but not entirely exact. In these cases, indirect statements and statements without quotation marks will be used.

8. We see here a common problem among professionals, especially among trainees, when they must learn from people of lower status but of greater knowledge.

9. I did not tell Carl what his patient said, and in general I did not tell either group what the other said. However, what I learned from one side of a case would lead me to ask questions of the other. Carl in particular became quite nervous about the fact that I talked with this patient. He insisted that I not tell him anything, but the existence of that talk bothered him continually. At one point he said that he was afraid that I might do something ruinous to the patient and her therapy.

10. The reader will find that a silence of even thirty seconds, especially with eight colleagues in a room, feels quite long.

11. This is a good example of psychiatric argument where all outcomes show it is correct. It also illustrates a nearly exact paraphrase but not a verbatim quote.

12. There are many ways to regard this process. If one takes Goffman's perspective, psychiatrists screen out marks who will be hard to cool out. A religious interpretation of psychiatry would suggest that both practitioner and subject seek a conversion experience, and those without soul are eliminated. Larry Rosenberg suggests that this selection of patients one likes, along with other forms of getting comfortable, can simply be seen as the residents' effort to get good talk. In terms of resident types, the family doctor and administrative types are more likely to seek patients they like, while the analytic residents seeks patients who are good theoretical objects. See Alan F. Blum and Larry Rosenberg, "Some Problems Involved in Professionalizing Social Interaction: The Case of Psychotherapeutic Training," *Journal of Health and Social Behavior*, 9 (1968), 72–85, esp. pp. 77–79. In an oral profession, good talk will be highly esteemed. Regardless of the conceptual frame, the selection of "successful" clients concerns all professionals.

13. Here we see Ned's analytic orientation setting him off from other residents. As a psychoanalytic resident, Ned did not look for cure or much progress in his patients.

14. To this I would add that residents also tend to keep their first two or three patients a long time, if possible. Regardless of the first patients' diagnosis or style, residents seem very attached to them. This reflects the great investment they put into their first cases.

15. Notice the nature of Adam's reply. The layman might expect a chief to reprimand Mike for malpractice and poor work. Rather, Adam is accepting and nondirective, the common features of psychiatric instruction and socialization.

16. Older residents interpreted remarks similar to Carl's as the frightened response of a new resident when confronted with the idea that he too may be crazy.

17. This comment implies the residents' view, that there is a basic condition of the patient onto which drugs are added.

18. Many examples such as this one indicate how peculiar is the information in a patient's record. For a conceptual analysis of this phenomenon, see Harold Garfinkel, *Studies in Ethnomethodology* (Englewood Cliffs, N.J.: Prentice Hall, 1967), chap. 6.

19. Notice that residents begin early to instruct other residents. This implies a pecking order. Any resident felt free to instruct Jeff. Ned was next from the bottom. At the top were Ken, Carl and Marc, who would also instruct each other, but in a different manner, as peers. Dave Reed seemed independent of this order.

20. Later, Ken said that his job and the reason he came here was "to relieve the pain," and he did all he could to make the patient feel better. Ironically, later Ken was criticized by nurses for being too soft with the patients, too kind-hearted. By the spring, he looked back and saw his earlier behavior the same way.

21. Marc's views are several months ahead of the others' in terms of socialization. Complaints against the hospital increased. Contrast this psychiatric view of hospitals to that of most nonpsychiatric physicians.

22. Some senior residents felt that psychiatric training, along with its required medical training, was so long that psychiatrists took out their anger on the patients, in terms of high fees, arrogance, and lack of sympathy.

23. See Blum and Rosenberg, "Social Interaction," 77–82. Marc was describing a very interesting process, the transfer of competence. When a patient first enters the psychiatric setting, he is the world's greatest expert on himself. The therapist can know nothing or very little. As the person talks about himself and acts, slowly the therapist takes over personal expertise until the therapist claims to know more about the person than that person himself. The ultimate mark of this process is not telling a person his diagnosis.

Notice that the patient must *talk*. If he merely *acts* on his feelings, the resident does not know what to do (aside from managing him) and will not tolerate him.

24. The circular reasoning here is typical, not of nurses, but of all members of the psychiatric team. An excellent analysis of this reasoning can be found in *Psychological Interpretation,* by L. Levy (New York: Holt, Rinehart & Winston, 1963).

Notice the incremental nature of the nurse's remarks. A patient earns his way out of the hospital, first by succumbing to the staff's definition of him at each stage and then by fulfilling the staf's expectations for progress.

25. The resident's suggestion indicates how central to professionalization is learning psychotherapeutic face. See Levy, *Psychological Interpretations,"* pp. 74–77.

26. Again, the words in quotations are verbatim; the others are close paraphrase.

27. Managerial residents seemed uniformly more balanced in their emotional relations with patients, a reflection of how they regard patients and their work. That the "problem" of controlled affectivity permeates the year reflects the great emotional involvement which residents experience with their patients.

28. Psychological interns usually carry only one or two patients.

29. Dr. Cohn's style with the residents was to listen very carefully and to make an occasional interpretation. The residents resisted its psychoanalytic character for much of the year, but by the end of the year most of them used psychoanalytic interpretations and were aware of Adam's influence. He had socialized them successfully.

30. Blum and Rosenberg ("Social Interaction," pp. 83–85) present a good discussion of these changes, considerably elaborated here.

31. One might see Carl and the others as having been "cooled out" of the failure they sense from coming into psychiatry. A very strong and popular chief of a service described his job as "helping the residents take the tremendous loss they experience."

32. DOC is the common term for Doctor-On-Call.

33. The maximum amount of time which residents reported seeing patients in therapy was twice a week for forty-five minutes or three times a week for thirty min-

utes, this only with their best therapy patients. This is less than reported in the winter, where the maximum could be daily for thirty minutes.

Residents of the previous year said that they had seen patients for much longer periods per week, about two to three hours each, and that they did this for all their patients, not just for one or two, as was the case with this cohort.

34. "Feelings Meeting" or "the chief's meeting" was where residents, chief and perhaps one or two others, talked about anything they wished in a private, leisurely meeting.

35. The audience laughed at this example of how one "takes care" of someone by giving her a severe or pessimistic diagnosis. Nothing could be more permanent and severe than to be psychotic by character.

36. "Group" refers to the Group Dynamic Seminar.

37. This is, of course, only one side of their feelings. Carl, especially, is very aware of his doctorhood. To some extent, the residents are indulging in very fashionable, one-upmanship remarks. In a psychiatric milieu, it is cool to make out normal people as sicker than they appear, and to show that patients are healthier than they seem.

38. In this passage, Carl Rabinowitz retreats from a moral stance against treatment to a personal objection based on his limited capacity for empathy. The conversation shows how moral issues are psychologized.

39. Notice how open the residents are with this noted figure. Never had they so explicitly expressed their doubts about the profession to a leading man. In part, the man's frank style invited frankness from the residents.

5. A Sociological Calendar of Psychiatric Socialization

1. For example, see *Boys in White,* by Howard S. Becker, Blanche Geer, Everett C. Hughes and Anselm L. Strauss (Chicago: Unitersity of Chicago Press, 1961).

2. This chapter builds on the pioneer work of Renée C. Fox, "A Dynamic Over-View of the Comprehensive Care and Teaching Program: Through the Medium of Participant Observation," typed, 1954; "A Sociological Calendar of the First Year in Medical School," typed, 1958; and "A Sociological Calendar on Medical School: Second Year, First Trimester," typed, 1956. I am indebted to Professor Fox for sharing her work with me and encouraging this analysis. A more scholarly presentation of the present chapter can be found in my article, "The Sociological Calendar: An Analytic Tool for Fieldwork Applied to Medical and Psychiatric Training," *American Journal of Sociology,* 80, 5 (March 1975), 1145–64.

3. For a comparative analysis of this phase, see "Learning the Ropes: Situational Learning in Four Occupational Training Programs," by Blanche Geer et. al., chap. 12 of *Among the Poor,* Irwin Deutscher & E. J. Thompson, eds., (New York: Basic Books, 1968).

4. For elaboration, see Alan F. Blum and Larry Rosenberg, "Some Problems Involved in Professionalizing Social Interaction: The Case of Psychotherapeutic Training," *Journal of Health & Social Behavior* (March 1968), vol. 9, 72–85; and Thomas J. Ungerleider, "That Most Difficult Year," *American Journal of Psychiatry* (1965), vol. 122, 542–45.

5. The elements of power and manipulation have been explored by two noted psychiatrists. See Judd Marmor, "The Feeling of Superiority: An Occupational Hazard in the Practice of Psychotherapy," *American Journal of Psychiatry,* vol. 110 (1953), 370–76; and Harold F. Searles, "Feelings of Guilt in the Psychoanalyst," *Psychiatry,* vol. 29 (1966), 319–23. These and other materials have been brought together for a larger analysis in my paper, "Omnipotent Tendencies in the Professions: The Case of Psychiatry" (1973), typed.

6. Psychiatrists have incorporated the spirit of business into their language. They speak of "getting down to work," "working in therapy," "getting into business" (i.e., forming a substantial bond with the patient and "working on" serious issues), and "productive" therapy.

7. Herbert C. Modlin et. al., "Growth of Psychiatrists During and After Residency Training: An Objective Evaluation," *American Journal of Psychiatry* 115 (June 1959), 1081–90.

In a letter to me dated March 24, 1971, Dr. Modlin wrote, "We were indeed surprised that the advanced residents did not score any higher than they did. In retrospect, we should not have been so surprised. I am enclosing a small summary article which suggests that the advanced residents are primarily concerned with developing and perfecting clinical technique with patients."

8. Modlin, "Growth of Psychiatrists," 1082–1083.

9. Rue Bucher and Joan Stelling, *Becoming Professional* (Beverly Hills, Cal.: Sage, 1977), 8.

6. Managing Patients

1. Rose Laub Coser, *Training in Ambiguity: Learning Through Doing in a Mental Hospital.* (New York: Free Press, 1979).

2. Ibid., p. 44. The following arguments for the T-A Split are found mainly between p. 22 and p. 52.

3. Ibid., p. 40.

4. Ibid., pp. 26, 47–48, 53–57, 65–67, 73–74.

5. Ibid., p. 54.

6. Ibid., pp. 27, 47–48, 53–57, 65–67, 73–74.

7. Ibid., p. 45.

8. Ibid., pp. 50, 68, 79–83, 92.

9. Ibid., pp. 90–91.

10. Ibid., chaps. 4 and 5.

11. David Van Buskirk, "Identity Development in the Beginning Psychiatrist," chap. 4 in *Teaching Psychotherapy of Psychotic Patients,* Elvin Semrad, ed. (New York: Grune and Stratton, 1969), p. 35. Buskirk adds that research suggests that the T-A split prolongs the patient's hospitalization.

12. Coser, pp. 55, 60, 127–31.

13. Robert K. Merton and Elinor Barber, "Sociological Ambivalence," in *Sociological Ambivalence and Other Essays,* by Robert K. Merton (New York: Free Press, 1976), pp. 3–31.

14. If one examines Merton and Barber's own material, their six types of socio-

logical ambivalence, their examples of apprenticeship and the doctor-patient relationship, or their four structural sources of ambivalence, one sees in each instance that
a person *might* become ambivalent, but it depends on the individual.

15. This analysis is derived from Robert K. Merton's insightful essay, "Social
Mechanisms for Articulation of Roles in Rolesets," in *Social Theory and Social Structure,* by Robert K. Merton (Glencoe, Ill.: Free Press, 1957), rev. ed., pp. 371–79.

16. Rose Laub Coser, "Insulation from Observability and Types of Social Con-
formity," *American Sociological Review* 26 (February 1961), 28–39.

17. Anselm Strauss, Leonard Schatzman, Danuta Ehrlich, Rue Bucher and Melvin Sabshin, "The Hospital and Its Negotiated Order," chap. 5 in Eliot Freidson, ed.,
The Hospital in Modern Society (New York: Free Press, 1963).

18. Despite the cautious phrasing here, one resident who read this wrote on the
margin, "rarely."

19. Erving Goffman, *Asylums* (New York: Doubleday Anchor, 1961).

20. Note the term, "raise," a physical image of raising a barrier, as opposed to
"increase."

21. Rose Laub Coser, "Evasiveness as a Response to Structural Ambivalence,"
Social Science and Medicine 1 (1967), 203–18; *Training,* chap. 6.

22. Coser, *Training,* p. 108.

23. Ibid. Compare p. 107 with p. 108 and what follows.

24. Ibid., p. 106.

25. Coser, "Evasiveness as a Response," p. 207.

26. The imbalance between the two interview questions makes it impossible to
accurately interpret the tables which fill the rest of Coser's article. In addition, she constructs from them an Evasiveness Index which has other troublesome qualities. The
first dimension, which rates the degree to which the resident handles the probe as his
own problem or as the patient's problem, is now rephrased as the degree to which the
resident "handles patient's statement at face value" versus "treats it as the patient's
problem" (p. 210). Thus Coser's subjectivity gets built into this dimension. The second dimension measures the degree to which the resident also clarifies the staff hierarchy involved in the question or evades it. But presumably this dimension applies only
when, on the first dimension, the resident handles the patient's statement "at face
value." If he responds by treating the question as the patient's problem, the second
dimension does not apply. Yet the index is constructed as if this were not the case.

27. Rose Laub Coser, "Insulation from Observability," 28–39.

28. Rose Laub Coser, *The Role of the Patient in a Hospital Ward,* Ph.D. dissertation in sociology, Columbia University (1957).

29. This attitude forms a striking contrast to the "miracle" of psychiatric drugs
which so impress the public. Residents at University Psychiatric Center also vehemently
opposed a computer program for clinical records.

30. These examples are the prime messages of advertisements from one issue of
the *International Journal of Psychiatry.*

31. It is quite dramatic that in a hospital with so many staff, almost no one was on
the ward at the time. Both the nurses and the residents were at different meetings elsewhere.

32. The resident was in supervision when he was first called by the chief. He said

that he wanted to finish the case discussed before coming, and he returned to his supervision while Jack was in the courtyard. Nurses and attendants thought this behavior was incredibly negligent, and I think other residents would not have done this.

33. Here we see the ward structure psychologically. The patients are anxious because the staff is (which is measured by anyone being out of control for more than a few minutes). The staff is anxious, because the doctors—and ultimately the patient's doctor—are upset. Even though they think they are more competent, the staff look to the doctors to define the situation with assurance and mastery.

34. This is typical of the psychologizing which residents learn and, especially after analysis, believe in.

35. This patient, like many long in therapy, thinks and talks like psychiatrists. Socialized patients create problems, such as the question of malingering discussed in the chapter on diagnosis.

36. The chief immediately assumes that the patient symbolically cut herself as a ploy for attention, an illustration of the almost paranoid defense against seduction by patients. Notice that no other reason for the patient's scratching herself is considered either by the resident (in his second week of residency) or the chief. This patient, moreover, was not prone to scratching and such activities.

37. See the chapter on case conferences. No diagnosis was given or considered, a strong sign of a discharge conference.

7. Diagnosis

1. Although this was one of the most intelligent and sensible residents, I found his diagnosis incredible, a grotesque exaggeration of what we had both heard and observed. In my notes at the time, I wrote that she had included all the elements to avoid such an interpretation by explaining why she would react so strongly. She had reacted, I thought, the way most middle-class parents would if they found marijuana around the house. I also liked her numerous stories; I thought she had a complex and artistic mind. As I understood her, she did not think the police were after her but simply observed that in her conflict-filled family, calling the cops was not extraordinary. Thus, "paranoid schizophrenic" struck me as reflecting a cultural gap which the resident could not bridge despite the efforts of the woman to help him. It also missed, I thought, the primary unit of problem, which was relations between members of the family.

This remark, by the way, reveals a temptation which most observers share, to diagnose the patient too. It is a game which everyone seems to enter, to see if they can piece the evidence together into a good formulation before anyone else. This was, for example, the pervasive atmosphere of case conferences devoted to diagnosis.

2. Erving Goffman, *Asylums* (New York: Doubleday, 1961), pp. 155–56.

3. Goffman, *Asylums,* p. 157. These examples are verbatim excerpts from patient files at St. Elizabeth's Hospital in Washington, D.C.

4. Goffman, "The Moral Career of the Mental Patient," *Asylums,* pp. 125–69.

5. For an extensive and striking example of noncommunication between psychiatrists, see the experience of Michael Wechsler as written by his father, James Wechsler. *In a Darkness* (New York: Norton, 1972).

6. This struck me as bizarre, creating from the start a psychotic situation where the psychiatrists would behave as if we were not there and would expect the girl to do likewise. In general, psychiatrists learn that it is professionally correct for them to break the normal rules of human intercourse and conversation whenever they see fit. Emerson found that judges in juvenile courts do similar things. They ask questions in such rapidity as to leave the victim stammering and stunned; they give short, curt answers to important questions; they use long pauses which undermine the conversation and build great tension; and they manage their face by, for example, looking without expression at the delinquent for a long time. The following interviews illustrate many of these techniques. Robert M. Emerson, *Judging Delinquents: Context and Process in Juvenile Court* (Chicago: Aldine, 1969).

7. This was the first question which seemed to set the girl off balance.

8. This is classic technique many residents learn early, to repeat a key word from the last few sentences uttered. Two variations were observed, repeating as a statement "Involved" and as a question "Involved?" Some psychiatrists use this technique of searching for associations exclusively.

9. This is a typical diagnosis and illustrates some fundamental features of that practice. A diagnosis is an agreed label that essentializes the patient. It suggests predictability, though psychiatric diagnoses are not noted for their predictive powers. This creates the problem of how to account for variations and changes in patient behavior, a problem common to most everyday language. (Precise, predictive language is rare in human affairs.) This problem is solved, argues Harold Garfinkel, with *et cetera* clauses (e.g., "with great counter noise") which allow one to make sense of unexpected changes "while retaining the perceived reasonableness of actual socially organized activities." Harold Garfinkel, "Studies in the Routine Grounds of Everyday Activities," *Social Problems* 11 (Winter 1964), 248.

10. "Object relations" is a very common term at Distinguished University, a very fashionable word. The "in" resident will speak of his own object relations and of those of his patients.

11. I was impressed by how perceptive this remark was among all of the diagnostic attempts.

12. Thomas J. Scheff, *Being Mentally Ill* (Chicago: Aldine, 1966), p. 175.

13. David Sudnow, "Normal Crimes: Sociological Features of the Penal Code in a Public Defender Office," *Social Problems* 12 (1963); 255–76.

14. See Peter Berger and Thomas Luckmann, *The Social Construction of Reality* (New York: Doubleday, 1966); and Garfinkel, "Routine Grounds of Everyday Activities," 225–50.

15. See *Diagnostic and Statistical Manual of Mental Disorders,* 2nd ed. (American Psychiatric Assoc., 1968).

16. See Goffman, *Asylums,* pp. 357–60.

17. While it is difficult to know exactly which terms should be counted as managerial diagnoses, I have chosen to underline only the more general words. For example, hallucinating and having delusions are considered specifics of the managerial term, to be disorganized; but one could argue that all three terms qualify as managerial diagnoses. Using the same approach below, I consider "getting higher" to be Mrs. R's diagnosis, and getting louder the description of that diagnosis.

18. Stephen R. Goldsmith and Arnold J. Mandell, "The Dynamic Formulation—A Critique of a Psychiatric Ritual." Paper read at the Annual Meetings of the American Psychiatric Association, Boston, May 13–17, 1968.

19. Ibid., p. 5.

20. Ibid., p. 7.

21. See E. B. Gallagher, M. R. Sharaf and D. J. Levinson, "The Influence of Patient and Therapist in Determining the Use of Psychotherapy in a Hospital Setting," *Psychiatry,* 28 (November 1965), 297–310; Richard I. Shader et. al., "Biasing Factors in Diagnosis and Disposition," *Comprehensive Psychiatry* 10:2 (March 1969); M. R. Sharaf and D. J. Levinson, "Patterns of Ideology and Professional Role-Identification Among Psychiatric Residents," pp. 263–385 in *The Patient and the Mental Hospital,* Milton Greenblatt, et. al., eds., (Glencoe, Ill.: Free Press, 1957); Hans H. Strupp, "Toward an Analysis of the Therapist's Contribution to the Treatment Process," *Psychiatry,* 22 (November 1959), 349–62.

22. Shader et al., "Biasing Factors in Diagnosis and Disposition," 81–89.

23. Ibid., p. 87.

8. Case Conferences

1. The resident is wary of being seduced by his patient. As always, quotation marks are reserved for exact wording, though paraphrases are very close to the original.

2. Notice how the exposé continues, regardless of the patient's embarrassment.

3. This sequence is a common way to refocus the patient and terminate the interview. The good interviewer should mentally and literally hand the patient back to her therapist.

4. That Blumberg, the classic analyst, suggested a different approach to this patient was a genuine shock to this analytic-type resident.

5. See the "Focus of Therapy" dimension in chap. 5.

6. See again, the "Focus of Therapy" dimension of the sociological calendar in chap. 5.

7. Note the language of suicide. Staff and residents also talk of a patient who committed suicide, when they mean a serious attempt.

8. This ideal is troublesome, because it values above all else the refinement of technique to the point where one can extract the most private and painful feelings and stories in a public arena without the patient getting upset. The cardinal value here is comfort.

Ironically, the unconscious or delayed effect of this ideal is ignored. One patient describes the effect at the end of this chapter.

9. Differences of opinion about techniques, exposing patients' lives in public, and the morality of probing always divided the therapeutic-type residents from the analytic and administrative types.

10. Here is another diagnosis, its smorgasbord character showing the symptomatic nature of the process. The comments on paranoia and mental content are striking.

11. "Really" is a key word in this culture, distinguishing as it does semblance from true reality. Residents in this program learn early that symptomatic or behavioral improvement does not mean the patient is "really" better and that drugs, shock, restrictions, or work programs do not get at the real dynamics of the patient's psyche. Only psychotherapy and "working through" various defenses can "really" get the patient better. Residents see the truth in this view when some patients discharged with symptomatic improvement after drugs or shock fall apart and return once again. On the other hand, when graduates of psychotherapy fall apart and return, the residents interpret this as showing that more therapy is necessary, or (eventually) that the patient is chronic and therefore unable to really get better.

12. This is a *hopeful* view of electroshock therapy. Note that senior psychiatrists loathe EST more than residents.

13. Note the phrasing. As with other failures, the blame is put on the patient, even though the idea of blocking electric shock while unconscious is plainly fantastic.

14. Note the change in diagnosis, reflecting a change in the resident. Senior staff members thought that the patient had not changed at all during this time.

15. Clearly the resident feels helpless too.

16. The residents at University Psychiatric Center view other state hospitals as chronic repositories for hopeless cases, a view they learn from their teachers. Here, the interviewer is suggesting that Mr. Downs can be transferred, relieving the staff of him, but that the doctors need not feel guilty for condemning him to a chronic hospital, because he will get himself out.

17. Notice the resentment, the feeling of being used. This attitude is the sequel to the basic instruction that one gives the patient what he wants. If he does not respond therapeutically, then residents learn to feel duped, manipulated, used. This feeling does not come naturally, and one hears psychiatrists constantly warning residents not to be manipulated or sucked in by their patients. See Alan Blum and Larry Rosenberg, "Some Problems in Professionalizing Social Interaction," *Journal of Health and Social Behavior* 9 (1968), 81.

18. A reasonable hypothesis to test would be that patients are more likely to decompensate or become upset within forty-eight hours after having a conference than to remain as before or seem behaviorally better. The main measure would be nurses' reports.

19. I thought this was an irrelevant and stupid opening. The interviewer's second question is a common probe which I always found an awkward reversal of roles.

20. While she may not have felt loved, I found this interpretation of the interview analogous to the one on p. 170.

21. See Erving Goffman, *Asylums* (New York: Doubleday, 1961), pp. 85–115.

22. This is a good example of how psychiatry commonly uses the "retrospective-prospective sense of present occurrence." Harold Garfinkel, *Studies in Ethnomethodology* (Englewood Cliffs, N.J.: Prentice-Hall, 1967), introduction.

9. Treating Suicide

1. E. C. Hughes, "Professions," *Daedalus* 12 (1962), pp. 655–68.

2. A. A. Stone and H. M. Shein, "Psychotherapy of the Hospitalized Suicidal

Patient," *American Journal of Psychotherapy,* 22 (1968), 15–25, (also opening epigraph); R. S. Mintz, "Basic Considerations in the Psychotherapy of the Depressed Suicidal Patient," *American Journal of Psychotherapy,* 25 (1971), 56–73; N. L. Farberow, "Crisis, Disaster and Suicide," *Essays in Self-Destruction,* E. Schneidman, ed., (New York: Science House, 1968), chap. 17; D. A. Schwartz, D. E. Flinn and P. F. Slawson, "Treatment of the Suicidal Character," *American Journal of Psychotherapy,* 28 (1974), 194–207; K. Glaser, "Suicidal Children-Management," *American Journal of Psychotherapy,* 25 (1971), 27–36, esp. 33; C. J. Frederick and H. L. P. Resnick, "How Suicidal Behaviors are Learned," *American Journal of Psychotherapy,* 25 (1971), 37–55, esp. 49; B. L. Danto, "Practical Aspects of Training of Psychiatrists in Suicidal Prevention," *Omega,* 7:1 (1976); H. M. Shein, "Suicide Care: Obstacles in the Education of Psychiatric Residents," *Omega,* 7:1 (1976); T. Bostock and C. L. Williams, "Attempted Suicide as an Operant Behavior," *Archives of General Psychiatry,* 31 (1974), 482–86, esp. 482–83; H. M. Shein and A. A. Stone, "Monitoring and Treatment of Suicidal Potential Within the Context of Psychotherapy," *Comprehensive Psychiatry,* 10 (1969), 59–70.

3. A. A. Stone, "Suicide Precipitated by Psychotherapy—A Clinical Contribution," *American Journal of Psychotherapy,* 25 (1971), 18–26.

4. D. A. Schwartz, E. E. Flinn and P. F. Slawson, "Suicidal Character," 194–207.

5. Robert E. Litman, "When Patients Commit Suicide," *American Journal of Psychotherapy,* 19 (1965), 570–76, esp. 574.

6. M. J. Kahne, "Suicide Among Patients in Mental Hospitals," *Psychiatry,* 31 (1968), 32–43; H. Perr, "Suicide and the Doctor-Patient Relationship," *American Journal of Psychoanalysis,* 28 (1968), 177–88; L. Kayton and H. Freed, "Effects of a Suicide in a Psychiatric Hospital," *Archives of General Psychiatry,* 17 (1967), 187–94; R. Noyes, Jr., "The Taboo of Suicide," *Psychiatry,* 31 (1968), 173–83; M. Rotov, "Death by Suicide in the Hospital," *American Journal of Psychotherapy,* 25 (1970), 216–27.

7. D. Light, Jr., "Treating Suicide: The Illusions of a Professional Movement," *International Social Science Journal,* 25 (1973), 475–88; Louis I. Dublin and Bessie Bunzel, *To Be Or Not to Be,* (New York: Harrison Smith & Robert Hass, 1933); Murray Levine and Peter F. O. Kay, "The Salvation Army's Anti-Suicide Bureau, London 1905," *Bulletin of Suicidology,* 5 (1971), 821–38; Chad Varah, ed., *The Samaritans* (New York: Macmillan, 1965); Louis I. Dublin, *Suicide: A Sociological and Statistical Study* (New York: Ronald Press, 1963); Norman L. Farberow and Edwin S. Schneidman, eds., *The Cry for Help,* (New York: McGraw-Hill, 1961); see also references in fn. 2.

8. V. Bloom, "An Analysis of Suicide at a Training Center," *American Journal of Psychiatry,* 123 (1967), 918–25; S. Basescu, "The Threat of Suicide in Psychotherapy," *American Journal of Psychotherapy,* 19 (1965), 99–105; W. A. Kelly, Jr., "Suicide and Psychiatric Education," *American Journal of Psychiatry,* 130 (1973), 463–68; E. F. El-Islam, "Mental Health of Students Receiving Clinical Psychiatric Training," *Lancet,* 2 (1968), 1184–85.

9. Shein, "Suicide Care," 75.

10. Mintz, "Basic Considerations," 56–73.

11. L. Moss and D. Hamilton, "The Psychotherapy of the Suicide Patient,"

American Journal of Psychiatry, 112 (1956), 814–20; P. M. Margolis, G. G. Meyer and J. C. Louw, "Suicidal Precautions," *Archives of General Psychiatry,* 13 (1965), 224–31; S. Lesse, "The Psychotherapist and Apparent Remissions in Depressed Suicidal Patients," *American Journal of Psychotherapy,* 19 (1965), 436–44; E. Robins, S. Gassner, J. Kayes et al., "The Communication of Suicidal Intent: A Study of 134 Consecutive Cases of Successful (Completed) Suicide," *American Journal of Psychiatry,* 115 (1959), pp. 724–33.

12. J. H. Davis, quoted in "Many Suicides Traced to Careless Prescribing of Drugs," *Journal of the American Medical Association,* 211 (1970), 1778.

13. J. A. Motto and C. Greene, "Suicide and the Medical Community," *Archives of Neurology and Psychiatry,* 80 (1958), 776–81.

14. Mintz, "Basic Considerations."

15. W. D. Wheat, "Motivational Aspects of Suicide in Patients During and After Psychiatric Treatment," *Southern Medical Journal,* 53 (1960), 273.

16. S. Lesse, "The Psychotherapist and Apparent Remissions."

17. Mintz, "Basic Considerations"; Stone, "Suicide Precipitated by Psychotherapy"; Margolis, Meyer and Louw, "Suicidal Precautions"; Bloom, "An Analysis of Suicide"; Rotov, "Death by Suicide"; N. Tabachnick, "Interpersonal Relations in Suicidal Attempts," *Archives of General Psychiatry,* 4 (1961), 16–21; N. Tabachnick, "Countertransference Crisis in Suicidal Attempts," *Archives of General Psychiatry,* 4 (1961), 64–70; G. C. Wilson, Jr., Suicide in Psychiatric Patients, *American Journal of Psychiatry,* 125 (1968), 752–57; H. Perr, Suicide and the Doctor-Patient Relationship, *American Journal of Psychoanalysis,* 28 (1968), 177–88.

18. V. Bloom, "An Analysis of Suicide."

19. Shein, "Suicide Care"; Tabachnick, "Interpersonal Relations"; Tabachnick, "Countertransference Crisis"; G. C. Wilson, Jr., "Suicide in Psychiatric Patients"; Perr, "Doctor-Patient Relationship"; C. Carter, "Some Conditions Predictive of Suicide at Termination of Psychotherapy," *Psychotherapy: Theory, Research and Practice,* 8 (1971), 156–57.

20. R. E. Litman, "When Patients Commit Suicide."

21. See the analysis in Donald W. Light, Jr., "Psychiatry and Suicide: The Management of a Mistake," *American Journal of Sociology* 77:5 (1972), 821–38.

22. This paragraph and several subsequent ones are excerpted from ibid., p. 830. The following analysis comes from pp. 824–25 and from L. Kayton and H. Freed, "Effects of a Suicide."

23. See Erving Goffman, *Asylums* (New York: Doubleday 1961), pp. 125–69.

24. H. Perr, "Doctor-Patient Relationship."

25. Rotov, "Death by Suicide"; N. Tabachnick, "Interpersonal Relations in Suicide Attempts"; Tabachinck, "Countertransference Crisis"; Basescu, "The Threat of Suicide"; Kelly "Suicide and Psychiatric Education"; El-Islam, "Mental Health of Students."

26. Shein, "Suicide Care."

27. Kai Erikson, *Wayward Puritans* (New York: Wiley, 1966), chap. 1.

28. Perr, "Doctor-Patient Relationship."

29. Charles L. Bosk, *Forgive and Remember* (Chicago: University of Chicago Press, 1979), p. 128.

10. Supervising Psychotherapy

1. This insight draws from and slightly modifies Charles L. Bosk's excellent book, *Forgive and Remember* (Chicago: University of Chicago Press, 1979).

2. Lewis R. Wolberg, "Supervision of the Psychotherapeutic Process," *American Journal of Psychotherapy,* V (April 1951), 147–71. The quotation is from page 148 of this classic article.

3. Wolberg, "Supervision," 150.

4. O. H. Mowrer, "Training in Psychotherapy," *Journal of Consulting Psychology,* 15 (August, 1951), 274–77. Quote from 275.

5. Page 273 of Richard D. Chessick, "How the Resident and the Supervisor Disappoint Each Other," *American Journal of Psychotherapy,* XXV (April 1971), 272–83.

6. Rose Laub Coser, *Training in Ambiguity* (New York: Free Press, 1979).

7. S. Nacht, "Reflections on the Evolution of Psychoanalytic Knowledge," *International Journal of Psychoanalysis,* 50 (1969), 597.

8. M. Grotjahn, "The Role of Identification in Psychiatric and Psychoanalytic Training," *Psychiatry* 12 (1949), 141.

9. This account is built on observations and interviews from many sources. I also attended supervision on the case every other week. When I asked to attend supervision, the resident said he would like to "start slow" and have me come every other week to see if my presence made a difference. I was determined to put the resident at ease, and after our first supervision we talked over what had been said. As was my rule, I contributed things already said, reserving any strong opinions I had. Nevertheless, the resident said that I had contributed to his understanding of the supervision, but he never invited me to come weekly and remained strictly aware of which weeks included me as an observer. Despite his caution in this manner, he was frank to me as few other residents were.

10. It developed that he was talking about Katherine and himself. Implicitly, I thought he was wondering if he could replace Katherine's earlier therapist. Can I fill the void? What am I worth? However, none of this was made explicit, and the other new residents told him what they thought.

11. ". . . to anyone else" means to another doctor, principally. Katherine related personally to several patients, an important fact which was ignored because in the pioneering hospital of open doors and milieu, residents were taught that for therapy, ward behavior is of secondary importance.

12. This contrasts with the resident's report in the fourth staff conference. It seemed to me that he was trying hard to be pleased with very little, one of the basic changes from medicine noted in chapter 5.

13. My own view was that she wanted to give her resident a message about trust, especially after the incident with her parents where she felt the resident had betrayed a confidence. Trust and loyalty are central to *The Little Prince,* but the resident did not know this and later interpreted the book in a more distant way.

14. To Katherine's friends, she was always this expressive. The report indicates how all behavior is watched for signs, a reason why sophisticated patients had Kafka visions of the total therapeutic environment in which they lived.

15. Was Katherine fooled by this *ad hoc* form of the T-A split? I do not know, but some patients were not, and these practices contributed to their strong sense of conspiracy around them.

16. I include this incident, because it is rare to hear a resident directly challenge or question a supervisor. The supervisor's response to me indicated that she, like most clinical workers, rely on hunches.

17. Again, quotation marks are reserved for times when I am sure I wrote down or remembered a passage verbatim. This, I thought, was an extraordinary sentence.

18. Generally, I found that certain patients were more accurate about how other patients were doing than the staff.

19. The strong cultural bias of the residents is transformed into the patient's pathology, because that culture itself is taken as symptomatic.

20. Other factors listed and more frequently checked by the resident included drugs, milieu, structure.

11. The Moral Career of the Psychiatric Resident

1. Page 286 in Samuel C. Klagsbrun, "In Search of an Identity," *Archives of General Psychiatry* 16 (March 1967), 286–89.

2. Page 339 in Seymour L. Halleck and Sherwyn M. Woods, "Emotional Problems of Psychiatric Residents," *Psychiatry* 25 (1962), 339–46.

3. On the premise that there is no one, final, true way to analyze the residency experience, this chapter offers another perspective from the interplay of professional issues and time.

4. See page 81 in Robert O. Pasnau and Stephen J. Bayley, "Personality Changes in the First Year of Psychiatric Residency Training," *American Journal of Psychiatry* 128:1 (July 1971), 79–83.

5. Page 22 in David R. Hawkins, chairman, *Conference on the Education of Psychiatrists-Preparatory Commission III: The Resident* (Washington, D.C.: American Psychiatric Association, mimeographed, about 1976).

6. Cited in ibid., p. 23.

7. Ibid., p. 24.

8. A. T. Russell, R. O. Pasnau, and Z. C. Taintor, "Emotional Problems of Residents in Psychiatry," *Am. J. Psychiatry* 132:3 (March 1975), 263–67.

9. Ibid., p. 265.

10. Ibid., p. 264.

11. Ibid., p. 263.

12. Halleck and Woods, "Emotional Problems," p. 339.

13. Alfred Stanton and Morris Schwartz, *The Mental Hospital* (New York: Basic Books, 1954).

14. Webster's *Third International Dictionary*.

15. Nor is it new to Erving Goffman, whose essay, "The Moral Career of the Mental Patient," inspired me to elaborate and extend his ideas to psychiatric training. Pages 125–69 of *Asylums* (New York: Doubleday, 1961).

16. Oswall Hall, "The Informal Organization of the Medical Profession," *The Canadian Journal of Economics and Political Science* 12 (1946), 30–44.

17. Leo Tolstoy, *Anna Karenina*.

18. See chap. 2.

19. Fred Davis, "Professional Socialization as Subjective Experience: The Process of Doctrinal Conversion Among Student Nurses," chap. 17 of *Institutions and the Person*, edited by Howard S. Becker, Blanche Geer, David Riesman, and Robert S. Weiss in honor of Everett Hughes (Chicago: Aldine, 1968), pp. 235–51. Kathleen Knafl and Gary Burkett, "Professional Socialization in a Surgical Specialty: Acquiring Medical Judgment," *Social Science and Medicine* 9 (1975), 397–404.

20. Page 375 in Cyril M. Worby, "The First-Year Psychiatric Resident and the Professional Identity Crisis," *Mental Hygiene* 54:3 (July 1970), 374–77.

21. Halleck and Woods, "Emotional Problems," 340.

22. Myron R. Sharaf and Daniel J. Levinson, "The Quest for Omnipotence in Professional Training," *Psychiatry* 27:2 (May 1964), 135–49, esp. 139. Citing a representative quote from his years of studying residents at Menninger, Robert R. Holt writes that a resident said, "I had just been through five years of long, hard medical training, but in this type of residency I couldn't even lean on my stethoscope. It's hard to be starting at the bottom of the heap again." Page 214 of "Personality Growth in Psychiatric Residents," *Archives of Neurological Psychiatry* 81 (1959), 203–15.

23. Edward E. Jones and Harold B. Gerard, *Foundations of Social Psychology* (New York: Wiley, 1967), chap. 9; Stanley Schachter and J. E. Singer, "Cognitive, social and physiological determinants of emotional states," *Psychological Review* 69 (1962), 379–99.

24. Elliot McGinnies, *Social Behavior: A Functional Analysis* (Boston: Houghton Mifflin, 1970), pp. 52, 306. Of residents, Halleck and Woods write, "It is well documented that new psychiatric residents tend to become obsessively preoccupied with conventional medical detail as a reaction to the impact of the first encounter with psychiatric patients." "Emotional Problems," p. 340.

25. Sir Frederick Bartlett, *Thinking* (New York: Basic Books, 1958).

26. Sharaf and Levinson, "Quest for Omnipotence," p. 139.

27. Page 194 of Lewis Merklin, Jr. and Ralph B. Little, "Beginning Psychiatric Training Syndrome," *American Journal of Psychiatry* 124:2 (August 1967), 193–97.

28. Halleck and Woods, "Emotional Problems," 340. See also Worby, "First-Year Psychiatric Resident," 374–75; Sharaf & Levinson, "Quest for Omnipotence," p. 139; Holt, "Personality Growth," 214; Joel Elkes, "On Meeting Psychiatry," *American Journal of Psychiatry* 122:2 (August 1965), 121–28; Gary Tischler, "The Transition Into Residency," *American Journal of Psychiatry* 128:9 (March 1972), 1103–06.

29. Merklin and Little, "Beginning Syndrome," p. 195.

30. Sharaf and Levinson, "Quest for Omnipotence," p. 139.

31. Halleck and Woods, "Emotional Problems," p. 341.

32. Merklin and Little, "Beginning Syndrome," p. 197.

33. Goffman, "Moral Career," pp. 131–32.

34. Ibid., p. 150.

35. Ibid., p. 153.

402 □ NOTES TO PP 248–254

36. Ibid., pp. 148–49.

37. Harold Garfinkel, "Conditions of Successful Degradation Ceremonies," *American Journal of Sociology* 61 (1956), 420–24. I have collapsed Garfinkel's eight conditions into five.

38. Sharaf and Levinson, "Quest for Omnipotence," pp. 139–40.

39. Fred Davis, "Professional Socialization."

40. Merklin and Little, "Beginning Syndrome," p. 195.

41. At this point and later on, I want to relate this model to the one developed by Fred Davis in "Professional Socialization." Ethnographically, Davis seems to be describing the same process among nurses as I am among psychiatric residents. However, his stages are a mixed bag, though better than Goffman's. His first two stages, "Initial Innocence" and "Labeled Recognition of Incongruity," cover material describing the confusion and exhaustion of nursing students. But "Initial Innocence" is a poor label, because it does not capture what the ensuing paragraphs describe and because "initial innocence" is the *institution's* point of view, not the individual's at the time. Initial innocence is a snap shot, a beginning moment, but not in itself the first movement toward change.

"Labeled Recognition of Incongruity" is something that happens, more in nursing than psychiatric residency and more there than brain washing, but it is a feature, not a phase of some settings. People go through what Davis describes (namely moral confusion and exhaustion) in isolation as well.

42. Robert Holt, "Personality Growth," p. 214.

43. Halleck and Woods, "Emotional Problems," p. 344.

44. Klagsbrun, "In Search," p. 286.

45. Ibid., p. 287.

46. Goffman, "Moral Career," pp. 164–65.

47. Halleck and Woods, "Emotional Problems," p. 344.

48. Klagsbrun, "In Search," p. 287–88.

49. Goffman, "Moral Careers," pp. 154–55.

50. Quoted from field notes in Gary Burkett, *The Self in Professional Socialization: Self-Evaluation in a Psychiatric Residency*. Dissertation in sociology, University of Illinois, 1974, p. 84.

51. Bartlett, *Thinking*.

52. The argument below follows Jerome Kagan in his synthesis of research about the process of identification, "The Concept of Identification," *The Psychological Review* 65 (1958), 296–305. Morris Rosenberg, in his study *Society and the Adolescent Self-Image* (Princeton: Princeton Univbersity Press, 1965), argues persuasively that anxiety produces low self-esteem, which makes a person highly vulnerable either to attack or to anyone offering anxiety-reducing mastery and support (299–301); Jones and Gerard, *Foundations,* p. 70; M. Sherif, *The Psychology of Social Norms* (New York: Harper & Row, 1966).

53. Gary Tischler, "The Transition Into Residency," *American Journal of Psychiatry* 129:9 (March 1972), 1103–06.

54. D. H. Lawrence and Leon Festinger, *Deterrents and Reinforcements: The Psychology of Insufficient Reward* (Palo Alto, Cal.: Stanford University Press, 1962).

55. Fred Davis's last two stages, Provisional Internalization and Stable In-

ternalization, are well labelled and include insightful discussion. My last two stages are very close to his. Preceding these are two other stages, Psyching Out and Role Simulation, which I have not used. This is not because I think they are not useful, but because I think they are not stages as much as techniques which are used at several stages. Davis explicitly excludes this interpretation of Psyching Out when he states that it cannot arise so long as the student group "is fixated on assessing performances and their motivational adequacy in terms of the lay imagery they bring with them" (244). I think, however, that students of professional socialization will find it more useful not to restrict Psyching Out in this way, but to recognize that trainees psyche out performances and motivations at different stages in different ways.

56. Jerome Frank, "Psychotherapists Need Theories," *Psychotherapy and Social Science Review,* 5 (14) (December 1971), 17–18.

57. Goffman, "Moral Career," p. 169.

58. Everett Hughes writes, "This technical—therefore relative—attitude will have to be adopted toward the very people one services; no profession can do its work without license to talk in shocking terms about its clients and their problems. Related to the license to think relatively about dear things and absolute values is the license to do dangerous things." *Men and Their Work* (Glencoe, Ill.: Free Press, 1958), p. 82.

59. See Tischler, "The Transition into Residency."

60. Davis, "Professional Socialization," 250.

61. This view is supported by the considerable research of Rue Bucher and her colleagues. See Bucher and Joan Stelling, *Becoming Professional* (Beverly Hills, Cal.: Sage, 1977).

62. William E. Henry, John H. Sims, and S. Lee Spray, *Public and Private Lives of Psychotherapists* (San Francisco: Jossey-Bass, 1973), p. 123.

63. Daniel J. Levinson, *The Seasons of a Man's Life* (New York: Knopf, 1978).

64. See, for example, previously cited works by Elkes, Halleck and Woods, Klagsbrun, Merklin and Little, Modlin, Sharaf and Levinson, and Worby.

65. Halleck and Woods, "Emotional Problems," 345.

12. The Structure of Psychiatric Residency

1. Observations by clinical psychiatrists include E. S. C. Ford, "Being and Becoming a Psychotherapist: The Search for Identity," *American Journal of Psychotherapy* 17 (1963), 472–82; Seymour L. Halleck and Sherwyn M. Woods, "Emotional Problems of Psychiatric Residents," *Psychiatry* 25 (1962), 339–46; Lewis Merkin, Jr. and Ralph B. Little, "Beginning Psychiatry Training Syndrome," *Am. J. Psychiatry* 124 (1967), 193–97; Samuel G. Klagsbrun, "In Search of an Identity," *Archives of General Psychiatry* 16 (1967), 286–89; Gary L. Tischler, "The Beginning Resident and Supervision," *Arch. Gen. Psychiatry* 19 (1968), 418–22; J. Thomas Ungerleider, "That Most Difficult Year," *Am. J. Psychiatry* 122 (1965), 542–45; H. Gaskill and J. Norton, "Observations on Psychiatric Residency Training," *Arch. Gen. Psychiatry* 18 (1968), 7–15; Robert R. Holt, "Personality Growth in Psychiatric Residents," *Archives in Neurology and Psychiatry* 81 (1959), 203–15; Rudolf Ekstein, "Omnipotence and Omni-Impotence: Phases of the Training Process," *International Journal of*

Psychiatry 4 (1967), 443–48; Martin Grotjahn, "The Role of Identification in Psychiatric and Psychoanalytic Training," *Psychiatry* 12 (1949), 141–51; Bertram D. Lewin, "Education or the Quest for Omniscience," *Journal of the American Psychoanalytic Association* V (1959), 389–412; Norman Kreitman, "Psychiatric Training," *Int. J. Psychiatry* 4 (1967), 451–52; D. E. DeSole, P. Singer and S. Aronson, "Suicide and Role Strain Among Physicians," *Int. J. Social Psychiatry* 15:4 (1969); C. S. Fleckles, "The Making of a Psychiatrist," *Am. J. Psychiatry* 128:9 (March 1972), 1111–15; J. W. Hamilton, "Some Aspects of Learning, Supervision, and Identity Formation in Psychiatric Residency," *Psychiatric Quarterly* 45:3 (1971), 410–19; S. H. Kardiner et al., "The Trainee's Viewpoint of Psychiatric Residency," *Am. J. Psychiatry* 126:8 (1970), 1132–38; W. A. Kelly, "Suicide and Psychiatric Education," *Am. J. Psychiatry* 130:4 (April 1973), 463–68; S. H. Kardiner & M. Fuller, "The First Born Phenomenon Among Psychiatric Residents," *Am. J. Psychiatry* 129:3 (September 1972), 350–52; D. H. Rosen, "Physician, Heal Thyself," *Clinical Medicine* 80 (Feb. 1973), 25–27; A. T. Russell, R. O. Pasnau and Z. T. Taintor, "Emotional Problems of Residents in Psychiatry," *Am. J. Psychiatry* 132:3 (March 1975), 263–67; J. M. Scanlan, "Physician to Students: The Crisis of Psychiatric Residency Training," *Am. J. Psychiatry* 128:9 (March 1972), 1107–10; B. W. Steiner, P. E. Garfinkel, R. C. A. Hunter, "The Processes of Psychiatric Residency Training," *Canadian Psychiatric Association Journal* 19 (1974), 193–200; C. M. Worby, "The First-Year Psychiatric Resident and the Professional Identity Crisis," *Mental Hygiene* 54 (1970), 374–77.

Studies by social scientists include Alan F. Blum and Larry Rosenberg, "Some Problems Involved in Professionalizing Social Interaction: The Case of Psychotherapeutic Training," *Journal of Health and Social Behavior* 9 (1968), 72–85; Rue Bucher, "The Psychiatric Residency and Professional Socialization," *J. Health Soc. Behavior* 6 (1965), 197–206; Rue Bucher, Joan Stelling and Paul Dommermuth, "Implications of Prior Socialization for Residency Programs in Psychiatry," *Archives of General Psychiatry* 20 (1969), 395–402; Myron R. Sharaf and Daniel J. Levinson, "Patterns of Ideology and Professional Role-Definition Among Psychiatric Residents," in Milton Greenblatt et al., eds., *The Patient and the Mental Hospital* (Glencoe, Ill.: Free Press, 1957), pp. 263–85; Myron R. Sharaf and Daniel J. Levinson, "The Quest for Omnipotence in Professional Training," *Psychiatry* 27 (1964), 135–49.

2. For a description of a residency that does not start the first year with inpatients, see Gaskill and Norton, "Observations."

3. Merklin and Little, "Beginning Syndrome," 194.

4. For an important refutation of this rule as reasonable, see chap. 4 of *Being Mentally Ill*, by Thomas Scheff (Chicago: Aldine, 1966). Two senior staff at a well-known residency explained to me their problem in starting new students with outpatients. The students could not "see" that the outpatients were sick at all and began arguing with the staff, who concluded that only inpatients would get their diagnostic point across.

5. See Scheff, *Being Mentally Ill;* and Bruce Ennis, *Prisoners of Psychiatry* (New York: Harcourt Brace Jovanovich, 1972).

6. Lawrence S. Kubie, "Traditionalism in Psychiatry," *Journal of Nervous Mental Diseases* 139 (1964), 6–19. Quote from p. 14.

7. Kubie, "Traditionalism," 14.

8. See Rachel Kahn-Hut, *Psychiatric Theory as Professional Ideology,* Ph.D. dissertation in Sociology, Brandeis University, 1974, pp. 81–82.

9. Halleck and Woods, "Emotional Problems," 340.

10. "Since in the great majority of cases of mental illness, the existence of this underlying illness is unproven, we need to discuss 'symptomatic' behavior in terms that do not involve the assumption of illness." Scheff, *Being Mentally Ill,* p. 31.

11. Richard Fisch, "Resistance to Change in the Psychiatric Community," *Arch. Gen. Psychiatry* 13 (1965), 359–66.

12. *Psychiatric Ideologies and Institutions,* by Anselm Strauss et al. (New York: Free Press, 1964), pp. 266–67. The authors are amazed that patients in this situation play games with their therapists, creating definitions of self and withholding information about their thoughts or activities. The authors seem unaware of Goffman's work or of the need the sane patients have, in these circumstances, to preserve their personal integrity and to keep the staff from manipulating their persona by wile or obstruction. The authors note that these patients will openly tell one another how they duped their therapist or hid an important truth from him, but seem to consider this a further sign of misguided behavior rather than of mental health.

13. The best-known work on how ideology influences professional behavior is the one just cited by Strauss and his colleagues.

14. Matthew P. Dumont, *The Absurd Healer: Perspective of a Community Psychiatrist* (New York: Science House), pp. 36–37.

15. Bucher, "The Psychiatric Residency."

16. See, for example, Marvin Kaplan, Richard Kurtz and William Clements, "Psychiatric Residents and Lower Class Patients: Conflict in Training," *Community Mental Health* 4 (February 1968), 91–97. See also Paul G. Cotton and Kyle D. Pruett, "The Affective Experience of Residency Training in Community Psychiatry," *Am. J. Psychiatry* 132:3 (March 1975), 267–70.

17. See the prophetic editorial by Eugene Pumpian-Mindlin, first presented in 1964 and published in the *Journal of Nervous & Mental Diseases* 144:8 (1967), 535–38.

18. See chap. 1, page 12.

19. Rue Bucher and Joan Stelling, *Becoming Professional* (Beverly Hills, Cal.: Sage, 1977).

20. Kathleen Knafl and Gary Burkett, "Professional Socialization in a Surgical Specialty: Acquiring Medical Judgment," *Social Science and Medicine* 9 (1975), 397–404.

21. Richard Coombs, *Mastering Medicine* (New York: Free Press, 1978).

22. Rose Laub Coser, *Training in Ambiguity* (New York: Free Press, 1978), chap. 10.

23. John W. Meyer, "The Effects of Education as an Institution," *American Journal of Sociology* 83:1 (July 1977), 55–77, esp. p. 65.

24. Anthony Giddens, *New Rules of Sociological Method: A Positive Critique of Interpretative Sociologies* (London: Hutchinson, 1976), p. 102.

25. John Van Maanen, "Experiencing Organization: Notes on the Meaning of Careers and Socialization," chap. 1 in John Van Maanen, ed., *Organizational Careers: Some New Perspectives* (New York: Wiley, 1977), p. 16.

26. Although Van Maanen takes a strong, individualistic stance toward socialization as symbolic interaction, more recently he and Edgar H. Schein have delineated the structural features of organizations and their tactics of socialization. Presumably these shape the process and outcome of socialization beyond the personal constructs of the individual. See their excellent article, "Toward a Theory of Organizational Socialization," *Research in Organizational Behaviour,* vol. 1 (1979), 209–64.

27. Van Maanen, *op. cit.,* pp. 36–37.

28. Giddens, *New Rules,* p. 82.

29. Ibid., p. 113.

30. Meyer, "Effects of Education," 65–66.

31. Ibid., p. 73.

32. Stanton Wheeler, "The Structure of Formally Organized Socialization Settings," pp. 51–116 in O. G. Brim and S. Wheeler, eds., *Socialization After Childhood* (New York: Wiley 1966). John Van Maanen, "People Processing: Major Strategies of Organization Socialization and Their Consequences," in J. Paap, ed., *New Directions in Human Resource Management* (Englewood Cliffs: Prentice-Hall, 1978).

33. Page 235 in John Van Maanen and Edgar H. Schein, "Toward a Theory of Organizational Socialization," *Organizational Behavior,* vol. 1 (1979), 209–74.

34. Ibid., p. 243.

35. This analysis is based on John W. Meyer's insightful article, "Effects of Education," 55–77.

36. Ibid.

37. Charles L. Bosk, *Forgive and Remember: Managing Medical Failure* (Chicago: University of Chicago Press, 1979).

13. Training for Uncertainty and Control

1. Everett Cherrington Hughes, *Men and Their Work* (Glencoe, Ill.: Free Press, 1958). Donald W. Light, Jr., "Psychiatry and Suicide: The Management of a Mistake," *American Journal of Sociology* 77 (March 1972), 821–38.

2. Renée C. Fox, "Training for Uncertainty," pp. 207–41 in Robert K. Merton et al., eds., *The Student-Physician* (Cambridge, Mass.: Harvard University Press, 1957). Since her original study, Fox has done important work on the special dilemmas and uncertainties of research physicians: *Experiment Perilous* (Glencoe, Ill.: Free Press, 1959), chaps. 2, 3, and 8; Fox and Swazey: *The Courage to Fail* (Chicago: University of Chicago Press, 1974). In some ways the problems of research physicians are similar to those of medical students (*Experiment,* pp. 237–38; *Courage,* pp. 317–18, and in many ways they are not (*Experiment,* pp. 28, 64, 240; *Courage,* pp. 40–41, 60–65, 144–46). Although both research physicians and medical students face the uncertainties arising from the limits of knowledge and their own mastery of that knowledge, the dual role of researcher and therapeutic clinician fundamentally alters the social organization around these uncertainties from that of medical training. Out of this dual role arise norms, rituals, and organizational safeguards that differ from those in medical training. This essay will leave aside the research physician to focus on the training process in medicine and other professions.

3. Fox, "Training," p. 208.

4. Blanche Geer et al., "Learning the Ropes: Situational Learning in Four Occupational Training Programs," in Irwin Deutscher and Elizabeth J. Thompson, eds., *Among the People: Encounters with the Poor* (New York: Basic Books, 1968), pp. 209–33.

5. Stephan J. Miller, *Prescription for Leadership: Training for the Medical Elite* (Chicago: Aldine, 1970).

6. Charles L. Bosk, *Forgive and Remember: Managing Medical Failure* (Chicago: University of Chicago Press, 1979).

7. Ibid., pp. 56–57.

8. Rue Bucher and Joan G. Stelling, *Becoming Professional* (Beverly Hills, Cal.: Sage, 1977), p. 65.

9. Ibid., p. 73.

10. Ibid., p. 72.

11. Fox, "Training," pp. 229–35.

12. Bucher and Stelling, *Becoming Professional;* Gary L. Burkett and Kathleen Knafl, "Judgment and Decision-Making in a Medical Specialty," *Sociology of Work & Occupations* 1 (1974), 82–109; Miller, *Prescription for Leadership;* Emily Mumford, *Interns: From Students to Physicians* (Cambridge, Mass.: Harvard University Press, 1970).

13. In Fox's original essay, training *for* uncertainty appears to be largely learning to appreciate and live with uncertain knowledge. The essay ends with a conference about a case that perplexes the staff, and one faculty member concludes, "There just aren't many 'ground rules' in this area. . . ." (p. 239).

14. Hughes, *Men and Their Work,* p. 54; Eliot Freidson, "The Impurity of Professional Authority," chap. 3 in Howard S. Becker et al., eds., *Institutions and the Person* (Chicago: Aldine, 1968).

15. Geer et al., "Learning the Ropes"; Miller, *Prescription for Leadership.*

16. Hughes, *Men and Their Work,* p. 90.

17. Anselm Strauss et al., *Psychiatric Ideologies and Institutions* (Glencoe, Ill.: Free Press, 1964).

18. Kathleen Knafl and Gary L. Burkett, "Professional Socialization in a Surgical Specialty: Acquiring Medical Judgment," *Social Science and Medicine* 9 (1975), 397–404, esp. 399.

19. D. W. Harding, "Leavis's Way," *The New York Review* XXV:9 (June 1, 1978), 36–40, esp. 36.

20. Knafl and Burkett, "Professional Socialization," 399–400.

21. Foreword to Bucher and Stelling, *Becoming Professional,* p. 12.

22. Rachel Kahn-Hut, *Psychiatric Theory as Professional Ideology,* Ph.D. dissertation, Brandeis University, 1974.

23. Bucher and Stelling, *Becoming Professional,* p. 283.

24. Joan Stelling and Rue Bucher, "Professional Socialization: The Acquisition of Vocabularies of Realism," *Social Science and Medicine* 7 (1973), 661–75.

25. Light, "Psychiatry and Suicide"; Bosk, *Forgive and Remember.*

26. Eliot Freidson, *Profession of Medicine* (New York: Dodd, Mead, 1970).

27. Marcia Millman, *The Unkindest Cut* (New York: Morrow, 1977); Bosk, *Forgive and Remember.*

28. Burkett and Knafl, "Judgment and Decision-Making," 94.

29. Freidson, "Impurity" and *Profession of Medicine*.

30. Howard B. Waitzkin and Barbara Waterman, *The Exploitation of Illness in Capitalist Society* (New York: Bobbs-Merrill, 1974).

31. Rolf Dahrendorf, *Class and Class Conflict in Industrial Society* (Stanford, Cal.: Stanford University Press, 1959).

32. Fox, "Training," 240.

33. Thomas Kuhn, *The Structure of Scientific Revolutions*, 2nd ed. (Chicago: University of Chicago Press, 1970).

34. Kuhn, *Revolutions*.

35. This study; Knafl and Burkett, "Professional Socialization;" Gary L. Burkett, *The Self in Professional Socialization: Self-Evaluation in a Psychiatric Residency*, Ph.D. dissertation, University of Illinois, Circle Campus, 1974.

36. Knafl and Burkett, "Professional Socialization," 401.

37. Ibid.; Burkett, *The Self*; Bosk, *Forgive and Remember*, p. 173.

38. Burkett, *The Self*, pp. 68–70.

39. Ibid., p. 67; this study.

40. Burkett, *The Self*; Alan F. Blum and Larry Rosenberg, "Some Problems Involved in Professionalizing Social Interaction: The Case of Psychotherapeutic Training," *Journal of Health and Social Behavior* 9 (1968), 72–85.

41. Renée C. Fox, "Is There a 'New' Medical Student? A Comparative View of Medical Socialization in the 1950s and 1970s," in Laurence R. Tancredi, ed., *Ethics of Health Care* (Washington, D.C.: National Academy of Sciences, 1974), pp. 197–220.

42. Bucher and Stelling, *Becoming Professional*.

43. Harold M. Schoolman, "The Role of the Physician as a Patient Advocate," *New England Journal of Medicine* 296:2 (1977); 103–05, esp. 104.

14. Narcissism and Training for Omnipotence

1. Susan Sontag, *Illness as Metaphor* (New York: Farrar, Straus & Giroux, 1978).

2. Otto Kernberg, *Borderline Conditions and Pathological Narcissism* (New York: Jason Aronson, 1975), p. 228. There are today two major schools of psychoanalytic theory concerning narcissism, one headed by Heinz Kohut. However, the debates between them concern issues peripheral to our use of the psychoanalytic concept here.

3. Ibid., p. 231.

4. Ibid., pp. 231–32.

5. Ibid., p. 235.

6. See Philip Slater's discussion of narcissistic withdrawal in his essay, "On Social Regression," *American Journal of Sociology* 28:3 (June 1963): 339–64, esp. 346–47.

7. See Clifford C. Clogg, "The Effect of Personal Health Care Upon Longevity in an Economically Advanced Population," paper presented at the Annual Meeting of the American Sociological Association, San Francisco, 1978.

8. See chapter 1.

9. The following argument is based on my paper, "Professional Superiority," read at the 1974 meetings of the American Sociological Association and derived from the writings of T. H. Marshall, Everett C. Hughes, and Eliot Freidson.

10. *Webster's New World Dictionary of the American Language* (Cleveland: World Publishing Co., 1960), College Edition, p. 1147.

11. Max Weber, "Types of Authority," in *Sociological Theory,* edited by Lewis Coser and Bernard Rosenberg (New York: Macmillan, 1964), pp. 129–34. Excerpted from H. H. Gerth and C. W. Mills, eds., *From Max Weber* (New York: Oxford, 1946).

12. David Mechanic, *Public Expectations and Health Care* (New York: Wiley Interscience, 1972), pp. 46–57.

13. Weber, "Types of Authority," p. 130.

14. See the important essay by John W. Meyer and Brian Rowan, "Institutionalized Organizations: Formal Structure as Myth and Ceremony," *Am. J. Sociology* 83:2 (September 1977), 340–63.

15. Ibid., p. 357.

16. Rachel Kahn-Hut, "Psychiatric Perspective on Powerlessness," mimeographed, 1971.

17. See Eliot Freidson and Buford Rhea, "Process of Control in a Company of Equals," *Social Problems* 11 (1963), 119–31; Gloria Engel, "The Effect of Bureaucracy on the Professional Autonomy of the Physician," *Journal of Health and Social Behavior* 10 (1969), 30–41; Mary W. Goss, "Influence and Authority Among Physicians in an Outpatient Clinic," *American Sociological Review* 26 (1961), 39–50; Mary W. Goss, "Patterns of Bureaucracy Among Hospital Staff Physicians," in Eliot Freidson, ed., *The Hospital in Modern Society,* (New York: Free Press, 1963) pp. 170–94; Richard W. Scott, "Reactions to Supervision in a Heteronomous Professional Organization," *Administrative Science Quarterly* 10 (1965), 65–81.

18. Freidson and Rhea, "Process of Control."

19. Richard D. Schwartz and Jerome H. Skolnick, "Two Studies of Legal Stigma," pp. 103–17 in Howard S. Becker, ed., *The Other Side,* (New York: Free Press, 1966).

20. Eliot Freidson, *Professional Dominance* (New York: Atherton, 1970), pp. 142–43.

21. Ibid., p. 121.

22. Sigmund Freud, "On Narcissism: An Introduction," (1914) in *Collected Papers,* translated under the supervision of Joan Riviere (London: The International Psycho-Analytic Press 1950): vol. IV, pp. 30–59.

23. Ibid., p. 51.

24. Harold Lasswell, *Power and Personality* (New York: Norton, 1948); Juliette and Alexander George, *Woodrow Wilson and Colonel House* (New York: Dover, 1964). This argument is indebted to Robert C. Tucker's insightful essay, "The Georges' Wilson Reexamined: An Essay on Psychobiography," *American Political Science Review* LXXI:2 (June 1977), 606–18.

25. Karen Horney, *Our Inner Conflicts* (New York: Norton, 1945), p. 100. This description of the narcissistic defense rests on Horney's work.

26. Ernest Jones, "The God Complex," in *Essays in Applied Psychoanalysis*, vol. II (London: Hogarth, 1951), pp. 244–65.

27. E. S. C. Ford, "Being and Becoming a Psychotherapist: The Search for Identity," *American Journal of Psychotherapy* 17 (1963), 472–82.

28. This theme is taken up in a number of other studies and essays. Ralph N. Zabarenko, Lucy Zabarenko and Rex A. Pittenger review a number of them in "The Psychodynamics of Physicianhood," *Psychiatry* (1969), 102–18. They explore both the doctor-patient relation and the psychological motivations for becoming a doctor as ways to handle aggression and infantile meglomania. Their own six-year study of primary-care physicians supports these themes.

29. Gary Tischler, "The Transition Into Residency," *American Journal of Psychiatry* 128:9 (April 1969), 1103–06, esp. 1103.

30. Myron R. Sharaf and Daniel J. Levinson, "The Quest for Omnipotence in Professional Training," *Psychiatry* 27 (1964), 135–49. Psychoanalytic training is even more omnipotent than psychiatric training. In his overview of psychoanalytic education, Robert Dorn wrote that many training analysts "point out that everything conspires to turn the training analyst into a master despite himself. . . . Present-day structuring of institutes and the relative social prominence of psychoanalysis in the field of psychiatry 'unwittingly conspire' to appeal to narcissistic defensive needs. . . . Our teacher and pupil relationship is closer to that of ruler and ruled." "Psychoanalysis and Psychoanalytic Education: What Kind of 'Journey'?" *The Psychoanalytic Forum*, vol. III.

31. Rudolf Ekstein, "Omnipotence and Omni-Impotence: Phases of the Training Process," *International Journal of Psychiatry* 4 (1967), 443–48, esp. 445.

32. This process is helped if the clients are of lower social status than the trainee, which is usually the case.

33. Harold Searles, "Feelings of Guilt in the Psychoanalyst," *Psychiatry* 29 (1966), 319–23, esp. 322.

34. Dan Rather, "Fifty Minutes," *60 Minutes* X:25 (February 19, 1978), CBS, Inc., p. 4.

15. The Nature of Professional Socialization

1. John Van Maanen, "Experiencing Organization: Notes on the Meaning of Careers and Socialization," chap. 1 in Van Maanen, ed., *Organizational Careers: Some New Perspectives* (New York: Wiley 1977), p. 18.

2. R. Day and J. Day, "A Review of the Current State of Negotiated Order Theory," *Sociological Quarterly*, 18 (1977), 126–42.

3. Anselm Strauss, *Negotiations: Varieties, Contexts, Processes, and Social Order* (San Francisco: Jossey-Bass, 1978).

4. Talcott Parsons, *The Social System* (Glencoe, Ill.: Free Press, 1951), pp. 207–08.

5. Robert K. Merton, "Some Preliminaries to a Sociology of Medical Education," in Robert K. Merton, George G. Reader and Patricia L. Kendall, eds., *The Student-Physician* (Cambridge, Mass.: Harvard University Press, 1957), pp. 40–41.

6. Ibid., p. 41.

7. Yet this emphasis is not entirely clear; for Professor Merton states that this study will *"temporarily"* focus upon attitudes and values and that skills and knowledge are central to the physician's role.

8. Orville G. Brim, Jr., "Adult Socialization," in John A. Clausen, ed., *Socialization and Society* (Boston: Little, Brown, 1968), p. 186. While Brim goes on to say this may not be the whole of socialization, he gives no indication what else it might involve.

9. Orville G. Brim, Jr., "Personality Development as Role-Learning," in I. Iscoe and H. W. Stevenson, eds., *Personality Development in Children* (Austin: University of Texas Press, 1960), p. 141.

10. Virginia L. Olesen and Elvi W. Whittaker, *The Silent Dialogue* (San Francisco: Jossey-Bass, 1968), pp. 5–6.

11. See, for example, Fred Davis, "Professional Socialization as Subjective Experience," in Howard S. Becker, Blanche Geer, David Riesman and Robert S. Weiss, eds., *Institutions and the Person* (Chicago: Aldine, 1968), chap. 17.

12. Wilbert E. Moore, "Occupational Socialization," in David Goslin, ed., *Handbook of Socialization Theory and Research* (Chicago: Rand McNally, 1969), chap. 21, p. 869.

13. Robert MacKay, "Conceptions of Children and Models of Socialization," in Hans Peter Dreitzel, ed., *Childhood and Socialization* (New York: Macmillan, 1973), chap. 1, p. 39.

14. Orville G. Brim, Jr., "Socialization Through the Life Cycle," in Orville G. Brim, Jr. and Stanton Wheeler, *Socialization After Childhood* (New York: Wiley, 1966). This quote is from p. 26; the other differences are presented on pp. 27–31.

15. Peter L. Berger and Thomas Luckmann, *The Social Construction of Reality* (New York: Doubleday, 1966).

16. Wilbert E. Moore, "Occupational Socialization," p. 878. Professor Moore's argument is also presented on pp. 76–79 of his book, *The Professions: Roles and Rules* (New York: Russell Sage Foundation, 1970).

17. Moore, "Occupational Socialization," p. 878.

18. Merton, Reader and Kendall, *The Student-Physician.*

19. Howard S. Becker, Blanche Geer, Everett C. Hughes, and Anselm L. Strauss, *Boys in White: Student Culture in Medical School* (Chicago: The University of Chicago Press, 1961). Howard S. Becker, *Sociological Work: Method and Substance* (Chicago: Aldine, 1970). The following two paragraphs first appeared on pp. 1161–62 of my article, "The Sociological Calendar," *American Journal of Sociology*, 80 (March 1975), 1145–64.

20. Stephen J. Miller, *Prescription for Leadership: Training for the Medical Elite* (Chicago: Aldine, 1970). Eliot Friedson, *Profession of Medicine* (New York: Dodd, Mead, 1970).

21. In Freidson's *Profession of Medicine*, compare his situational argument (pp. 15–18, 56, 65) with passages about underlying values (pp. 85, 141, 146–51, 160).

22. Becker, *Sociological Work*, p. 280.

23. Ibid., p. 283.

24. Ibid., p. 261.

25. Ibid., p. 265.

26. Ibid., p. 266.

27. E. Abramson et al., "Social Power and Commitment: A Theoretical Statement," *American Sociological Review* XXIII (February 1958), pp. 15–22. Quotation is from p. 16.

28. *The Random House Dictionary of the English Language,* unabridged (New York: Random House, 1967), p. 296.

29. Becker, *Sociological Work,* p. 284.

30. Daniel J. Levinson, "Medical Education and the Theory of Adult Socialization," *Journal of Health and Social Behavior* 8 (December 1967), 253–65.

31. Levinson, "Medical Education," p. 257.

32. Kai T. Erikson's review of *Outsiders* by Howard S. Becker, *American Journal of Sociology* 69 (1964), 417–19.

33. Glen H. Elder, Jr., "On Linking Social Structure and Personality," *American Behavioral Scientist* 16 (July/August 1973), 790–91.

34. Of course, both situational adjustments and internalized traits exist; one need not choose between them. The prevalence of one or the other depends on the individual and the environment, but these authors believe internalization is on the wane.

35. Herbert C. Kelman, "Process of Opinion Change," *Public Opinion Quarterly* 25 (January 1961), 57–78.

36. See Oswall Hall, "The Informal Organization of the Medical Profession," *Canadian Journal of Economics and Political Science,* XII (1946), 30–41.

37. Van Buren O. Hammett and George Spivack, "What Residents Do After Graduation," *Archives of General Psychiatry,* 33 (April 1976), 414–17.

38. Rachel Kahn-Hut, *Psychiatric Theory as Professional Ideology,* Ph.D. dissertation at Brandeis University, 1974.

39. William E. Henry, John H. Sims and S. Lee Spray, *Public and Private Lives of Psychotherapists* (San Francisco: Jossey-Bass, 1973).

40. Ibid., pp. 45 and 91.

41. See chap. 1, "The Psychiatric Domain."

42. Kahn-Hut, *Psychiatric Theory,* p. 189.

43. Ibid., p. 221.

44. Eliot Freidson, *Profession of Medicine,* chap. 7.

45. See Yi-Chuang Lu, "The Collective Approach to Psychiatric Practice in the People's Republic of China," *Social Problems* 26:1 (October 1978), 2–14. A good overview of Chinese medicine is provided in the book by Victor and Ruth Sidel, *Serve the People* (Boston: Beacon, 1974). See also Victor Sidel, "Medical Care in the People's Republic of China," *Archives of Internal Medicine,* 135 (July 1975), 916–26; Ruth Sidel, *Women and Child Care in China: A Firsthand Report* (Baltimore: Penguin, 1973); Peter K-M New and Mary L. New, "The Links Between Health and the Political Structure in New China," *Human Organization* 34 (Fall 1975), 237–51.

46. Penelope Gilliatt's review of *Face to Face* in *The New Yorker,* April 5, 1976, p. 121. The symptoms and causes of this postresidency identity crisis is beautifully described by Kenneth A. Fisher's "Crises in the Therapist," *The Psychoanalytic Review* 54 (Spring 1967), 81–98.

At first glance, this idea of further self-doubt may seem to contradict the socialization process as I have described it and the omnipotent tendencies inherent in the structure of training. But in many ways psychiatry seems to fit the narcissistic personality, with its combination of grandiosity and inauthenticity. Even its origins seem analogous. As John Murray Cuddihy argues in *The Ordeal of Civility: Freud, Marx, Lévi-Strauss and the Jewish Struggle with Modernity* (New York: Basic, 1974), Jews were forced in a gentile world to internalize a bad image of themselves by repressing natural desires and sources of gratification that made up their Jewishness. Freud fought back, building a theory showing that everyone is Jewish—aggressive, vulnerable, driven by sex, hungry for love. Psychiatry became the agent of this revenge, the profession that was superior to all others in its pretensions of civility; yet, argues Cuddihy, the profession by this fact stands apart and is born from a sense of unworthiness. Psychiatry is often noted for its lack of cooperation or meaningful contact with allied professions, for the analytic technique's emotional distance and manipulative approach to patients, for its intellectual powers, for its uneasy sense that the rest of the world does not love it and is trying to destroy it. These are all described by Otto Kernberg in *Border-line Conditions and Pathological Narcissim* (New York: Jason Aronson, 1975). See also Robert T. Morse, "A Serious and Little-Recognized Deficit in Post-War Psychiatric Resident Training," *Am. J. Psychiatry* 115 (10) (April 1959), 899–904, esp. 903; Eugene B. Piedmont, "Referrals and Reciprocity: Psychiatrists, General Practitioners, and Clergymen," *J. Health Soc. Behavior* (1968), 29–41; and especially Christopher Lasch, "The Narcissistic Society," *The New York Review of Books* XXIII (15), (September 30, 1976), 5–13.

47. This analysis follows in part Kenneth A. Fisher's insightful article, "Crisis in the Therapist," *The Psychoanalytic Review* 54 (Spring 1967), 81–98.

48. Tracey McCarley, "The Psychotherapist's Search for Self-Renewal," *Am. J. Psychiatry* 132:3 (March 1975), 221–23, esp. p. 222.

49. These questions come from the rows of the sociological calendar in chapter 5.

50. Merton et al., *The Student-Physician*, p. 77.

51. Anthony R. Harris and Lorene L. Conto, "Negation and Identity," paper presented at the August 1976 meetings of the American Sociological Association, New York City. See also H. Schein, *Coercive Persuasion*. (New York: Norton, 1971); and "Learning to be Healthy," by Gary Easthope (University of East Anglia, typed, 1978).

52. Rosabeth M. Kanter, "Committment and Social Organization: A Study of Committment Mechanisms in Utopian Communities," *American Sociological Review* 33:4 (1968).

16. Professional Training and the Future of Psychiatry

1. This perspective on professions was suggestively described by Rue Bucher and Anselm Strauss in "Professions in Process," *American Journal of Sociology* (1961) 66: 325–34.

2. Personal communication.

3. Donald G. Langsley, Alfred M. Freedman, Melvyn Haas, and James H. Grubbs, "Medical Student Education in Psychiatry," *American Journal of Psychiatry* 134 (1977), 15–20.

4. Charles W. Patterson, "Psychiatrists and Physical Examinations: A Survey," *Am. J. Psychiatry* 135:8 (L978), 967–68.

5. Specifically, 7 percent of the national sample did family therapy with 50 percent or more of their patients, while 22 percent never used it at all. Ten percent did group therapy on half or more of their patients, and 48 percent never used it at all. Donald G. Langsley, "Psychiatry and Mental Health Manpower," 1978, typed, from the American Psychiatric Association, p. 14.

6. Eliot Marshall, "It's All in the Mind," *The New Republic*, August 5–12, 1978, 18.

7. Joseph W. Schneider, "Deviant Drinking as Disease: Alcoholism as a Social Accomplishment," *Social Problems* 25:4 (1978), 361–72.

8. Nancy Roeske, M.D., "Women in Psychiatry," the American Psychiatric Association's *Conference on the Education of Psychiatrists, Commission I*, James N. Susses, M.D., chairman, 1975, typed, pp. 17–42, esp. p. 26.

9. The A.P.A.'s *Conference on the Education of Psychiatrists, Commission III*, David R. Hawkins, M.D., chairman, 1975, typed, p. 34.

10. The A.P.A.'s *Conference*, David R. Hawkings, M.D., chairman, pp. 39–40. See also Chester M. Pierce, M.D., "Teaching Cross-Racial Therapy," pp. 56–62 in the A.P.A.'s *Conference, Commission IV*, Milton Greenblatt, M.D., chairman.

11. David F. Musto, "Whatever Happened to Community Mental Health?" *Psychiatric Annals* 7:10 (1977), 30–55.

12. On the last point, see Andrew Scull, *Decarceration* (Englewood Cliffs, N.J.: Spectrum, 1976).

13. Musto, "Whatever Happened," p. 43.

14. Ibid., p. 50.

15. See, for example, Jonathan F. Borus, "Issues Critical to the Survival of Community Mental Health," *Am. J. Psychiatry* 135:9 (1978), 1029–35.

16. Musto, "Whatever happened"; Ellen L. Bassuk and Samuel Gerson, "Deinstitutionalization and Mental Health Services," *Scientific American* 238:2 (1978), 46–53.

17. Langsley et al., "Medical Student Education," 23.

18. Borus, "Survival of Community Mental Health," 1031.

19. Table 13 of Langsley's report shows that, aside from prescribing medications and managing inpatients, psychiatrists do not spend their time differently at community mental health centers than psychologists and social workers.

20. Thomas Kuhn, *The Structure of Scientific Revolutions*, revised edition (Chicago; University of Chicago Press, 1970). See Allen W. Imershein's explication of Kuhn in his suggestive article, "Organizational Change as a Paradigm Shift," *The Sociological Quarterly* 18 (Winter 1977), 33–43.

21. Bassuk and Gerson, "Deinstitutionalization," p. 52.

22. Park Elliott Dietz and Jonas R. Rappaport, "Professional Activities of Maryland and U.S. Psychiatrists," typed, 1976.

23. Borus, "Surival of Community Mental Health," 1032.

24. William E. Henry, John H. Sims, and S. Lee Spray, *Public and Private Lives of Psychotherapists* (San Francisco: Jossey-Bass, 1973).

25. Morton O. Wagenfeld and Stanley S. Robin, "Social Activism and Psychiatrists in Community Mental Health Centers," *American Journal of Community Psy-*

chology 6 (3) 1978; 253–64, esp. 263. See also the authors' article, "Structural and Professional Correlates of Ideologies on Community Mental Health Workers," *Journal of Health and Social Behavior* 15 (1974), 199–210.

26. For a precise analysis of the different models underlying psychoanalysis and community mental health, see Miriam Seigler and Humphrey Osmond, "Models of Madness," *The British Journal of Psychiatry*, 112:493 (1966), 1193–1203.

27. Judith Lorber and Roberta Satow, "Creating a Company of Unequals: Sources of Occupational Stratification in a Ghetto Community Mental Health Center," *Sociology of Work and Occupations* 4 (1977), 281–302. For a professional analysis of these problems, see *Racism, Elitism, Professionalism: Barriers to Community Mental Health*, Israel Zwerling et al., eds., (New York: Jason Aronson, 1976).

28. Eugene Pumpian-Mindlin, "Problems of Professional Identity in Training Psychiatrists," *The Journal of Nervous and Mental Disease* 144:6 (1967), 535–138.

29. Marvin L. Kaplan, Richard M. Kurtz, and William H. Clements, "Psychiatric Residents and Lower Class Patients: Conflict in Training," *Community Mental Health* 4:1 (1968), 91–97.

30. Paul G. Cotton and Kyle D. Pruett, "The Affective Experience of Residency Training in Community Psychiatry," *Am. J. Psychiatry* 132:3 (March 1975), 267–69.

31. Roy G. Grinker, "The Future Educational Needs of Psychiatrists," *American Journal of Psychiatry* 132:3 (1975), 259–62.

32. Ibid., p. 260.

33. Francis J. Braceland, "Psychiatry and the Third Revolution," *Psychiatric Annals* 7:10 (1977), 4–5.

34. James J. Strain, "The Medical Setting: Is it Beyond the Psychiatrist?" *Am. J. Psychiatry* 134:3 (1977), 253–56.

35. Rosemary Stevens, *American Medicine and the Public Interest* (New Haven: Yale University Press, 1971).

36. Philip A. Berger, "Medical Treatment of Mental Illness," *Science* 200:4344 (26 May 1978), 974–81, esp. 974–75.

37. Ronald R. Fieve, "The Revolution Defined: It is Pharmacologic," *Psychiatric Annals* 7:10 (1977), 10–28.

38. Andrew Scull, *Decarceration,* chap. 5.

39. G. E. Crain, "Clinical Psychopharmacology in Its Twentieth Year," *Science* 181 (1973), 124–28; R. F. Prien and C. J. Klett, "An Appraisal of the Long-Term Use of Tranquilizing Medication with Hospitalized Chronic Schizophrenics: A Review of the Drug Discontinuation Literature," *Schizophrenia Bulletin* 5 (1972), 64–73.

40. P. Allen, "A Consumer's View of the California Mental Health Care System," *Psychiatric Quarterly* 48 (1974), 1–13.

41. E. Laska et al., "Patterns of Psychotropic Drug Use for Schizophrenia," *Diseases of the Nervous System* 34 (1973), 294–305.

42. H. L. Lennard et al., *Mystification and Drug Misuse: Hazards in Using Psychoactive Drugs.* (San Francisco: Jossey-Bass, 1971).

43. H. R. Lamb and V. Goertzel, "Discharged Mental Patients: Are They Really in the Community?" *Archives of General Psychiatry* 24 (1971), 29–34; U. Aviram and S. P. Segal, "Exclusion of the Mentally Ill: Reflections on an Old Problem in a New Context," *Archives of General Psychiatry* 29 (1973), 126–31.

44. Fieve, "Revolution Defined," 13.

45. T. J. Scheff, "Medical Dominance: Psychoactive Drugs and Mental Health Policy," *American Behavioral Scientist* 19: 3 (1976), 299–317, esp. 301.

46. Ibid., pp. 305–06.

47. Ibid., p. 307.

48. Fieve, "Revolution Defined." A new book which purports to teach nonmedical therapists what they need to know about medicine to diagnose emotional problems with physiological aspects is *Primer for the Nonmedical Psychotherapist,* by Joyce A. Backar (New York: Wiley Spectrum, 1976).

49. Herbert C. Modlin et. al., "Growth of Psychiatrists During and After Residency Training: Objective Evaluation," *Am. J. Psychiatry* (June 1959), 1081–90.

50. Ibid., p. 1088.

51. Some argue that residents should receive a salary for the services they provide. This is the central debate in American Psychiatric Association's 1975 *Conference on Education of Psychiatrists: Economic Issues in the Education of Psychiatrists, Commission VI,* Herzl R. Spiro, chairman. In 1972 it was estimated that residency training cost $21,053 per year. If residents were paid $20 an hour for twenty hours of services a week, they would make almost this amount. In my opinion, those who write for this approach make better arguments than those against it.

52. The APA's *Conference on the Education of Psychiatrists, Commission VII,* Eric Pfeiffer, M.D., chairman (1975, typed), p. 20.

53. Ibid., p. 20.

54. Ibid., p. 24. In all there were nine criteria, eight of them without substance and tautological.

55. Herbert C. Modlin, M.D., "An Evaluation of the Learning Process in a Psychiatric Residency Program," *Bulletin of the Menninger Clinic,* vol. 19 (September 1955), 139–59, esp. 157.

56. This analysis comes from Perry London's article, "The Future of Psychotherapy," *The Hastings Center Report,* vol. 3, no. 6 (December 1973), 10–13. See also Richard Sennett, *The Fall of Public Man* (New York: Knopf, 1976).

57. Gene M. Abroms and Norman S. Greenfield, "A New Mental Health Profession," *Psychiatry,* vol. 36 (February 1973), 10–21.

58. Samuel Martin, "Factors Influencing the Future of Financing Psychiatric Residency Education," in the A.P.A.'s *Conference on the Education of Psychiatrists Commission VI,* Herzl R. Spiro, M.D., chairman (1975, typed), pp. 10–13.

59. See Peter L. Berger, "Towards A Sociological Understanding of Psychoanalysis," *Social Research* 32 (Spring 1965), 26–41; and Christopher Lasch, "The Narcissistic Society," *The New York Review of Books* XXIII (15), (September 30, 1976), 5–13.

Appendix II. Methods

1. Martin Trow, "Comment on 'Participant Observation and Interviewing: A Comparison'," *Human Organization* 16:3 (1957), 33–35.

2. Robert S. Weiss, "Alternative Approaches in the Study of Complex Situations," *Human Organization* 25:3 (1966), 198–206.

3. Ibid., 199.

4. See Appendix III.

5. George J. McCall and J. L. Simmons, *Issues in Participant Observation: A Text and Reader* (Reading, Mass.: Addison-Wesley, 1969), pp. 5, 61–64.

6. See Florence R. Kluckhohn, "The Participant-Observer Technique in Small Communities," *American Journal of Sociology* 46 (1940), 331–43. See also page 32 of Arthur J. Vidich and Gilbert Shapiro, "A Comparison of Participant Observation and Survey Data," *American Sociological Review* 20 (1955), 28–33.

7. The following argument and the literature on which it is based is found in Albert J. Reiss, Jr., "Systematic Observation Surveys of Natural Social Phenomena," in H. Wallace Sinaiko and Laurie A. Broedling, eds., *Perspective on Attitude Assessment: Surveys and Their Alternatives* (Washington, D.C.: Smithsonian Institution, 1975), pp. 132–50.

8. Barney G. Glaser and Anselm L. Strauss, *The Discovery of Grounded Theory* (Chicago: Aldine, 1967).

9. McCall and Simmons, *Participant Observation*, pp. 20–26.

10. Clifford Geertz, *Interpretation of Cultures*. (New York: Basic, 1973), p. 27.

11. In the scheme presented by Morris and Charlotte Schwartz, I was an active participant observer. The authors describe well my main experience in this role, shuttling back and forth from participating to observing what has just happened. They correctly imply that one should enjoy this style or not do it. "Problems in Participant Observation," *Am. J. Sociology,* LX, 4, (1955), 343–53.

12. In the spectrum between a casual, easy style used by Elliot Liebow and a structural and channeled style described by Alfred Stanton and Morris Schwartz in *The Mental Hospital* (New York: Basic Books, 1954), my approach was close to Liebow's. See the appendix of Elliot Liebow's *Tally's Corner* (Boston: Little, Brown, 1967). William F. Whyte concludes, "Whether it was a good thing to write a book about Cornerville depended entirely on people's opinions of me personally." (*Street Corner Society,* Chicago: University Chicago Press, 1955), p. 300.

13. Like Liebow, I found that by the time a few objected, my right to be doing my work was clearly established, even in their minds. (*Tally's Corner,* pp. 247–48.)

14. When I chanced to drop by the hospital for something dressed like a student—sports shirt and sandals—I felt very uncomfortable and wary of meeting residents there. I looked like an attendant. Only a tie separates a resident from a college student attendant, a fine line which threatens residents. See ibid., p. 255.

15. Stanton and Schwartz, *The Mental Hospital,* pp. 427, 429–30, 447.

16. Simmel pinpoints this problem in "The Sociology of Sociability." While sociable interaction centers upon persons, it can occur only if the more serious purposes of the individual are kept out, so that it is an interaction not of complete but of symbolic and equal personalities." *Am. J. Sociology* (November 1949), 254.

Not only did I find Simmel's observation a constant experience but more profoundly I discovered that people often would not tolerate inquiry. Garfinkel discusses this in terms of how people make sense of the world, by features of common understanding which are understood to be shared and are not to be questioned.

17. Although low morale has its dangers (Schwartz and Schwartz, "Participant Observation," 351), I forced myself to work steadily regardless of mood. I soon dis-

covered the harmony between what the residents experienced and what I did, adding immensely to my understanding of what I observed.

18. My practices and experiences in methods are shared and expressed by Stanton and Schwartz, *The Mental Hospital,* pp. 437–38.

19. Ibid., pp. 344–45.

20. See Stanton and Schwartz "The Observer's Effect on the Observed," in ibid., 346–47. See also John Lofland, *Analyzing Social Settings: A Guide to Qualitative Observation and Analysis* (Belmont, Cal.: Wadsworth, 1971), pp. 102–09.

21. Thus, I tried to separate out the "covert transactions in the process of participant observation." Schwartz and Schwartz, pp. 343–46.

22. Schwartz and Schwartz took many fewer notes, seeing them as a secondary aid for review; for me the notes were the core of the data, a discovery which they learned at the end of their project. Ibid., pp. 343–44.

23. This approach and the parallel between countertransference in participant-observation and in psychotherapy is suggested by Schwartz and Schwartz, ibid., 351–53. See also Lofland, *Social Settings,* and McCall and Simmons, *Participant Observation,* pp. 63, 99–100.

24. Lofland, *Social Settings,* p. 92.

Appendix III. The Problem of Typing Residents by Ideology

1. M. R. Sharaf and D. J. Levinson, "Patterns of Ideology and Professional Role-Definition among Psychiatric Residents," in *The Patient and the Mental Hospital,* M. Greenblatt, D. J. Levinson, R. H. Williams, eds., (Glencoe: Free Press, 1957), pp. 263–85.

2. A. Strauss, L. Schatzman, R. Bucher et al., *Psychiatric Ideologies and Institutions* (Glencoe: Free Press, 1964), chap. 4.

3. R. Bucher, J. Stelling and P. Dommermuth, "Implications of Prior Socialization for Residency Programs in Psychiatry," in *Archives of General Psychiatry* 20 (1969), 395–402.

4. On a range of 10 to 70, Sharaf and Levinson got a mean of 54 and a high score of 58. Since the test was administered at an analytically oriented program, these figures cast doubt on the validity of the instrument. The revised scales of Strauss's group also appear to slice reality into jumbled pieces, as evident in Ehrlich and Sabshin's study, especially pp. 469–77. Danuta Ehrlich & Melvin Sabshin, "A Study of Sociotherapeutically Oriented Psychiatrists," *American Journal of Orthopsychiatry* 34: 3 (1964), 469–80.

5. This is also clear in Ehrlich and Sabshin's study.

6. T. Kuhn, *The Structure of Scientific Revolutions* (Chicago: University of Chicago Press, 1962).

Index